INTELLECTUAL DISABILITY

MANCHESTER
1824
Manchester University Press

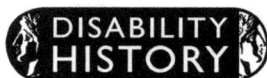

DISABILITY HISTORY

Series editors
Dr Julie Anderson, Professor Walton Schalick, III

This series published by Manchester University Press responds to the growing interest in disability as a discipline worthy of historical research. The series has a broad international historical remit, encompassing issues that include class, race, gender, age, war, medical treatment, professionalisation, environments, work, institutions and cultural and social aspects of disablement including representations of disabled people in literature, film, art and the media.

Already published
Deafness, community and culture in Britain: leisure and cohesion, 1945–1995
Martin Atherton
Rethinking modern prostheses in Anglo-American commodity cultures, 1820–1939
Claire L. Jones (ed.)
Destigmatising mental illness? Professional politics and public education in Britain, 1870–1970
Vicky Long
Fools and idiots? Intellectual disability in the Middle Ages
Irina Metzler
Framing the moron: the social construction of feeble-mindedness in the American eugenics era
Gerald V. O'Brien
Recycling the disabled: army, medicine, and modernity in WWI Germany
Heather R. Perry
Worth saving: disabled children during the Second World War
Sue Wheatcroft

INTELLECTUAL DISABILITY

A CONCEPTUAL HISTORY, 1200–1900

Edited by Patrick McDonagh, C. F. Goodey,
and Tim Stainton

Manchester University Press

Published by Manchester University Press
Altrincham Street, Manchester M1 7JA
www.manchesteruniversitypress.co.uk

British Library Cataloguing-in-Publication Data is available

ISBN 978 1 5261 2531 6 hardback
ISBN 978 1 5261 5164 3 paperback

First published by Manchester University Press in hardback 2018

This edition first published 2021

Typeset by Servis Filmsetting Ltd, Stockport, Cheshire

To our families

Contents

List of figures

List of contributors

Katie Branch is a member of Openstorytellers, where she helps to manage the gigs for the storytelling group and to deliver training courses.

Janina Dillig is currently a Post-Doc in Medieval German Literature at the University of Bamberg, Germany. She wrote her dissertation on identity and masks in the Middle High German versions of the Tristan story, and while she approached the question of identity with methods from gender studies, disability studies is another important focus of her recent research in medieval literature. More specifically, she is interested in the use of disability as a tool for the creation of the hero in Middle High German literature.

Clemma Fleat was born with Fragile X Syndrome. She writes poetry and is collecting a book of favourites. At Openstorytellers she tells stories, trains people, and works on computers, and she plans to carry on hearing, writing and sharing stories and poems.

D. Christopher Gabbard is Associate Professor of English at the University of North Florida. His work has appeared in *PMLA, Eighteenth-Century Studies, SEL, Restoration,* and *The Disability Studies Quarterly.* He has just finished a book-length manuscript, *The Boy Who Broke The Enlightenment: Disability, Medicine, and Fatherhood,* which tells the story of raising a child with significant impairments. His entry 'Human' appeared in *Keywords for Disability Studies* (New York University Press, 2015), and his chapter, 'From Custodial Care to Caring Labor: The Discourse of Who Cares in *Jane Eyre*' appeared in *The Madwoman and the Blindman: Jane Eyre, Discourse, Disability* (Ohio State University Press, 2012). Currently he is co-editing volume four (Age of Enlightenment) of a six-volume Bloomsbury series, *A Cultural History of Disability.* His new project is titled, 'Who Cares? Representations of Caregiving'. And he serves on the editorial board of the *Journal of Literary and Cultural Disability Studies.*

C. F. Goodey holds a PhD from the Department of History and Philosophy of Science, University of Cambridge. He formerly held research and teaching posts at UCL Institute of Education and The Open University, and is currently Honorary Fellow at the Centre for Medical Humanities, University of Leicester. He is the author of *A History of Intelligence and 'Intellectual*

Disability': The Shaping of Psychology in Early Modern Europe (Ashgate, 2011) and *Learning Disability and Inclusion Phobia: Past, Present, Future* (Routledge, 2016).

Nicola Grove lectured at City University, London in Speech and Language Therapy, then left to set up the company of Openstorytellers. She holds an honorary senior lectureship at the Tizard Centre, University of Kent.

Simon Jarrett is a historian, writer, university teacher, and editor of *Community Living* magazine, the UK's only print magazine about learning disability. His doctoral thesis at Birkbeck, University of London explored the changing notion of idiocy in the eighteenth and early nineteenth centuries. He is the author of 'The History of Intellectual Disability: Inclusion or Exclusion?' (in *Community Care and Inclusion for People with an Intellectual Disability*, Floris Books, 2016) and 'Laughing About and Talking About the Idiot in the Eighteenth Century' (in *The Variable Body in History*, Peter Lang, 2016). He has also written numerous articles about the history and culture of people defined as having intellectual disabilities.

Tim Lumley-Smith is a storyteller and disability officer with Openstorytellers, where he has been doing performances for five years.

Patrick McDonagh is a part-time faculty member in the Department of English at Concordia University, Montreal, and the author of *Idiocy: A Cultural History* (Liverpool University Press 2008). He has written a number of articles exploring literary, cultural, philosophical, medical, and other discourses engaging with ideas of intellectual disability, autism, and precursor notions such as idiocy, with an emphasis on the socio-symbolic labour performed by these concepts. He holds an interdisciplinary PhD in Humanities from Concordia, and is co-founder of the Vancouver-based Spectrum Society for Community Living.

Robin Meader is a storyteller and artist for Openstorytellers. His role is to illustrate the stories and publicity for events, book, and training courses. Robin also has his own art business where he draws pictures for meetings and conferences, and sells work to the general public.

Irina Metzler currently holds a Wellcome Trust University Award at Swansea University, working on a research project concerning disability among the later medieval clergy. She is a leading expert on cultural, religious, and social aspects of physical and mental disability in the European Middle Ages. Her books on these topics, including *A Social History of Disability in the Middle Ages: Cultural Considerations of Physical Impairment* (Routledge 2013), *Disability in Medieval Europe: Thinking About Physical Impairment During the High Middle Ages, c.1100–1400* (Routledge 2016), and *Fools and Idiots? Cognitive Disability in the Middle Ages* (Manchester University Press), cover theoretical and socio-cultural aspects of disability in medieval Europe. Her wider research interests revolve around perceptions of the natural world and historical anthropology in the Middle Ages, such as hot climate in cosmography and travel literature.

Murray Simpson is Reader at the School of Education and Social Work at the University of Dundee. He has published a monograph, *Modernity and the Appearance of Idiocy*, plus various articles and chapters on the history of intellectual disability. In addition, he has published on a variety of contemporary topics relating to theoretical and other aspects of intellectual disability. His current interests are in signification, disability, and cinema.

Tim Stainton is Professor at the School of Social Work and Director of the Centre for Inclusion and Citizenship, University of British Columbia. He holds a PhD on disability rights and social policy from the London School of Economics. He has published widely on history, ethics, rights-based social service structures, and disability rights.

Wendy J. Turner, PhD, is a graduate of UCLA and Professor of History at Augusta University. She is the author of *Care and Custody of the Mentally Ill, Incompetent, and Disabled in Medieval England* (Brepols 2013) and the editor of several books, most recently, edited with Sara Butler, *Medicine and the Law in the Middle Ages* (Brill 2014). Turner generally works on the intersection between law and medicine or science in medieval England. She has written articles on many topics concerning medieval English forensic investigation, mental health, intellectual disabilities, treatment of the disabled, trauma, alchemy, and the brain-mind question.

Series editors' foreword

You know a subject has achieved maturity when a book series is dedicated to it. In the case of disability, while it has co-existed with human beings for centuries the study of disability's history is still quite young.

In setting up this series, we chose to encourage multi-methodologic history rather than a purely traditional historical approach, as researchers in disability history come from a wide variety of disciplinary backgrounds. Equally 'disability' history is a diverse topic which benefits from a variety of approaches in order to appreciate its multi-dimensional characteristics.

A test for the team of authors and editors who bring you this series is typical of most series, but disability also brings other consequential challenges. At this time disability is highly contested as a social category in both developing and developed contexts. Inclusion, philosophy, money, education, visibility, sexuality, identity and exclusion are but a handful of the social categories in play. With this degree of politicisation, language is necessarily a cardinal focus.

In an effort to support the plurality of historical voices, the editors have elected to give fair rein to language. Language is historically contingent, and can appear offensive to our contemporary sensitivities. The authors and editors believe that the use of terminology that accurately reflects the historical period of any book in the series will assist readers in their understanding of the history of disability in time and place.

Finally, disability offers the cultural, social and intellectual historian a new 'take' on the world we know. We see disability history as one of a few nascent fields with the potential to reposition our understanding of the flow of cultures, society, institutions, ideas and lived experience. Conceptualisations of 'society' since the early modern period have heavily stressed principles of autonomy, rationality and the subjectivity of the individual agent. Consequently we are frequently oblivious to the historical contingency of the present with respect to those elements. Disability disturbs those foundational features of 'the modern.' Studying disability history helps us resituate our policies, our beliefs and our experiences.

Julie Anderson
Walton O. Schalick, III

Acknowledgements

This collection could not have been completed – indeed, could not have begun – without the engagement and support of a number of individuals. Initial discussions about compiling a collection of works exploring the conceptual history of intellectual disability began some years ago, and included not only the current editors but also Murray K. Simpson and M. Lynne Rose, and we would like to thank them both for their help in these early stages. We would also like to acknowledge the insights offered by Manchester University Press's anonymous reviewer, whose commentaries helped improve the chapters included here. Patrick McDonagh would like to express his thanks for the support (and the welcome distractions) offered by his family: Lynne Peters, Graeme Peters, and Anne McDonagh.

Patrick McDonagh
C. F. Goodey
Tim Stainton

INTRODUCTION:
THE EMERGENT CRITICAL HISTORY OF
INTELLECTUAL DISABILITY

Patrick McDonagh, C. F. Goodey, and Tim Stainton

In 1861, as the concept of 'idiocy', and authority over those designated 'idiots', was in the process of being transported into the medical sphere, the English physicians Martin Duncan and M. B. Lond lamented that 'The terms used in the literature of idiocy complicate the first steps of practical inquiry greatly, and different writers, regardless of the necessity for unanimity, use the same words to describe various classes of idiots'.[1] The fluid terminology that worried Duncan, Lond, and their peers has often appeared as both an obstacle to understanding idiocy (and related concepts), and as an indication of its universality. Edouard Séguin opens his 1846 *Traitement Moral, Hygiène et Éducation des Idiots* with a multi-linguistic and cross-cultural list of synonyms for 'idiocy', and his implication was clear: if everyone has a word for it – or indeed, many words – then 'idiocy' must be a universal condition that crosses time and culture. But at the same time, the slipperiness of the key terms noted by Duncan and Lond might equally point to an accompanying slipperiness of the concept itself, as well as to the struggles of medical and other professionals in the nascent 'idiocy' industry as they sought to define the object of their attention.

Anyone exploring the history, or pre-history, of intellectual disability is faced immediately with a question similar to that which frustrated Duncan and Lond: what *does* the term 'intellectual disability' or, for that matter, 'learning disability' refer to? And what, glancing further back in time, of idiocy? Or folly? We can assume a smooth transhistorical continuity in which one term substitutes for another, but there is another possibility, one supported by critical historical research: that intellectual disability and related concepts are products of and contingent upon specific social and intellectual environments, and perform specific functions within those environments. The questions then become 'How and why do these concepts form? How do they connect with one another? Under what historical circumstances might these connections have taken place?' The objective of this collection is to explore and expand the question of how and why the category of 'intellectual disablity' was defined or, to use the slightly more loaded term, 'constructed'. The disciplinary range covered in this collection – legal, educational, literary, religious, philosophical, and psychiatric histories among others – was not chosen so that sources could be easily filleted for references to some trans-historical human type, but so that each might inform a specifically modern concept, intellectual disability, from their own *sui generis* perspective as forces which shaped definitions and responses at various points in time and place. In so choosing, however, we do not neglect the consequences of these defining forces for the actual people encircled by the shifting definitional field, and who contribute a further perspective to this volume.

In putting together this collection, we seek to chart a course between the Scylla of assuming a trans-historical subject, whose definition was gradually revealed over time to emerge as the modern-day 'person with an intellectual disability', and the Charybdis of extreme post-modern constructionism which ultimately dissolves into a fog of isolated contingencies. There is a connection between the early modern and the modern intellectually disabled subject; but the nature of that connection, however, is not readily defined or discerned. We can say what it is not: it is not one simply of terminology, underdeveloped ontological understanding, or epistemological refinement. And what is clearer is that the historical treatment of the subject requires certain considerations in order for that connection to emerge as free from retrospective taint as possible. This introductory chapter will review some of the key areas of contention in delineating the role and relationship of history to the present-day subject and will set out the broad organizing principles for this volume.

The challenges of language and terminology

If, as we argue, there is no definitive trans-historical concept of intellectual disability, then it is no surprise that language used to describe it is remarkably unstable, even in this age of presumptive certainty that 'we know what intellectual disability is'. This very volume could easily be marketed to the same audience under at least three different labels (intellectual disability, developmental disability, and – in the UK at least – learning disability). Anne Digby, in discussing the choice to use the terminology of the historical period under study, notes that its multiplicity has confused the subject matter, and that both political correctness and the desire to reduce stigma associated with terminology has accelerated the rate of terminological change.[2] While not inaccurate, this observation seems to imply the kind of historical continuity of the subject which has plagued much of the scholarship in the area and does not fully address the implications of that multiplicity. Rather than confusing the subject matter, the plethora of terms *is*, in part, the subject matter, and certainly the starting-point for research. Understanding their meaning in context, their roots and implications, and the social forces which brought them to this association is a critical site for historical inquiry. Is 'political correctness' the only or primary reason for changing terminology? To what extent can we posit an essential core underlying the labels used, or does this shifting sand in fact imply the lack of any essential core? These questions do not have simple or singular answers.

On one level the most concrete problem is that, in many cases, terms assumed to directly mirror contemporary 'intellectual disability' in fact do not do so, or least not in a linear fashion. The philosopher John Locke, for example, author of some of the founding texts of modern psychology, used at least four different terms which have been presumed to reference intellectual disability. Locke used 'idiot' when describing the purely intellectual realm of the human understanding (the ability to 'abstract') and its absence; on the other hand, when he was discussing natural history and species difference, he used 'changeling'. He also used 'fools' or 'naturals' (an abbreviation for 'natural fools') interchangeably with both, though possibly referring only to the 'lower' end of that category. 'Idiots' would have likely covered a broader group than the one we would today consider as persons with intellectual disabilities, and would also have encompassed the uneducated and uncultured (one of the earlier definitions of the term). In his differentiation between madness and idiocy, Locke situates 'idiots' apart from the mentally ill and alongside 'brutes', the general category for animals, which 'abstract not'.

While clearly there is some overlap, we cannot assume a direct correlation either among these terms or to our modern subject: Locke's idiot is not the same as his changeling, and neither can be equated with a person labelled as intellectually disabled today. But, critically, these usages can tell us much about the process of constructing the subject as well as the broader social positioning. The term 'brute', for instance, recalls the longstanding association of intellectual disability with non-human animals. Indeed Locke directly suggests that 'changelings' represent an interstitial species: 'Here every body will be ready to ask, if Changelings may be supposed something between Man and Beast, "Pray what are they?" I answer, Changelings, which is as good a Word to signify something different from the signification of Man or Beast'.[3] 'Changeling' itself has a long and complex history reaching well beyond an association with anything remotely related to intellectual disability, ranging from children with physical disabilities, to Christian nonconformists, to Jews. A good example of this comes from the interpretation of Luther's *Table Talk*, a standard reference-point where he suggests that a 'changeling' child be drowned because he is a 'mass of flesh' having no soul. This has led the period to be seen as the worst in history for people with an intellectual disability.[4] On closer examination, however, it is not clear that this was an intellectually disabled child as we would recognize one today; it is also unclear whether the story itself is even Luther's.[5]

While complete misassociations are rare, uncritical assumptions that these terms represent a trans-historical subject persist, most notably in the recent craze for retrospective diagnosis of the 'Mozart had Asperger's' or 'caveman had autism' variety (in Ch. 8 this question is addressed briefly, as the writers discuss the possibility – and its potential relevance – that 'Peter the Wild Boy' had Pitt Hopkins Syndrome). This is not to suggest that the trisomy 21 associated with Down's Syndrome, for instance, did not exist prior to the actual discovery of the chromosomal variation. We merely warn against jumping to the conclusion that it would have placed you in any of the categories suggested by the above historical labels at any given point in time, or that having the physical appearance of such a chromosomal variation would have meant the same thing as it does today in terms of social position, recognition or responses. What this means for historians is not that there is a complete lack of association between terms, but that we must treat them as signifiers that are highly contingent and context-dependent. Indeed, language is a critical site of historical inquiry that can tell us much about the nature of the subject and the forces constructing it, as well as the contemporary social responses to it.

On a more contemporary front, to dismiss the rapidly changing terminology as simple 'political correctness' misses the more critical point of language as a site of struggle and identity – similar to what we have seen in the civil rights movement (negro, black, African American, person of colour, etc) or the women's movement (girls, ladies, women, wymyn, wimmin, etc); such a simple dismissal also ignores the continued instability of the concept itself. It is not insignificant that the movement of people *currently* bearing the various labels and who advocate for recognition of their rights has chosen to reject the label altogether, and to replace it with 'People First'. This is a recognition of the fact that there is no essential subject in social terms, and also of the more politically relevant position that it does not matter why or how you came to be excluded or marginalized: it is the marginalization itself which defines you as 'other'.

The notion of othering is also useful in understanding the approach we propose here. As Digby notes, 'Implicit in the language used to describe these individuals is the notion of the Other'.[6] Clearly there was a both an implicit as well as often an explicit purpose to label and define people as 'not like us'. The example from Locke is perhaps most explicit in taking this so far as to tie the description to an interstitial species difference that forms a stable item in natural history (though even he suggests that category definitions are ultimately arbitrary). But if we accept this notion of othering, then does it not imply that to understand the nature of the other we must understand those doing the othering and their context? And if the independent variable in the equation is the dominant actor, then surely there is also great scope for mission creep. In other words, there is a risk that categories used to identify anyone 'not like us' may have a broader scope than what the term may imply on first reading. As discussed above, 'changeling' was applied at different points in history to a broad range of persons 'not like us'. A more recent example can be drawn from the first wave of eugenics, when 'women of loose morals', indigenous people, and immigrants often found themselves classified as part of the feebleminded or idiot class. We cannot understand the category without understanding the social and cultural circumstance of those doing the classifying; thus, understanding the 'history of intellectual disability' requires not an understanding of the march of science so much as an investigation of changing socio-cultural contexts. This applies equally to the present as to the past, and as such implies in addition a different *future* for how we conceptualize and respond to people currently categorized as 'intellectually disabled'.

Intellectual disability and historiography

Our topic has received comparatively little attention from historians and the humanities in general. But in recent years there has been, if not a torrent of historical treatments of intellectual disability, at least a steady stream. For many years, the standard works on the history of intellectual or learning disability were those by by Leo Kanner and Richard Scheerenberger, which charted the 'progress' in definition and services and implicitly assumed a trans-historical intellectually disabled subject that has gradually been revealed through scientific progress.[7] But since the early 1990s there has been a shift from these Whiggish histories, or in Noll and Trent's words 'achievement histories',[8] to works exploring the social, cultural, and intellectual history of idiocy, learning disability, intellectual disability, and related concepts. Not coincidentally, the appearance of these new histories has been paralleled by shifts in the social position of people identified as having intellectual or learning disabilities. The 1980s and 1990s witnessed the closure of many long-term institutions, with formerly segregated people being moved (with varying degrees of integration) into community-based settings. At the same time, People First and other grass-roots self-advocacy groups of people labeled as having learning or intellectual disabilities have sought to make heard the voices of the profoundly margin-alized, and while these groups may have little mainstream political impact, they have gained some small measure of recognition within the disability community and the professions engaged with that community.

A first wave of critical histories – primarily social, institutional, and policy histories – appeared in the mid-1990s, with James Trent's *Inventing the Feeble Mind* (1994), Philip Ferguson's *Abandoned to Their Fate* (1994), Steven Noll's *Feeble-Minded in Our Midst* (1995), and Wright and Digby's collection *From Idiocy to Mental Deficiency* (1996). These works suggested new ways of approaching the idea of intellectual disability, analysing the forces that gave shape to the notion and engaging with questions of the status of people identi-fied as idiots according to their sociocultural environment.

Fundamental to Trent's thesis is the Foucauldian notion that 'care' is a central tool of 'control', and he argues that 'mental retardation is a construc-tion whose changing meaning is shaped both by individuals who initiate and administer policies, programs and practices, and by the social context to which these individuals are responding'.[9] Drawing on the examples of 'madhouse' histories such as those by Roy Porter and Andrew Scull,[10] Trent tracks the early asylum movement in the US, from Samuel Gridley Howe and Edouard Séguin through to the 'normalization' movement and the deinstitutionaliza-tion advocacy of the late twentieth century, focusing primarily on the means by which a professional medical and scientific class sought to assert control over people identified as 'feeble-minded' in order to cement its own authority.

Trent's work was not alone in focusing on the US, with his study being published at roughly the same time as Ferguson's history of the American institutionalization movement, which focused on the Rome State Custodial Asylum for Unteachable Idiots (later the Rome Developmental Center) as its prime exemplar,[11] and Noll's analysis of the development of the eugenic agenda within institutions in the southern US from 1900 to 1940, which explored the influence of class, race, and gender in determining who would be incarcerated and, further, who would be subjected to eugenic procedures, notably sterilization.[12] Of these three works focusing on the institutionaliza-tion of people labeled as 'idiots' or 'feebleminded', Trent casts the widest net, surveying 150 years of institutionalization in America, and is the most asser-tive in arguing the socially constructed aspects of 'feeble-mindedness'. Noll and Trent also edited a collection of essays, *Mental Retardation in America: A Historical Reader*, reaching back to the mid-nineteenth century but with most contributions being institutional or policy histories focusing on twentieth-century issues of eugenics, segregation, education, and policy development; some contributions, however, explored the ideological and cultural construction of intellectual disability.[13]

Across the Atlantic, Wright and Digby's 1996 collection explored the place of learning disability in the UK, with contributions representing social, legal, institutional and intellectual histories from the medieval period to the twentieth century.[14] This broad-ranging collection – necessarily more eclectic than a single-author monograph – can be credited with opening even further avenues of research into the idea of learning disability or intellectual disability (terms which in UK usage are roughly synonymous). In her introduction to the collection, Digby expressed the hope that the book would 'stimulate further studies into the history of these individuals',[15] and in the five years following its publication, three of its contributors published their own book-length studies: Mathew Thomson's *The Problem of Mental Deficiency* (1998), Mark Jackson's *The Borderland of Imbecility* (2000), and David Wright's *Mental Disability in Victorian England* (2001).[16] Thomson examines the development and application of mental deficiency laws in the UK from 1913 to the 1946 National Service Health Act; the bulk of his analysis focuses on policy development, and of the forces acting on it, with an emphasis on the work of the Royal Commission on the Care and Control of the Feeble-Minded and the 1913 Mental Deficiency Act that came out of the Commission's recommendations. In tracking the relations of these laws to movements in political theory, health care, and eugenics, Thomson argues that 'to understand why the problem of mental deficiency has become acute by the early twentieth century we need to go beyond an explanation which rests on the eugenic threat posed by the feeble-minded, to consider how this fear ineracted with anxieties about regulating the boundaries of responsible citizenship and managing an increasingly sophisticated network of welfare instiututions'.[17]

Jackson's history of the creation of the liminal category of the feeble-minded focuses on Mary Dendy's Sandlebridge schools and her related writings to explore how this group was presented as a threat to the health of the nation; he argues that 'late Victorian and Edwardian conceptions of [feeble-mindedness] and its boundaries were clearly fabricated under the influence of profound, predominantly middle-class, anxieties about race, class, criminality, and sexuality' that were 'reconfigured through the window of contemporary biological explanations of mental deficiency'.[18]

Meanwhile, Wright delved into the Earlswood archives to present a comprehensive institutional story of the Royal Earlswood Asylum from its mid-nineteenth-century foundation to the end of the century, touching on the policies and practices that characterized the first large British institution for people identified as 'idiots' from the 1840s to the end of the nineteenth century. While this work focuses specifically on institutions and their operations, Thomson and Jackson are more particularly concerned with the creation of a new group, the 'feeble-minded', lying on what Jackson identifies as 'the borderland of imbecility'. Thus they investigate social forces – notably anxieties around urban poverty, moral degeneracy, and ethnic and race relations shaping these late nineteenth- and early twentieth-century categories – with the deeper aim of showing how these intersect with medical and scientific discourses and result in the formation of a new group of outcast undesirables who could be controlled through segregation (Jackson) and social policy (Thomson).

More recent studies have undertaken a critical interrogation of the concept itself, exploring less the question of 'how the intellectually disabled were treated and/or managed', and moving beyond the immediate social forces and towards how the concept was formed and took shape. These histories analyse the cultural discourses and intellectual currents that helped give shape to intellectual disability; further, they investigate the symbolic labour performed by the idea of idiocy: that is, they ask *what* people mean when they refer to idiocy or intellectual or learning disability, and they ask *why* these concepts assume significance in a particular historical time and place, whether this significance is expressed within a cultural product or a social event.

The first book-length cultural study of idiocy, Martin Halliwell's *Images of Idiocy: The Idiot Figure in Modern Fiction and Film* (2004), explores the use of 'idiot' characters in novels and in films based on these novels, focusing on 'the way in which idiot figures have been constructed to propel narratives in a particular direction or to act as a counterpoint to other characters';[19] however, Halliwell's work is not a history, and further is limited by his choice not to explore the idea of idiocy beyond the parameters of these cultural products, and by his implicit assumption of a trans-historical materiality to idiocy.

Two of the editors of the present collection have also published books engaged with tracking the history of ideas of intellectual disability, both arguing that the concept, and its various precursor concepts, are given shape and meaning by their historical context, connecting these notions to the social and intellectual tensions of their specific time and place. Patrick McDonagh's *Idiocy: A Cultural History* (2008) takes an explicitly historical approach in exploring the discursive and symbolic function of the 'idiot' figure in cultural products – primarily plays, poems, and novels, from the sixteenth to the early twentieth century – in order to illuminate more fully the symbolic labour performed by the image of the idiot in other discourses – legal, theological, scientific, and medical – and to use this evidence to track the historical and ideological development of the idea of idiocy.[20]

Chris Goodey's *A History of Intelligence and 'Intellectual Disability'*: *The Shaping of Psychology in Early Modern Europe* (2011) further demonstrates that the history of intellectual disability is also the history of intelligence, and is interwoven with a wide range of other histories across disciplines, including legal, theological, philosophical, and aesthetic discourses.[21] Goodey's research, focusing on Europe from the late medieval period to the early eighteenth century, argues that ideas of intelligence developed in a bid for social authority and status in competition with other status modes, those of the 'honour' and 'grace' societies; in this formulation, the 'idiot', as the outsider group enabling the creation of a society characterized by 'intelligence', stands in direct relation to the 'vulgar' and the 'reprobate' – the outsider groups that helped defined the 'honour' and 'grace' societies, respectively.

Gerald O'Brien's *Framing the Moron: The Social Construction of Feeble-Mindedness in the American Eugenic Era* (2013) looks at the different metaphors – including the moron as animal, as pathogen, and as enemy force – used to give shape to the idea of the 'moron' in the US in the first four decades of the twentieth century.[22] Murray K. Simpson's *Modernity and the Appearance of Idiocy: Intellectual Disability as a Regime of Truth* (2014) presents a Foucauldian 'archaeology of intellectual disability',[23] exploring the intellectual discourses shaping ideas of intellectual disability from the eighteenth-century Enlightenment through the development of Édouard Séguin's pedogy in the nineteenth century, the medicalization of idiocy and classification of its different types, and the creation of idiocy as a problem of development: all of these function as means towards a kind of 'conceptual exclusion' that isolates idiocy as an objective phenomenon.[24] Simpson's analysis argues that idiocy is a 'discursive contingency' that is symptomatic of contemporary anxieties rather than a constant and transhistorical state of being.

Most recently, Irina Metzler's *Fools and Idiots? Cognitive Disability in the Middle Ages* (2016) marks the first book-length exploration of the idea of cognitive disability in the medieval period.[25] This work in particular demonstrates historians' increasing recognition of the significance of ideas of idiocy to the trajectory of other, more mainstream narratives – philosophical, theological, and educational, rather than purely medical or scientific. It is in this burgeoning context that the history of the idea of intellectual disability and related notions, while still sparsely represented in the catalogues, is making its presence and importance felt.

Why we need a conceptual history of intellectual disability

In the gradual emergence of this critical history, and particularly one that targets conceptual foundations, a wide range of disciplines has become relevant: the history of medicine, literary and cultural history, social history, legal history, the history of religion, the history of education, and latterly (with the closure of the institutions) oral history. A tension remains between the history of medicine and those other disciplines, however, inasmuch as residual notions of a trans-historical subject linger on in them. Under 'medicine' come too psychiatry and psychology, often operating in its name and drawing from it a scientific cachet. Professionals in these latter fields were once well represented on the list of authors who have written histories of intellectual disability, including Kanner and Scheerenberger, and they must be distinguished from professional historians whose area of interest just happens to be the history of psychology. Offsetting such quasi-medical professional motives, however, which might be seen as favouring the scientific or 'medical model' of a trans-historical subject, there has also been a high incidence of authorial motives that spring from a direct, non-professional knowledge of people with intellectual disabilities, either as family members or as advocates. This latter motive tends to be 'biased', if one may use such a term, in a different direction, towards asserting the full humanity of the people thus labelled – though such is the contradictoriness of our topic that neither motive necessarily excludes the other.

Disability studies, meanwhile, starts off from its direct opposition to that medical model, and some of the recent work cited above would claim disability history rather than the history of medicine as its reference-point. Of course this discipline is more sophisticated than we have space to discuss,[26] but a parallel problem occurs here too. To put it crudely, disability studies tends to take the ontological status of 'impairment' more or less for granted. Grounded as the discipline is in studies of physical and sensory conditions, it sees 'disability' as the *social* consequence of an underlying *natural* impairment.

Two different, though not entirely contradictory, possibilities ensue. Many people before the modern era, and some people still, have taken physical or sensory impairment as external signs of an impaired intellect. The classic reference here is the person whose partner or friend is asked 'Does she take sugar?' Consequently, in response to this calumny, the 'social model' retains space for a tacit belief that some intellectually disabled nature does indeed truly exist: that there are people whose real essence constitutes the thing which people with physical and sensory impairments are not, and which they vehemently deny being. Equally, though, the social model retains space for the fact that across history a missing limb is always a missing limb; hence physical disability contains some sort of 'natural' bedrock through which critical analysis prob-ably cannot penetrate, and this *contrasts* with the fundamental lack of histori-cal stability or conceptual permanence in intellectual disability – thus raising the question whether the latter can be considered to have any such natural bedrock.

In short, is intellectual disability an impairment at all? The sheer range of primary conceptual sources and their dislocated character, evident from research in our field and in the chapters presented here, is a pointer to the thought that, in the long historical sweep, it is not. The obvious demur would be that despite this historical and conceptual shape-shifting, some actual people at this present moment are lacking in certain specific abilities that everyone else takes for granted as a mode of their social functioning. And of course that is true. All academic sophistication aside, it is no good denying it or one might create a situation where it seems a good idea to ditch people's social supports along with their labels. However, while this objection may confirm something as a disability in the 'social model' sense (i.e. it is forms of social organisation that create discrimination and the very need for support), the nature of any notionally trans-historical 'impairment' beneath it remains unclear.

Consequently, while both history of medicine and disability studies have given rise to work on our topic that is both critical and sound, we venture to suggest that for the purposes of future research some additional disciplinary reference-points are necessary.

First of all, it seems obvious that one avenue through which the history of *intellectual* disability should be pursued is *intellectual* history. This is a discipline whose various schools (there is also 'history of ideas' and 'con-ceptual history') research large ideas not ahistorically but in the context of specific historical cultures and actors. It asks: what questions were men and women of a particular time asking of each other, how did they perceive each other, and what do their conceptual and theoretical apparatuses owe to this? Moreover, it tends to specialize in the early modern era, from late medieval to Enlightenment, with which this present volume too is concerned, and this means that it engages inevitably and especially with something historically specific, namely the emerging concepts and centrality of a secular human reason, of intelligence and intellectual ability. The study of the corresponding *dis*ability surely has some vital connection to this. Yet the 'reason' on which intellectual history has focused consists mainly of philosophical, political, and economic ideas. It tends to leave knowledge of the psychological kind out of the frame, perhaps partly convinced by the latter's characteristic claim to be a 'hard' science by association with biology. And it has touched only in passing on our topic: for example, by tracing forwards from the classical era the theory of 'natural slavery', in which intellectual inferiority is inseparable from political subordination.[27]

This might be seen as an avoidance tactic, in psychoanalytic terms a 'resistance': would one really want to expose oneself to the kind of evidence from intellectual *dis*ability which might detract from the intellectual ability that is the foundation of one's own discipline and its assumptions? If so, then something similar applies to a discipline like the history of the human sciences, which ought to be particularly receptive to our topic and in which psychology does indeed form one strand. As its leading critical authorities point out (and as routine accounts of the history of psychology do not), the subject and the object of study here are made of the same primary materials as each other. The mind studies the mind. And if even physics has a notorious subject-object problem (in quantum physics both the object and the instruments measuring it consist of quantum systems), so much the more problematic must it be in psychology, whose constituents are not even material ones. It is especially necessary and especially difficult, therefore, to 'look at it "from outside"'.[28] Neither intellectual history nor the history of the human sciences is simply a lens through which a particular historical culture observes some primary conceptual entity that otherwise has a permanent and natural existence; rather, the conceptual entity is also itself the lens. The critical study of such a core consistuent as intelligence and its absence should surely form part of intellectual history and contribute to it.

Secondly, it ought not to be necessary to add that another avenue through which the history of intellectual disability must be pursued is *history*, as a discipline with its own theories and methodologies that have to be respected. Its leading theorists have insisted that, rather than rush immediately to 'what happened in the past' and thereby risk only holding it up as a static and distorted mirror to the present, the historian should recognize before even setting out that the relationship is a dynamic one. R. G. Collingwood famously pointed out that each past era has had its 'absolute presuppositions' which, though unfamiliar to us now, were once beyond question and which there had been a prior and unwitting decision to believe. These presuppositions constitute, so to speak, the metaphysics of the particular era. The historian's job is to get round the back of them. Collingwood also said that doing so makes it easier to get round the back of our own.[29] The dynamic element consists in a living tension between past and present, in which 'without historical knowledge of the beliefs held about the nature of being human, we are ignorant of what it is to be human'.[30] And so one question vital to the historian in our field, at the outset of their research, is as follows: What, in the absolute presuppositions of past eras about the essence of what it is to be human, occupied the key position which cognitive-type intellectual ability occupies today, and by what concrete historical processes did the former become the latter?

Also called for is the appropriate historical methodology: a modicum of something akin to scientific method. For example, it is standard practice in the history of medicine to cross-check the *label* a primary source has for some bodily disease against the symptoms or *characteristics* which are attached to it in that same source. This is all the more crucial for intellectual disability, in view of psychology's subject-object problem. As indicated above, when the source contains a label such as 'mental defective' or 'feeble-minded', or earlier 'idiot' or 'imbecile', or earlier still 'innocent' or 'natural fool' (or indeed Latin and other foreign-language equivalents, whose translation introduces yet further chances of semantic slippage), the same procedure needs to be followed. In setting down to work, then, another vital question will be: Do the specific descriptive characteristics with which the adjacent context defines that label correspond with the characteristics which define today's 'intellectually disabled' people? The cognitive critieria of the latter can be found in any current textbook and are very specific indeed.

If they do not, and if all possible alternative meanings are not researched first, then modern criteria will travel back through time to slip cosily and ghostlike into the vacant slot. And when this happens, it may have something to do with the absolute presuppositions of our own that result from both the (relatively recent) sacralized social status of intelligence and its seemingly indispensable place in the mutual recognition and self-esteem of individuals. Collingwood's dictum implies moreover that the further away in time the presuppositions are, the stranger they will seem to the twenty-first-century eye, and therefore the more difficult to interpret or even detect. In addition, in the special case of intellectual disability, the further away they are, the greater too the degree of cultural *variety* there will be even across one and the same period. This is yet another contrast with today's outlook which is monolithic, and derives from the Baconian or Kantian idea of a universal human history with a universal human reason or intellectual ability at its core.

Finally, in noting and recommending the emergence of a distinctively 'conceptual' approach to historiography, we cannot leave it floating freely above the hard realities of social existence. As Reinhart Koselleck has pointed out, neither social history nor conceptual history are singular branches of the discipline as are (say) economic history, diplomatic history, or church history. Rather they constitute, in tandem, a *general* claim, 'so to speak, an anthropological claim', that encompasses all special histories. Researchers confronted with the plethora, ambiguity and, at times, sheer contradictoriness of labels and concepts in our particular field will grasp the salience of this, and the correspondingly restricted 'specialness' of medical or disability history. Yet the social-conceptual relationship itself is not straightforward. Transformations over the course of social history occur at a different rate from those occuring in conceptual history, and the 'structures of repetition' in each are likewise mutually distinguishable. The terminology of social history remains dependent on the history of concepts because it needs to access 'linguistically stored experience', while conceptual history remains dependent on social history because it has to keep an eye on the 'unbridgeable difference between vanished reality and its linguistic evidence'.[31] All this plays havoc with periodisation, as we shall see. The problem is that while labels and concepts in psychology are unstable by comparison with the facts of social history, their respective timescales are different *and* connected.

From the middle ages to the great confinement

We have suggested above the possible extension of scholarly research as far as certain disciplines that are already intrinsic or adjacent to our subject matter, rather than into social theory in general. Without them, 'theory' itself, even in its most radical forms, would be ill-equipped to stand fully outside our absolute presuppositions about people who, being socially invisible, are largely invisible to theory too.

That is not to argue against the importance of theory. Michel Foucault's identification of 'the great confinement' (*le grand enfermement*) has shaped much research into the history of 'unreason', and while we would certainly employ caveats to our use of this phrase, it remains relevant to the conceptual history of intellectual disability. Foucault himself had nothing to say about intellectual disability as such, and in comparison with the broad historical sweep implied in his use of *le grand enfermement*, in the history of intellectual disability it refers to a specific moment: the onset of the long-stay hospital institutions in the last third of the nineteenth century. Of course, with intellectual disability, as with mental illness, the majority of people affected always remained in the wider community or at least in the family home, not in the institutions.[32] Nevertheless, the image of confinement remains central: the institutions *did* in fact sweep into a more or less single remit a range of human conditions, and drew their inmates from community and family situations whose immediate causes cannot easily be categorized.[33]

In so doing, they helped to create the climate of labelling in which the modern (albeit, as always, provisional) definition – the *conceptual* confinement

– of intellectual disability arose. Although physicians were centrally involved in the creation of the first long-stay institutions and continued to be so, others, such as psychiatrist Wilhelm Griesinger and the polymath statistician and psychologist Francis Galton, were soon visiting, and from their preocuppations would inevitably come a sharper delineation of categories that reciprocally reinforced their own 'mind-science' specialisms. The combined medical model that ensued finally removed the organic identity of individuals and imposed its own upon them, stealing from them who they were and dictating who they would become.

That is why we stop in the mid-nineteenth century, with the onset of the institutions. The relative abruptness of our end-point helps to highlight the historical contingency of what would subsequently be presented to the public as a scientific category. Moreover, for scholarly purposes, the decisiveness of that break opens out whole fields of enquiry prior to 1850. Instead of hunting down pre-modern examples of modern intellectual disability, one enquires instead across all pre-modern forms of 'othering' and beyond for the conceptual ingredients that would go into the creation of intellectual disability as a specifically modern concept. And this sets new conditions for historical research, since the most widely read and discussed research work thus far has focused chiefly on the nineteenth and twentieth centuries; as we have said, the conceptual pre-history is much less well known. Could this very choice and limitation of subject matter confine the intellects of potential historians, or at least block our field of vision? The more critical of the studies we discussed at the outset recognize intellectual disability's cultural contexts. Yet it is a step considerably further to suggest that it is a cultural category at its very root, rather than a natural kind. And that, as the articles in this volume show, is what is proved to be the case once the pre-modern field, along with its terms of enquiry, is opened out.

At the same time, that very breadth of field poses a more difficult problem: where to start. Periodisation is always a notoriously difficult task. *Any* year zero for our topic would be purely notional. But we can say with some assurance that going back much further would have finally rendered this collection incoherent, and made it impossible to have psychology's state-of-the-art term 'intellectual disability' in the title. Let us suppose some notional point in the far distant past where there was no such thing. At what point did the concept come about? Is it not arbitrary to begin as we do with the late medieval era? As Irina Metzler's chapter in this volume shows, apposite resonances, in a restricted sense, appear in primary source texts earlier than that; one can begin to detect them at the height of the Roman Empire, and with the start of Christianity. In the philosophy of that period, it is possible to find descriptions of what look like modern 'intellectual' deficiencies if not in a discrete type, then attached to sensory impairment, to blind and deaf people.[34] Disconcertingly for the historian, though, people labelled 'fool' or 'innocent', familiar though the labels as such may look, tend *not* to be defined by deficiencies of that particular sort. And this continues to be the case well into the sixteenth century.

It is not an easy chronological ride, then. What we can say, however, is that the late medieval era was witnessing a huge expansion in the social administration of church and state ('Empire' in its broadest sense), and with this came the rise of a written bureaucratic culture among the *literati*. Thus our collection starts with the sightings of a modern concept among a precise social caste which specialized in the writing and application of the law or had been educated accordingly. As Brian Stock's seminal work on the history of literacy demonstrates, in the late middle ages *idiota* was the term for a broad sector of the population: the illiterate in general (if only illiterate in Latin, knowledge of which was what the term *literatus* indicated), or simply an ordinary lay person who, even if able to read, was unversed in a particular profession; in ecclesiastical contexts, *idiota* referred to a novitiate.[35]

This semantic matrix survived well into the seventeenth century. Yet alongside it, within the professional niche of the *literati*, alarm bells had already begun to ring. What if that broadly interpreted *idiota* were spotted within the sphere (however demographically restricted) of property inheritance, or of an education system whose function was to form the administrative elite doing the classifying? There, the non-expert status was more evidently problematic. Even so, if in this one label out of many we have discovered forward connections and the beginnings of a 'shaping' role for the modern profile of intellectual disability, nevertheless its presence in legal theory was not understood at all clearly even then – not even by practising lawyers, as Wendy Turner's chapter in this volume illustrates.

Its eventually crucial historical role thus originated from what has rightly been called 'a strange place', one that was at the time esoteric.[36] Important as property law may have been to late medieval socio-economic functioning, this restricted kind of idiot did not yet have a central position in broad cultural discourses, since today's universally dominant idea of a general, species-specific human intelligence had still to acquire its now sacred status. Nevertheless, from that point on, an unbroken line can start to be traced (on which medicine for a long time remains in the rearguard) – a line that would lead one day to the embodiment of deficiency concepts in a human or, more often, sub-human *type*.

Overview of chapters

We begin this collection, accordingly, with Wendy Turner's investigation of medieval responses to 'intellectual disability', which supplies the appropriate vantage-point for seeing how an existing set of labels (*idiota, fatuus, stupidus* etc) started to become relevant to the courts. The skills of perception, cogitation, and memory were needed to learn and act appropriately in a social environment – albeit one restricted by membership to an elite class (to the other social classes these labels might apply across the board). Lawyers and clerical experts who had studied at the first universities would have learned about such mental operations in their theological and philosophical studies of the soul and intellect; they then used them for practical administrative purposes, in the bureaucracy needed to cope with the burgeoning feudal property system. Officials challenged individuals who seemed unable to cope with their landholding obligations and material goods. New laws based on primogeniture imposed a greater need to distinguish permanent incapacity from temporary mental illness. As in modern tests for head injury, they tested people on everyday things they should be familiar with, such as counting money. The main dividing line across the spectrum of abilities thus focused on whether people could handle their social responsibilities. It leaves us to wonder, was their deficiency some natural condition *recognized* first in jurisprudence, or a predominantly social construct that first begins to be *invented* there, at a specific Western historical conjuncture?

Irina Metzler deals with education, starting from a standard categorization within medieval thought that separated the reasoning faculty from the will – a division whose themes still pervade subdisciplines such as educational psychology. 'Will-nots', as the name suggests, were able but reluctant to learn, or obstreperous enough to willfully sabotage their learning objectives. Following clues in the Roman writer Quintilian, she describes how this aspect of medieval educational theory surfaces particularly in that widely studied teaching manual, the *Didascalicon* of the twelfth-century theologian Hugh of St Victor. Making more detailed differential analyses of learning ability than before, in a context where the important areas of study were theology and philosophy, Hugh, like most other writers, assumed that disabilities were malleable and improvable. The more important problem for him was the distinction between people regarded as not wanting to learn something and people incapable of doing so despite perhaps wanting to, between 'pretend fool' and 'genuine fool'. Metzler discusses also the beginnings of a greater concern with what would later become the mind-body problem, through the relationship between physical physiognomy and difficulties with learning.

Janina Dillig looks at how these ideas and practices were reflected in literature. Using the legend of Parsifal as her central reference, Dillig demonstrates medieval ideas of what it meant to be a fool in a literary context, and shows how that literature embraces an entire range of concepts regarding 'intellectual disability' which have in common only how much they differ from modern ideas about the intellect. These examples of fools in medieval literature, by no means a complete list, nevertheless exhibit the sheer variety of depictions prior to foolishness becoming a popular literary theme from the sixteenth century onwards. Above all, foolishness was not simply contrasted with reason as we now understand it. On the contrary, it could indicate sainthood or mere innocence (where the primary discourse was about sin rather than reason), or a simple lack of knowledge or awareness of social mores. Moreover, these were also the basis for comical situations in which foolishness could be greeted with or without malice; these were contextually related to the court jester, whose occupation represented the socially acceptable form of the will fool. On the widest cultural kind of evidence then, that of fictional literature, medieval discourses on intellectual disability cannot be reduced to one type, but can be seen to have interacted with each other.

Taking us into the early modern era, Chris Goodey directs our attention to some of the dominant actors, those doing the classifying of people. In his focused reading of a debate from the 1650s, he describes how sections of the church, faced with the social, political, and denominational chaos of the English civil wars and revolution, developed an obsession with the formal, codified assessment of human types. The church catechism was the diagnostic manual by which a pastor would assess the understandings of his flock and grant them access to holy communion, or, conversely, deny it. In the latter case, driven by circumstance and the dialectic of religious dispute, a novel type of 'idiocy' was singled out that differed from madness inasmuch as it was permanent and promised no lucid intervals, and differed from the 'reprobation' of sinners and hypocrites inasmuch as idiocy was not willful as theirs was. 'Idiots', then, marked a category that should be *excused* but *not included*. In this sense they were direct precursors of those pathological minority 'idiots' who by the nineteenth century would be featuring in a modern science of the mind, as a stage on the almost seamless journey from elimination by excommunication to elimination by pre-natal testing, and from the catechism to the IQ test.

Turning to literary articulations of intelligence and 'defects of the mind', Chris Gabbard explores the fourth and final section of Jonathan Swift's 1726 satire *Gulliver's Travels*, in which Lemuel Gulliver, Swift's protagonist, finds himself in the land of the Houyhnhnms, a society governed by rational horses but also infested with the 'cursed race of *Yahoos*'. Eventually Gulliver comes to recognize the Yahoos as bestial humans. Gabbard argues persuasively that Swift here develops a thought experiment based upon John Locke's distinctions between rational 'persons' and those lesser humans lacking rational capacity, also identified by Locke as 'changelings' – instances of Locke's investment in what the philosopher Licia Carlson has called 'cognitive ableism'.[37] Swift applies Locke's notions to the world of Houyhnhnms and Yahoos; Gulliver, himself a character whose rationality is ambiguous, slowly recognizes himself to be a 'yahoo' – at least so far as his equine hosts are concerned – and all he can succeed in negotiating is most-favoured-beast status. In the end, having been driven from the land of the Houyhnhnms, Gulliver too would like to establish a society based on 'cognitive ableism', albeit narcissistically around himself. But he must settle for a parody of that world, and upon his return to eighteenth-century England he shuts himself up in his stable with his horses. In Swift's satirical inversion, Gulliver's need to exclude the animalistic 'other' results in his retreat from human society.

Like Chris Gabbard, Tim Stainton also tracks the profound impact of the work of John Locke, but in this case focusing on the theory of sensationalism – the theory that knowledge comes not from innate ideas or principles but from sensory experience and our intellect's capacity to interpret that experience. While sensationalism predates Locke, Stainton explores how Locke's articulation of it refined the notion. He then traces the permutations of Lockean sensationalism through the writings of Jean-Jacques Rousseau, especially his *Émile*, a discourse on pedagogy, and the philosophy of the senses and their role in intellectual development presented by Étienne Bonnot de Condillac in his *Essay on the Origin of Human Knowledge*, which Condillac saw as a 'supplement' to Locke's work. While these thinkers further developed the theory of sensationalism and created thought experiments to elaborate upon it – exemplified by Rousseau's developing child character Émile and Condillac's 'statue' who acquires senses one by one – it was not until Jean Itard's famous pedagogical experiments with Victor, the 'Wild Boy of Aveyron', that philosophers found a means by which they could apply and test these theories. As we know, Itard's attempts to instruct Victor met with mixed results, and in the end Itard admitted failure, not of the theory of sensationalism itself but rather of his own capacity to construct proper tests, and of Victor's appropriateness as a test subject. But this apparent failure did not diminish the impact of Itard's work; Stainton demonstrates how Itard's development of the ideas of Locke, Rousseau and Condillac formed the foundation for the hegemonic control later exercised by medicine over both the idea of idiocy and the care and control of those individuals so labelled.

In the following chapter, Openstorytellers, a collective of people with learning difficulties, put their own labelling under the historical microscope. In the early eighteenth century two exotic individuals were brought to England from Hanover, the second on the orders of the first; both were outsiders, and both found it difficult to communicate with the society around them. The Elector of Hanover, brought over in 1714 to be England's King George I, was responsible a decade later for bringing 'Peter the Wild Boy', recently discovered in the woods outside Hanover. Peter was as famous among cultural commentators of the later eighteenth century as Victor, the 1800s' 'Wild Boy of Aveyron', is among today's, and can thus be seen as Victor's precursor in establishing a modern science of idiocy. The discussants place 'fellow-feeling' (to use an eighteenth-century term), rather than cognitive ability, at the core of what it is to be human, situating it in the tangible context of Peter's life experiences rather than in rhetorical generalities. This fellow-feeling stands in contrast to the formal, unfeeling scientific categories that tie human difference to the materiality of genes and 'syndromes', and shows how the abuse undergone by outsiders exhibits a greater degree of historical continuity than the shifting conceptual frameworks behind their various constructions and historical manifestations. This chapter is not, therefore, an entry in some intelligence-related 'special olympics' where any offering, however slight, has the role of fulfilling the quota demands of an inclusive methodology. Rather, the parallel is with oral history. Life stories, for the purposes of social research, constitute primary sources of equal value with others. The same can be true of conceptual history; the discussants' choice of focus, in keeping with the scholarly aims of the rest of the volume, supplies a privileged and necessary perspective from which more needs to be heard in future.

The complex interplay of medical, legal, and lay knowledge in legal definitions of idiocy, imbecility, and related terms forms the focus of Simon Jarrett's chapter. Jarrett documents the shifts in legal theory and, drawing on a series of compelling case histories, illustrates the tensions that would transform legal notions of what might constitute idiocy. Legal definitions of idiocy relied heavily on a set of traditional formulae to determine one's capacity to manage oneself and one's estates, but in practice eighteenth-century case histories employed a mix of popular notions about idiocy alongside these formulae to determine the status of individuals brought before the court. Jarrett also shows how legal developments took place in shifting social contexts, as the crown relinquished authority for the protection of the rights of 'idiots' and families began to look to the courts to provide this protection instead. A further transformation begins at the start of the nineteenth century, as medical authorities lay claim to knowledge offering clearer and more consistent understandings and definitions of idiocy. However, these claims are not tested in court until the second half of the nineteenth century, and even then the tensions between reputed medical knowledge, the historically developed opinions of law-makers, and popular lay beliefs continued to shape the understanding of 'idiocy' and 'imbecility' in the courtroom – rather than the others simply capitulating to medical knowledge. Indeed, as Jarrett shows, when appearing in the court, medical authority often simply repeated established lay and legal notions of idiocy rather than extending an understanding of the concept, formalizing as medical knowledge what had previously been dismissed as the ignorance of lay folk.

Murray Simpson's chapter examines an overlooked issue, the place of idiocy in psychological theories in the late eighteenth and the nineteenth centuries. Too often historians of psychology ignore the presence of idiocy in psychological schemata, dismissing it as irrelevant to post-Freudian understandings of the mind. As Simpson shows, this elision obscures our understanding of how these early psychological theorists imagined the mind to work. Simpson tracks the idea of idiocy in the 'conceptual economy of madness' to illuminate how it interacts with notions such as madness, melancholy, and mania in the frameworks of mental conditions as developed by William Cullen, Philippe Pinel, John Conolly, Henry Maudsley, A. F. Tredgold, and others whose ideas shaped the development of psychology through the nineteenth century. In the twentieth century idiocy becomes separated from the mainstream of psychology and psychiatry – and from its historiography – as Freudian and other forms of ego-based theories of psychology displace the apparently 'ego-less' idiot; Simpson's research re-inserts the idiot into this history, and in so doing provides insights into the role of professional authorities in defining pathologies and, ultimately, what it means to be human.

In the final chapter, Patrick McDonagh turns to literary evidence to explore the shaping of not only idiocy but the notion of a separate world – both conceptual and actual – that is occupied by those bearing the label. He investigates a number of travelogues written by visitors to the Royal Earlswood Asylum for Idiots in the 1850s and 1860s in order to track how these writings gave shape to a new idea of the idiot. Asylum travelogues portrayed a parallel world in which this isolated person, cared for by benevolent, enlightened medical authorities, was able to grow and prosper. In most cases, these travelogues were public-relations tools, often connected to fund-raising for the institution; in all cases, they reinforce the idea of the idiot as an individual apart from the rest of society, even while emphasizing his (and, less often, her) humanity. McDonagh's chapter provides a critical anatomy of these writings, exploring their shared rhetoric and content to demonstrate how they set out to form a new idea of idiocy for readers, contributing to the transformation of the popular understanding of idiocy.

Conclusion

While these chapters draw on varying forms of evidence and theoretical approach, they share an interest in tracking the processes by which the ideas of idiocy, stupidity, folly, imbecility, and related pre-modern terms are given shape and apparent substance, and how these shift across time and place. In their interdisciplinarity they demonstrate the breadth of forces operating in any historical period on the notion of what it is to be human. At the present historical moment, for people bearing the labels, as well as for the rest of us, recognition of how strange and different the past is can help with imagining a future that is also different. The conceptual confinement of 'intellectual disability' – the dominance of the cognitive model of what it means to be human – continues today in places where physical confinement is still the norm, but it thrives too in countries like Canada and the UK, which have taken deinstitutionalisation furthest.

Notably in these countries, structured forms of community support for independent living through 'person-centred planning' were first introduced as a matter of sheer existential necessity: what were these people going to do once suddenly liberated? The person-centred plan was not premised on what was wrong with people; they were no longer told who they were and who they would become. Rather, they could say it for themselves, and as the oral histories of people liberated from the institutions show, they have wanted all along the same things as everyone else: friendships, independence, a job.[38] The formerly piecemeal practice of person-centred planning has recently entered national legislation in these leading-edge countries, in schools and colleges as well as in adult social policy. Making it work within long-standing professional and administrative structures and, where necessary, dismantling or transforming them, is, of course, a more difficult enterprise. Nevertheless, this practice and its enshrinement in law are historically of great significance inasmuch as they signal the first change for a century and a half in how identities are formed and conceived.

Not only does knowing that things were different in the past prompt the imagining of a different future, imagining that future is itself a historical event, an intervention by historical actors. It is what people do, sooner or later. And if those people happen to be historical researchers, imagination can be an aid to scholarship. It may be a cliché to say that you cannot know where a society is going if you do not know where it came from, but it is also the case that you will not be able to know where it came from without also having some feel for where it might now be going, and for your own place in that trajectory.

Notes

1 P. Martin Duncan, M. B. Lond, et al. 'Notes on Idiocy', *Journal of Mental Science* 7 (1861), 236.

2 Anne Digby, 'Contexts and Perspectives', in *From Idiocy to Mental Deficiency: Historical Perspectives on People with Learning Disabilities*, edited by David Wright and Anne Digby (London: Routledge, 1996), 2–3.

3 John Locke, *An Essay Concerning Human Understanding* [1689], edited by Peter Nidditch (Oxford: Clarendon Press, 1975), 569; Bk. IV, Ch. IV, S. 14.

4 See, for example, Richard Scheerenberger, *A History of Mental Retardation* (Baltimore: P. H. Brookes, 1983).

5 M. Miles, 'Martin Luther and Childhood Disability', *Journal of Religion, Disability and Health* 5.4 (2001); C. F. Goodey and T. Stainton, 'Intellectual Disability and the Myth of the Changeling Myth', *Journal of the History of the Behavioral Sciences*, 37.3 (2001).

6 Digby, 'Contexts and Perspectives', 3.

7 Leo Kanner, *A History of the Care and Study of the Mentally Retarded* (Springfield: C. C. Thomas, 1964).

8 Steven Noll and James Trent, eds. *Mental Retardation in America: A Historical Reader* (New York: New York University Press, 2004), 7.

9 James Trent, *Inventing the Feeble Mind: A History of Mental Retardation in the United States* (Berkeley: University of California Press, 1994), 2.

10 See, for example, Roy Porter, *A Social History of Madness: The World Through the Eyes of the Insane* (New York: Dutton, 1989) and Andrew Scull, *Museums of Madness: The Social Organization of Insanity in Nineteenth-Century England* (London: Allen Lane, 1979).

11 Philip Ferguson, *Abandoned to Their Fate: A History of Social Policy and Practice Toward Severely Retarded People in America, 1820–1920* (Philadelphia: Temple University Press, 1994).

12 Steven Noll, *Feeble-Minded in Our Midst: Institutions for the Mentally Retarded in the South, 1900–1940* (Chapel Hill: University of North Carolina Press, 1995).

13 For works in this collection exploring the ideological and social construction of intellectual disability see Janice Brockley, 'Rearing the Child who Never Grew: Ideologies of Parenting and Intellectual Disability in American History', 130–164; Gerald Schmidt, 'Fictional Voices and Viewpoints for the Mentally Deficient, 1929–1939', 186–206; and Karen Keely, 'Sexuality and Storytelling: Literary Representations of the "Feebleminded" in the Age of Sterilization', 207–222. All in Steven Noll and James Trent, eds. *Mental Retardation in America: A Historical Reader* (New York: New York University Press, 2004).

14 David Wright and Anne Digby, eds. *From Idiocy to Mental Deficiency: Historical Perspectives on People with Learning Disabilities* (London: Routledge, 1996).

15 Digby, 'Contexts and Perspectives', 1.

16 Mathew Thomson, *The Problem of Mental Deficiency: Eugenics, Democracy, and*

Social Policy in Britain c.1870–1959 (Oxford: Oxford University Press, 1998); Mark Jackson, *The Borderland of Imbecility: Medicine, Society and the Fabrication of the Feeble Mind in Late Victorian and Edwardian England* (Manchester: Manchester University Press, 2000); David Wright, *Mental Disability in Victorian England: The Earlswood Asylum* (Oxford: Oxford University Press, 2001).

17 Thomson, *The Problem of Mental Deficiency*, 35.

18 Jackson, *The Borderland of Imbecility*, 11.

19 Martin Halliwell, *Images of Idiocy: The Idiot Figure in Modern Fiction and Film* (Aldershot: Ashgate, 2004), 14.

20 Patrick McDonagh, *Idiocy: A Cultural History* (Liverpool: Liverpool University Press 2008).

21 C. F. Goodey, *A History of Intelligence and 'Intellectual Disability': The Shaping of Psychology in Early Modern Europe* (Farnham and Burlington VT: Ashgate, 2011).

22 Gerald O'Brien, *Framing the Moron: The Social Construction of Feeble-Mindedness in the American Eugenic Era* (Manchester: Manchester University Press, 2013).

23 Murray K. Simpson, *Modernity and the Appearance of Idiocy: Intellectual Disability as a Regime of Truth* (Lampeter: Edwin Mellen, 2014), 8.

24 Ibid., 7.

25 Irina Metzler, *Fools and Idiots? Intellectual Disability in the Middle Ages* (Manchester: Manchester University Press, 2016).

26 See, for example, Dan Goodley, 'Learning Difficulties, the Social Model of Disability and Impairment: Challenging Epistemologies', *Disability and Society* 16.2 (2001), 207–231.

27 See, for example, Don Herzog, *Happy Slaves: A Critique of Consent Theory* (Chicago: University of Chicago Press, 1989).

28 Roger Smith, *Between Mind and Nature: A History of Psychology* (London: Reaktion Books, 2013), 7.

29 R. G. Collingwood, *The Idea of History*, revised edn (Oxford University Press, 2005).

30 Roger Smith, *Being Human: Historical Knowledge and the Creation of Human Nature* (Manchester: Manchester University Press, 2007), 9.

31 Reinhart Koselleck, *The Practice of Conceptual History: Timing History, Spacing Concepts* (Stanford, CA: Stanford University Press, 2002), 20, 37.

32 Peter Bartlett and David Wright, *Outside the Walls of the Asylum: The History of Community Care 1750–2000* (London: The Athlone Press, 1999).

33 Deborah Cohen, *Family Secrets: Living with Shame from the Victorians to the Present Day* (Oxford: Oxford University Press, 2013).

34 C. F. Goodey and M. Lynn Rose, 'Mental States, Bodily Dispositions and Table Manners: A Guide to Reading "Intellectual Disability" from Homer to Late Antiquity', in *Disabilities in Roman Antiquity: Disparate Bodies a Capite ad Calcem*, edited by C. Laes et al. (Leiden: Brill, 2013).

35 Brian Stock, *The Implications of Literacy: Written Language and Models of Interpretation in the Eleventh and Twelfth Centuries* (Princeton: Princeton

University Press, 1983). See also M. T. Clanchy, *From Memory to Written Record: England 1066–1307* (Chichester: Wiley-Blackwell, 2013), 226ff.

36 Eliza Buhrer, '"But What is to be Said of a Fool?" Intellectual Disability in Medieval Thought and Culture', in *Mental Health, Spirituality, and Religion in the Middle Ages and Early Modern Age*, edited by Albrecht Classen (Berlin: De Gruyter, 2014), 314–343.

37 Licia Carlson, *The Faces of Intellectual Disability: Philosophical Reflections* (Bloomington: Indiana University Press, 2009).

38 See, for example, the 'Life Stories' materials gathered on The Open University's Social History of Learning Disability website: www.open.ac.uk/health-and-social-care/research/shld/resources-and-publications/life-stories, accessed 8 August, 2016.

2

CONCEPTUALIZATION OF INTELLECTUAL DISABILITY IN MEDIEVAL ENGLISH LAW

Wendy J. Turner

In 1286, the Exchequer sent an escheator – an investigator of escheats, lands that could revert to the king – to inquire about Peter Seyvill, a man said to be 'incapable of managing his lands or affairs', a *freneticus idiota*. If Peter was mentally 'incapable', the escheator was to grant guardianship of Peter, his wife, children, and property to Peter's brother-in-law, John Dychton. The escheator found Peter to be 'unable to manage', a condition that in the twenty-first century, depending on his exact symptoms, would be called an 'intellectual disability'. The escheator sent John Dychton to Westminster with written documentation that would give him guardianship over his 'idiotic' and 'frenetic' relative; however, John became lost on the way to Westminster and returned without having delivered the paperwork. The escheator now described *John* as 'incapable' of taking on further responsibilities since he was 'weak in knowledge and reason'. To be certain he was not judging out of frustration, the escheator had his findings concerning John Dychton confirmed by a jury of knights from the area.[1]

What did these ideas mean to the escheator as he described these two men, one 'incapable of managing' as well as 'a frenetic idiot', and the other 'weak in knowledge and reason'? Was the escheator describing different conditions or similar? Did he know the differences between various intellectual disabilities?

The focus of this study is the different terminologies concerned with learning and intelligence in the English Middle Ages, and the medieval understanding of these concepts. This understanding is difficult to pin down since they used their own terminology, which was quite different from the vocabulary of today. They had no need to define their terms *per se* since they understood what they meant among one another. After much study of medieval English terms and use of vocabulary, the medieval discussions at court and in the royal administrative records of individuals with 'incapacity to manage', 'weakness in reason', and 'lack of understanding', among other phrases, can be shown to describe those individuals having deficiencies of memory, difficulties managing responsibilities, issues of behavioural discretion, and weaknesses of intellectual functioning – in essence, the learning disabled.[2]

Studies of medieval mental health

Until recently, the history of medieval mental health was not as rich or well researched as similar histories for the periods of the early modern,[3] modern,[4] and beyond. There were only a handful of scholarly works about medieval mental health before the 1960s,[5] but much more scholarship began to trickle out in the late twentieth century as part of the effort to understand the so-called 'fringe' of society, including works beginning in the 1960s by Michel Foucault,[6] Judith S. Neaman,[7] H. H. Beek,[8] Hellmut Flashar,[9] Michèle Ristich de Groote,[10] Thomas Graham,[11] Heinrich Schipperges,[12] and Donald W. Sutherland.[13] Many of these scholars wrote only one article on the topic of medieval mental health as part of their individual attempts to understand the actions (or reactions) of medieval society. Beek's monograph is probably the most thorough study within this group of scholars, although his work (written in Dutch) was never translated into English and did not have the wide readership of Foucault or Neaman. The collective work of these 1960s scholars became something of a movement. Work in the area of early mental health developed into the beginnings of its own field in the 1970s with numerous monographs and major articles by Penelope Reed Doob,[14] Stanley W. Jackson,[15] Richard Neugebauer,[16] Robert S. Kinsman,[17] Basil Clarke,[18] E. S. Gurdjuan,[19] E. Ruth Harvey,[20] and Vieda Skultans.[21] While some of those working in this new field continued to publish into the 1980s and 1990s, new scholars emerging in this period began asking different questions of the records about treatment, legal standing, and medicine, leaving behind philosophical and literary discussions over whether medieval communities saw the mentally impaired as punished by God, tormented by demons, or protected by God as innocents. Some of these new historical studies, while admitting they were basically 'social' or 'cultural' in scope, began to emulate science rather than traditional humanities. Those advocating these new approaches include Roy Porter,[22] Sander L. Gilman,[23] and Simon Kemp[24] writing in the 1980s, and F. Fandery,[25] Jean-Marie Fritz,[26] David Roffe,[27] George Rosen,[28] John Southworth,[29] Allen Thiher,[30] and Judith Weiss[31] in the 1990s.

A new wave of interest in mental health and disabilities generally in the Middle Ages emerged in the twenty-first century. Many of this new generation of scholars 'have not only brought an innovative set of questions to bear upon material from medieval literature and history, but they have also had to confront issues of "presentism" in disability theory, modifying it to suit the cultures of the European Middle Ages'.[32] It is not simply that these new scholars are looking at medieval materials in a different way, but that they are re-examining materials for things either medieval or contemporary authors missed or buried. They are, at last, tracing meanings behind the medieval vocabulary – once used quite haphazardly by scholars – precisely, and finding that medieval society had a decent working knowledge of the differences between what modern physicians and psychiatrists have distinguished as neurotic, psychotic, and learning disorders.

Medieval understanding of mental health

English legal and administrative records – including but not limited to Chancery records, court records, inquisitions post mortem, plea records, accounts of fines, deeds, and warrants – used a variety of terms to describe and categorize mental health conditions. Additionally, medieval physicians had their own commonplace books (personal records of patients and/or diagnoses) and vocabulary – the great difference being not in conditions, but that their words for these conditions came from Greek roots rather than Latin, as they were in law. The medical community recognized at least three general categories of brain function and realized that epilepsy and migraine were separate conditions of the brain.[33] The church had its own way of discussing mental health conditions and generally used the mentally disabled in particular as a trope, warning parishioners that loss of mental faculties might be because of sin in the mind.[34] Court representatives – including local officials such as sheriffs and jury members, along with crown officials such as escheators, commissioners, lawyers, and judges – did not call for assistance from physicians or clergy to aid in their determinations; they had their own 'tests' for cognitive abilities, discussed in more detail below.

In the Middle Ages, intellectual ability was a matter of carrying out responsibilities. If a man or woman could not intellectually do so *and* his or her responsibilities mattered to the community, the individual would have been tested as to his or her ability and, if lacking, given into the care of a guardian or keeper or both, which is how many medieval English ideas about mental health generally and intellectual disability more specifically can be uncovered today.[35] Many of those without responsibilities that mattered never made it to pen and parchment. For the most part, only intellectually weak heirs or lawbreakers found their way into the records. Still, those few records tell a larger story about the medieval English understanding of the intellect.

In the case that opened this article, Peter Seyvill might have had some issues with interpersonal situations, since he was described as *frenetic*, which suggests uncontrolled action. He was certainly weak in intelligence since he could not 'manage his lands or affairs'. He understood enough to come this far in life as a farmer, husband, and parent. He had not been in trouble with the law. Peter must have started to make mistakes, perhaps became overwhelmed by his responsibilities, due to age or some factor that exacerbated his condition. Whatever the reason, though, he came to the attention of the escheator. His brother-in-law, John, functioned a bit more within an acceptable range, well enough to be left in control of his own property and entrusted, however briefly, with the guardianship documentation. When John returned, still carrying the parchment, the escheator came to the conclusion that John was weak in intelligence.

Medical understanding of the brain

Although legal and administrative officials did not call on medical experts for advice on mental health questions, at least by the end of the thirteenth century, the medieval medical community had several working theories on how the brain functioned, and postulated ideas of how the brain could be corrected, if not functioning properly. The brain, they theorized, held three 'chambers' that governed from front to back the senses, cogitation, and memory. Input from the world entered the front of the brain through the senses, the theory said, and people cogitated about what their senses told them in the middle, remembering what was important in the back.[36] Bartholomeus Anglicus wrote:

> in the brain there are three chambers. In the front most, the imagination works. There, the things that the senses ['utter wit'] perceive in the world are ordered and put together in the mind, as says Johannicus. There is also a middle chamber hosting logistics. There, the sensibility of reason or estimation virtue is a master. Finally, there is the third and last [chamber], which holds the memory, the virtue of the mind. That virtue holds things that are mentally perceived and that the mind understands [already] from imagination or reason.[37]

Later in the Middle Ages, physicians identified five functions along with the senses and linked them to locations in the brain. There was even accounting for an exchange between memories and current thinking.[38]

If there was a problem, physicians would suggest treatments to rebalance humours through diet, medicines, or other remedies – including baths, extra sleep, dark rooms, or change in living conditions. Medieval physicians said little, even when using their own terminology, about learning disorders or intellectual disabilities. Yet, they describe areas of the brain responsible for various conditions, which, at times, overlapped from one category to the next, blending perception, cogitation, and memory. Alongside these therapies, they gave possible reasons for malfunction, including both humoural and environmental causes.

Medieval tests for intellectual ability

The medieval social, legal, and administrative understanding and categorization of mental health conditions was related to the medical organization of brain functions. Clerks and lawyers used a highly structured spectrum of conditions from active to passive and simultaneously violent to non-violent, which corresponds logically to the same symptoms and conditions physicians describe from anterior to posterior in the brain.[39] Legal and administrative officials used tests for cognitive and sensory function, much as the twenty-first century individual might in cases of head trauma.

Individuals were tested when and if their responsibilities were neglected or questioned. The community became concerned when a person 'forgot' his or her responsibilities to society. For example, in 1342, Thomas Grenestede, sane, was tested when someone reported that he had neglected his responsibilities. The escheator verified Thomas's intellectual functioning by asking him to do a variety of tasks, among others 'counting money' and 'measuring cloth'. The escheator found Thomas to be 'of good mind and sane memory in word and deed'.[40] The investigator's questions brought to light an individual's abilities at verbal and active tasks as well as examining his or her aptitude in terms of common sense, discernment, critical thinking, calculating, and remembering.

Responsibility and memory speak to the pragmatic side of life in the mostly illiterate and community-oriented Middle Ages. Responsibility and memory were of a practical and upmost concern, while understanding an individual's cognitive ability was not necessarily important; however, when an individual stopped upholding responsibilities or forgetting, court representatives questioned his or her intelligence. Emma Beston provides an excellent case study, highlighting her weakness in these skills.[41] She could not remember the name of her town or of her son. She did not know where she was. This lack of awareness left her vulnerable and in potential danger, which was the responsibility of the community. She knew she had been married three times, but could only remember the name of one of her husbands. 'Being asked whether she would rather have twenty silver groats than forty pence, she said they were of the same value'.[42] The royal officials examining her concluded that Emma had 'neither sense nor memory nor sufficient intelligence to manage herself, her

lands or her goods. As appeared by inspection, she had the face and countenance of an idiot'.[43] What exactly this last statement means is hard to know, but
it probably had something to do with lack of embarrassment at not knowing
the answers or of a general aspect of vacancy.

The term *idiota*, idiot, is an ancient Latin term for an uneducated com-
moner. In the Middle Ages, it carried three meanings: 'weak intelligence',
a 'charlatan', and sometimes a 'fool', as in a sane person who acts unwisely.
Officials conducted tests for weak intelligence at various times and at different
levels of authority, which included but was not limited to local sheriffs, juries,
escheators, the Exchequer, the king's council, parliament, or the king. Their
diligence was in part because the crown claimed guardianship over all mentally incapacitated landholders. In the *Prerogativa Regis*[44] and late medieval
English legal commentaries,[45] there was a perception of a qualitative difference
between those born mentally incapacitated (*fatui naturales*) and those who
became incapacitated later (*non compotes mentis*), which foreshadowed the
modern difference between a learning disorder and a mental weakness with
a moment of onset. These also led to a difference in how the crown held an
individual's lands in guardianship.

Deficient in memory

Medieval tests for memory[46] included questions as to whether an individual
knew the names of his or her relatives, where the court was being held, and
where he or she normally resided. These tests might also include identification of
practical objects, such as coins. If an individual could not correctly identify coins
and their associated value, he or she could not be trusted with money or account
records. For example, the crown sent a commission of three men, later expanded
to five, to investigate Ralph Bolmere in 1352. Someone reported to the king that
Ralph was 'not of sound memory' (*non bone memorie*).[47] The commission found
that Ralph had problems with memory; furthermore, he had 'alienated a great
quantity of land [...] in the counties of York and Northumberland', which the
commission restored to Ralph's estate, seizing it from those who purchased it
while Ralph was not in his right mind. The commission acted 'without delay' to
return the lands to Ralph, since the holders of the lands might damage the properties.[48] In the case of Ralph, the commission labeled him *non bone memorie*, not
of sound memory. In other instances, royal officials used terms such as *non sane
memoria*, not of a healthy memory, listed in medieval medical works as conditions associated with lethargy and the posterior of the brain.[49]

Giving away or selling (quitclaiming) land reduced an individual's holding
and could also destroy an inheritance, which was of importance to heirs and

the crown alike. A poor memory for details such as family rights and responsibilities could spell disaster for future generations. Those persons with poor
memories, called *non sane memoria* or some variant, came to also bear the
label of *non compos mentis*. For example, Roger Blick was listed as 'mentally
incapacitated' (*non fuit compos mentis sue*) after he gave a parcel of land to the
local chaplain in 1248, prompting the complaint of his heirs (his sisters and
their husbands). The jurors of the case examined and tested Roger, finding him
'of good memory and sound mind' (*fuit bone memorie et compos mentis sue*).[50]
Although Roger might well have been thinking of the church and his eternal
soul, his heirs called his action into question because it weakened their future
standing socially and economically.

Other cases bear out the connection between a sound mind and a healthy
memory. Much like Roger Blick, William de Clamberge was 'not of sound
mind or good memory' and granted land to another party, which aggravated
his heirs. In this case the recipient of the land was the king. The council for the
king told the opposite story: William was sane at the time of the transaction,
and the council wanted William's relatives punished for slander against the
crown. At the next parliament, the relatives laid out their case that the royal
officials making the transaction knew that William was 'neither mentally sound
nor of good memory' (*non fuit sane mentis sue aut bone memorie*), and it was the
officials that should be punished.[51] In another example, investigators found
Elizabeth Strange 'feeble ... and without a good memory' (*debilis ... et non
bone ... memoria*).[52] In this case the terminology was not *non compos mentis*,
but *debilis*, 'feeble', yet the meaning is much the same. To have a poor memory
meant that an individual was also weak in the eyes of medieval society, which
relied heavily on memory in their mostly illiterate world.

A final example of weak memory highlights a man who might not be intellectually weak, but rather have other issues; the differences are subtle but important. 'Thomas the husband of Margery Gernet' died and a witness said that
John Gernet killed him. The account also claimed that John 'was outlawed, and
having become an idiot of deficient memory, [he] alienated [his lands]'.[53] A
couple of things strike the reader as odd – both for a modern audience and presumably for the medieval judge as well. Running away, becoming an outlaw, is
a likely response from a person in panic – something either an intelligent or an
intellectually weak person might do. And, if an 'idiot' was away long enough,
this person might lose his lands. Yet, the record implied he 'became' an idiot
because of the murder, and if so, why would someone so overly emotionally
affected take the time to sell, 'alienate', his property? If he was cognizant of the
situation, he was not *that* affected, and he was *not* an 'idiot'. The medieval judge
had good reason to question this unlikely story. The escheator, who protected

the lands while awaiting a decision, eventually located John Gernet, learning that he had not killed anyone and he was not mentally incapacitated; he had sold (quitclaimed) the lands 'about Michaelmas'. John was acquitted of all wrongdoing. The reason this case is important as a study is that it demonstrates the power of both investigation in the Middle Ages into possible mental health conditions and breaking of the law, and the potential for disruption of lives if falsely accused of being learning disabled or having another mental affliction.

Managing responsibilities

Two interconnected phrases that describe the phenomenon of the inability of an individual to care for self, property, and family were an inability to 'rule his lands' or 'manage his affairs', or variants of 'rule' and 'manage'. Landholders so described were seen to have low mental abilities in cognition and cogitation. They could not think rationally enough to be entrusted with property. John Bryt, for example, was an 'idiot from birth, unable to manage himself or his lands'.[54] He was given a guardian, as were Ralph Clendon, who was 'incapable of managing',[55] and Gilbert atte Hale, described as 'an idiot and incapable of managing his lands and goods'.[56] John Harpesfeld was 'an idiot from birth with insufficient sense to administer his lands and tenements'.[57] And Emma Beston had not the 'intelligence to *manage* herself, her lands or her goods' (emphasis added).[58] Others have similar problems. Royal officials found Peter Seyvill's ability 'insufficient to rule his lands';[59] Ralph Trelewith could 'not manage his affairs';[60] and John Bertelot was 'incapable of administering his property'.[61] All of these people lacked enough intelligence to cope in medieval society and were not to be trusted with property, lands, or goods.

Others were found to have such low intelligence that they could not be left alone, as they could not care for themselves. Geoffrey Aston found Roger, for example, unable to live without care, after he 'personally examine[d] Roger de Kyngeford who is said to be an idiot and not sufficient for the rule of himself or his lands'.[62] Joan Wantyngg, another example, was found to be 'entirely without sense'[63] to the point that she 'may not have governance of herself'.[64] The records say not only that she was 'incapable of managing her affairs',[65] but also that she 'has not her reason' (*sensum racionabilem*).[66] Henry Appleford, 'an idiot from birth with insufficient intelligence to administer his lands and tenements',[67] was given a royal guardian, as were many of these property holders – as much to help them as to help the crown. Those like John Martyn, 'an idiot since his birth, so that he is incapable of managing himself or his lands',[68] and Roger Stanlak, 'an idiot from birth so that he was not capable of ruling himself or his lands',[69] could bring money to the guardian and Exchequer.

Medieval use of the term *idiota*

The question remains: did English medieval administrators using the word *idiota* mean that those who were described as 'idiots' were by definition also *ignorant* or was *idiota* something else? In one case of 1308, William Maureward was brought 'before the king's council at Westminster' to be interrogated as to his mental ability. There was doubt in the mind of the other officials – sheriffs, escheators, or others – who initially investigated his mental capacity, and they sent him to the council. The councilmen questioned him until they 'found that he is not a madman and an idiot, but is wise and sufficient for the government of his affairs, and so he is dismissed'.[70] His level of intelligence was 'sufficient' to govern his affairs; he was not an *idiota* but 'wise'. These were cleverly written as if opposites, idiot and wise.

Of the individuals in the administrative accounts called *idiota*, some were intellectually weak, while others were not. John Heton, for example, had 'good sense and [was] quite sane' until about twenty-four.[71] In 1353, a jury examined him and found him to be 'an idiot, insensible to his surroundings, having a fancy in his head, whereby he remains unconscious of his own personality (*ipsius negligens*) and paying no heed to anything at all'.[72] Certainly this could be a decent description of a modern intellectually disabled person, except for the fact that this condition would not have onset when an individual was twenty-four. John married before the onset of his affliction, which might indicate that he had something akin to the modern conditions of schizophrenia or a personality disorder, or that he had a stroke and was not simply intellectually or learning disabled. Therefore, rather than count up all of those persons described as *idiota* as a way to identify those medieval persons with what the DSM-5 today would label as having learning disorders and intellectual disabilities specifically, caution must be taken not to treat all those described in the Middle Ages as *idiota* the same. Those cases of 'idiots' with descriptions of a lack of memory, self-neglect, property neglect, or having signs of cognitive difficulties are those that could be included among the medieval intellectually weak.

Lack of discretion

The modern understanding of a person lacking discretion invokes deficiencies of social skills or of interpersonal skills. Such individuals today may not understand the social conventions of embarrassment, regard for others, waiting in turn, or even non-literal references, such as the phrase, 'someone is pulling my leg', taking it to mean that someone is literally touching my leg. Medieval

accounts of persons lacking discretion often called them 'fools' or more specifically 'fatuous'. Use of the term 'fool' ran the gamut in medieval England, as
it does in the twenty-first century. Some people were called 'fools' (often, for
some reason, the clerks used the French term *sot* or *fol*, even in the Latin court
records, probably to avoid confusion with and distinguish between the various
meanings of *idiota*) who were in no way intellectually weak, but rather rational
and sane individuals who made poor decisions. At other times the word fool,
fatuus, especially in conjunction with *idiota*, meant 'fatuous', a socially inept
person, lacking interpersonal skills and social poise. For example, a clerk in the
Miscellany role described Elizabeth Chambernon as 'a fool and an idiot since
birth' (*fatuus et idiota a nativitate*).[73] She clearly did not understand the world
around her, allowing her to be taken advantage of by the leading men of the
town. She was 'married within three days of her said father's death to William
Polglas', and, within days of the death of William, she married John Sergeaux.
With William she had a son, Richard, who was also a 'fool and idiot from birth',
as well as a daughter, Margaret, whom the medieval records treat as 'normal'
in her thinking and countenance. These records portrayed Elizabeth as completely unaware that her daughter's husband, John Herle, worked with his new
father-in-law, John Sergeaux, to gain control of Margaret's learning disabled
brother, Richard, who would one day be heir to four fortunes. John Sergeaux
moved the 'foolish and intellectually weak' Richard out of the area to keep the
king from finding him when Elizabeth died.

Other examples in administrative rolls used the phrase 'by reason of his
foolishness and idiocy' (*ratione fatuitatis et idiocie*) as motivation to intercede
with a guardian for an estate. These cases were fairly common in the post
mortem records of the fourteenth and fifteenth centuries, such as with John
Aleyn, who was described as 'a mere fool and idiot since birth',[74] and William
Brekore, part of whose lands 'belongs to the king' since William was 'a fool and
an idiot'.[75] William Venour was also said to be 'a fool and idiot', but when the
escheator examined him in 1328, he found William 'sufficiently discreet',[76]
letting him live on his own and continue to control his own affairs. In the eyes
of medieval court representatives, foolishness and lack of discretion, then,
pointed to a behavioural aspect of weakness in personality often linked to a
weak intellect.

Weak intellectual functioning

The medieval tests for intellectual functioning examined a person's ability to
calculate and think critically – to cogitate – about an issue put to them. Could
they, for example, make change or measure cloth? Emma Beston, mentioned

above, did not know the difference between silver coins and copper ones. This might have been an example of poor memory, but it also spoke to an inability to think critically about coinage, to note differences – copper versus silver – even when she knew they were coins.

Used quite precisely, the term *ignorant*, 'unintelligent', meant having a low cognitive ability and lacking insight or any ability to think critically. Several examples of persons described as *ignorant* will illuminate the medieval English understanding of this disabling mental state. In 1420, Thomas atte Wode,[77] was described as 'ignorant by reason of his fatuousness and idiocy' (*ignorant ratione fatuitatis et idiocie*),[78] connecting the ideas of a low cognitive ability and lack of discretion to weak intellectual functioning. The abbot accused of holding Thomas's property illegally said that Thomas was 'a demented unintelligent person' (*demencia ignorans*) and tried to explain that he was only helping poor Thomas.[79] Yet, the link is there – to be labeled an 'idiot' in the administrative records meant that the person was, in particular instances, intellectually weak and, therefore, disadvantaged. Another example of an *ignorant* is Joan Jordan, also known as Joan Spencer, from 1399. She was a London heiress to many shops and properties; her guardians were not keeping her in 'sufficient sustenance' and a few of her properties were not in good repair. In the *post mortem* records she is listed as an *idiote* or *fatua et idiota*,[80] but in the Exchequer enrollments of inquiry of 1401, Joan is identified as *ignorant*.[81] In 1396, another example, the escheator found John Berghdon also to be *fatuitatis* (in a state of foolishness) and at the same time *ignorant*;[82] he became a ward of the crown. About 1465, the description of Alice Fyssh, the daughter of John Saltby, is most telling as to the medieval connections between the intellectual capacity of an 'idiot' and that of being 'ignorant' when the escheator reported that Alice was born in her condition: 'she is a natural fool and idiot ... inwardly ignorant' (*naturalis fatua et ydiota ... penitus ignorant est*).[83] There were others, such as Thomas Erons, who admitted to killing a person when 'effecting dementia ... while ignorant' (*demens effectus sint ... quod ignorant*).[84] All of these instances of being in a state of poor cognition, *ignorant*, appear severe and were qualified by other words, such as 'inwardly', 'by reason of fatuousness', 'an idiot from birth (natural)', or 'effecting dementia'. A person of low cognitive ability to the medieval official, then, was someone who could outwardly act demented or fatuous but also inwardly had difficulty thinking, remembering, and decision-making. Some of these individuals, such as Alice Fyssh, probably had the medieval equivalent of a learning disorder, while others, like Joan Jordan, may have had something like modern cortical dementia, such as Alzheimer's or Creutzfeldt-Jakob disease, since in her longer recorded history she grew worse over time.

Conclusions

In the Middle Ages, responsibility for tasks, goods, property, and other things was important to the success and well-being of the community and family as a whole. To that end, the crown's representatives examined and sometimes protected and removed from positions of authority, no matter how insignificant that authority might seem today, those persons who neglected their responsibilities. The process of examination and civil 'diagnosis' of ability included an individual's intelligence, memory, cognitive ability, discretion, and, at times, appearance. Although the English medieval administrative arm of the crown did not use the term 'intellectually disabled', they certainly recognized differences in intellectual ability and used vocabulary appropriate for each condition depending on whether the individual had a faulty memory, weak intelligence, difficulty managing property or goods, issues with 'managing', or acted without discretion. The medieval legal and administrative community had their own set of standards by which to judge these individuals, and they understood a wide variety of intellectual conditions, having categories of mental health conditions and learning disabilities that within the medieval record remain consistent in use and meaning.

Notes

1 The National Archives, Public Record Office division (Kew, England) manuscript, (hereafter TNA: PRO), C 133/46, m 2; *Calendar of Inquisitions Post Mortem and Other Analogous Documents Preserved in the Public Record* Office, 26 vols. (Vols. I–XXI: London: HMSO, 1904–95; Vols. XXII–XXVI: Woodbridge: Boydell, 1987–2010), hereafter *CIPM*, v. 2, no 611 (pp. 373–374); and *Calendar of the Fine Rolls Preserved in the Public Record Office*, 22 vols. (London: HMSO, 1916–2003), hereafter *CFR*, 1272–1307, p. 230 (John's name is listed as John de Eton). For more on the escheator's implied frustration, see: Wendy J. Turner, 'Silent Testimony: Emotional Displays and Lapses in Memory as Indicators of Mental Instability in Medieval English Investigations', in *Madness in Medieval Law and Custom*, edited by Wendy J. Turner (Leiden, Boston: Brill, 2010), 81–96, pp. 86–87.

2 For current equivalencies, see: *Diagnostic and Statistical Manual of Mental Disorders, Fifth Edition, DSM-5*, 'Section II: Diagnostic Criteria and Codes' under 'Neurodevelopmental Disorders' (Arlington, VA: American Psychiatric Association, 2013) available online at http://dsm.psychiatryonline.org, accessed 9 September, 2014, see: 'Intellectual Disability (Intellectual Developmental Disorder)'. The medieval concept of 'managing' is similar in many ways to the current concept of an inability for 'personal independence and social responsibility'. Likewise, the medieval concept of what I am calling 'behavioural discretion', they would have called a 'fatuous' person, which appears to be similar to

the idea today of lacking social and interpersonal skills. In modern English, a 'fool'.

3   Most notable is the work of H. C. Erik Midelfort, 'Madness and Civilization in Early Modern Europe: A Reappraisal of Michel Foucault', in *After the Reformation*, edited by B. C. Malament (Philadelphia: University of Pennsylvania Press, 1980); *Mad Princes of Renaissance Germany* (Charlottesville and London: University Press of Virginia, 1994); and *A History of Madness in Sixteenth-Century Germany* (Stanford, CA: Stanford University Press, 1999).

4   Two examples that have had reverberations within the community writing about the history of disabilities include Sharon L. Snyder and David T. Michell, *Cultural Locations of Disability* (Chicago and London: The University of Chicago Press, 2006) and Sara Newman, *Writing Disability: A Critical History* (Boulder and London: First Forum Press, 2013).

5   Daniel Hack Tuke, *Chapters in the History of the Insane in the British Isles* (London: Kegan Paul, Trench & Co., 1882); Tuke, *Insanity in Ancient and Modern Life, with chapters on its prevention* (London: Macmillan & Co, 1878); Edith A. Wright, 'Medieval Attitudes towards Mental Illness', *Bulletin of the History of Medicine* 7 (1939), 352–356; Gregory Zilboorg, *A History of Medical Psychology* (New York: Norton, 1941); Enid Welsford, *The Fool: His Social and Literary History* (New York: Farrar and Rinehart, n.d. [c.1942?]); E. Renier, 'Observations sur la terminologie de l'aliénation mentale', *Revue Internationale des droits d'antiquité* 4 (1956); and Gennaro J. Sesto, *Guardians of the Mentally Ill in Ecclesiastical Trials: A Canonical Commentary with Historical Notes*, Canon Law Studies 358 (Washington, DC: Catholic University of America Press, 1956).

6   *Histoire de la Folie* (Paris: Librairie Plon, 1961), later published as *Madness and Civilization: A History of Insanity in the Age of Reason* (1965), translated by Richard Howard (New York: Vintage Books, 1988).

7   'The Distracted Knight: A Study of Insanity in the Arthurian Romances', unpublished doctoral dissertation (Columbia University, 1968); *Suggestion of the Devil: The Origins of Madness* (New York: Doubleday Anchor Books, 1975); and 'Possessed by the Spirit: Devout Women, Demoniacs, and the Apostolic Life in the Thirteenth Century', *Speculum* 73.3 (1998), 733–770.

8   *Waanszin in de Middeleeuwen: Beeld van de Gestoorde en bemoeininis met de Zieke.* Haarlem (De Toorts: Nijkerk, G. F. Callenbach, 1969).

9   *Melancholie und Melancholiker in den medizinischen Theorien der Antike* (Berlin: De Gruyter, 1966).

10   *La folie: A travers les siècles* (Paris: Robert Laffont, 1967).

11   *Medieval Minds: Mental Health in the Middle Ages* (London: Allen and Unwin, 1967); and *Stars and Shadows: Mental Health in Ancient Times* (Akron: Beacon-Bell Books, 1967).

12   'Der Narr und sein Humanum im islamischen Mittelalter', *Gesnerus* 18 (1961), 1–12.

13   'Peytevin v. La Lynde', *Law Quarterly Review* 83 (1967), 527–546.

14 *Nebuchadnezzar's Children: Conventions of Madness in Middle English Literature* (New Haven: Yale University Press, 1974). Doob continued with similar topics for another 15 or more years, writing: 'Medieval and Early Modern Theories of Mental Illness', *Archives of General Psychiatry* 36.4 (1979), 477–483; and *The Idea of the Labyrinth from Classical Antiquity through the Middle Ages* (Ithaca and London: Cornell University Press, 1990).

15 'Unusual Mental States in Medieval Europe. I. Medical Syndromes of Mental Disorder: 400–1100 A.D.' *Journal of the History of Medicine* 27 (1972), 262–297. Jackson, like Doob, continued his scholarship in this direction for another 20 years, writing two monographs on the subject: *Melancholia and Depression from Hippocratic Times to Modern Times* (New Haven and London: Yale University Press, 1986) and *Care of the Psyche: A History of Psychological Healing* (New Haven and London: Yale University Press, 1999).

16 'Mental Illness and Government Policy in Sixteenth and Seventeenth Century England', unpublished doctoral thesis (Columbia University, 1976); 'Treatment of the Mentally Ill in Medieval and Early Modern England', *Journal of the History of the Behavioural Sciences* 14 (1978), 158–169; 'Medieval and Early Modern Theories of Mental Illness', *Archives of General Psychology* 36 (1979), 477–483; and 'Mental Handicap in Medieval and Early Modern England: Criteria, Measurement and Care', in *From Idiocy to Mental Deficiency: Historical Perspectives on People with Learning Disabilities*, edited by David Wright and Anne Digby (London: Routledge, 1996), 22–43.

17 Editor of *The Darker Vision of the Renaissance: Beyond Fields of Reason* (Berkeley: University of California Press, 1974); his article in this volume is 'Folly, Melancholy and Madness: A Study in Shifting Styles of Medical Analysis and Treatment, 1450–1675'.

18 *Mental Disorder in Earlier Britain: Exploratory Studies* (Cardiff: University of Wales Press, 1975).

19 *Head Injury from Antiquity to the Present with Special Reference to Penetrating Head Wounds* (Springfield, IL: Charles C. Thomas, 1973).

20 *The Inward Wits: Psychological Theory in the Middle Ages and the Renaissance* (London: Warburg Institute, University of London, 1975).

21 *English Madness: Ideas on Insanity, 1580–1890* (London: Routledge, 1979).

22 *Mind-Forg'd Manacles: A History of Madness in England from the Restoration to the Regency* (Cambridge, MA: Harvard University Press, 1987); *A Social History of Madness: Stories of the Insane* (London: Weidenfeld and Nicolson, 1987); *A Social History of Madness: A World through the Eyes of the Insane* (New York: Weidenfeld and Nicolson, 1988); 'Margery Kempe and the Meaning of Madness', *History Today* 38 (February, 1988): 39–44; 'Madness and its Institutions', in *Medieval Attitudes towards Mental Illness*, edited by Andrew Wear (Cambridge: Cambridge University Press, 2009), 277–301.

23 While Gilman continued in the vein of a philosophical discussion, he is using the new methods of Porter and others in his works. *Difference and Pathology:*

Stereotypes of Sexuality, Race and Madness (Ithaca: Cornell University Press, 1985); and *Disease and Representation: Images of Illness from madness to AIDS* (Ithaca: Cornell University Press, 1988).

24 'Modern Myth and Medieval Madness: Views of Mental Illness in the European Middle Ages and Renaissance', *New Zealand Journal of Psychology* 14.1 (1985), 1–8; and *Medieval Psychology* (New York: Greenwood Press, 1990).

25 *Krüppel, Idioten, Irre. Zur Sozialgeschichte behinderter Menschen in Deutschland* (Stuttgart: Silberburg-Verlag, 1990).

26 *Le discours du fou au Moyen Age: XIIe-XIIIe siècle: étude comparée des discours littéraire, médical, juridique et théologique de la folie* (Paris: Presses universitaires de France, 1992).

27 'Perceptions of insanity in medieval England'. Body and Mind Seminar, Department of Geriatiric Medicine, Keele University, April 1998, Internet publication, David Roffe, 2000, www.roffe.freeserve.co.uk/keel.htm, accessed 18 June, 2003; and with Christine Roffe, 'Madness and Care in the Community: A Medieval Perspective', *BMJ* 311 (1995), 1708–1712, accessed 18 June, 2003 at BMJ.com.

28 'The Mentally Ill and the Community in Western and Central Europe During the Late Middle Ages and the Renaissance', *Journal of the History of Medicine* 19 (1964), 377–388; *Madness in Society: Chapters in the Historical Sociology of Mental Illness* (Chicago: The University of Chicago Press, 1968); *A History of Public Health* (London and Baltimore: Johns Hopkins University Press, 1993).

29 *Fools and Jesters at the English Court* (Stroud: Sutton, 1998).

30 *Revels in Madness: Insanity in Medicine and Literature* (Ann Arbor: The University of Michigan Press, 1999).

31 'The Metaphor of Madness in the Anglo-Norman Lives of St Mary the Egyptian', in *The Legend of Mary of Egypt in Medieval Insular Hagiography*, edited by Erich Poppe and Bianca Ross (Dublin: Four Courts Press, 1996), 161–174.

32 Edward Wheatly, 'Afterword', in *The Treatment of Disabled Persons in Medieval Europe: Examining Disability in the Historical, Legal, Literary, Medical, and Religious Discourses of the Middle Ages*, edited by Wendy J. Turner and Tory Vandeventer Pearman (Lewiston: Mellen, 2010), 347. These 'new scholars' comprise a long list studying medieval disabilities, including those producing works specifically on mental health issues: this includes my own *Care and Custody of the Mentally Ill, Incompetent, and Disabled in Medieval England*, Cursor Mundi 16 (Turnhout: Brepols, 2013), and many articles; Aleksandra Pfau, 'Protecting or Restraining? Madness as a Disability in Late Medieval France', in *Disability in the Middle Ages: Reconsiderations and Reverberations*, edited by Josh Eyler (Surrey: Ashgate, 2010), 93–104; Sari Ktajala-Peltomaa and Susanna Niiranen, eds, *Mental (Dis)Order in Later Medieval Europe* (Surrey: Ashgate, 2014); Irina Metzler, *Fools and Idiots? Cognitive Disability in the Middle Ages* (Manchester: Manchester University Press, 2016); Susan Koslow, 'The Impact of Hugo van der Goes's Mental Illness and Late-Medieval Religious Attitudes on the Death of the Virgin', in *Healing and*

History: Essays for George Rosen, edited by Charles E. Rosenberg (Kent: Dawson, 1979), 27–50; Anne E. Bailey, 'Miracles and Madness: Dispelling Demons in Twelfth-Century Hagiography', in *Demons and Illness: Theory and Practice from Antiquity to the Early Modern Period*, edited by Siam Bhayro and Catherine Rider (Brill, forthcoming); Eliza Buhrer, 'Law and Mental Competency in Late Medieval England', *Reading Medieval Studies, Special Issue – Law's Dominion in the Middle Ages: Essays for Paul Hyams*, XL (2014), 82–100; and Sylvia Huot, *Madness in Medieval French Literature: Identities Lost and Found* (Oxford: Oxford University Press, 2003).

33 Gilbertus Anglicus, *Healing and Society in Medieval England: A Middle English Translation of the Pharmaceutical Writings of Gilbertus Anglicus* [c.1230–50], edited by Faye Marie Getz (Madison: University of Wisconsin Press, 1991), see p. 4 for migraine, which Gilbertus called 'demegreyn', and pp. 20–27 for epilepsy.

34 Sabina Flanagan, 'Heresy, Madness, and Possession in the High Middle Ages', in *Heresy in Transition: Transforming Ideas of Heresy in Medieval and Early Modern Europe*, edited by Ian Hunter et al. (Aldershot: Ashgate, 2005), 29–41; Huot, *Madness in Medieval French Literature*; Jerome Kroll and Bernard Bachrach, *The Mystic Mind: The Psychology of Medieval Mystics and Ascetics* (New York: Routledge, 2005); Peter Kwasniewski, 'Transcendence, Power, Virtue, Madness, Ecstasy – Modalities of Excess in Aquinas', *Mediaeval Studies*, 66 (2004), 129–181; and Stephen Harper, *Insanity, Individuals, and Society in Late-Medieval English Literature: The Subject of Madness*, Studies in Medieval Literature, 26 (Lewiston: Mellen, 2003).

35 For recent historical studies of mental health in the Middle Ages, see: Beth Allison Barr, 'Madness', in Margaret Schaus ed., *Women and Gender in Medieval Europe: An Encyclopedia* (New York: Routledge: 2006), 503–504; C. F. Goodey, *A History of Intelligence and 'Intellectual Disability': The Shaping of Psychology in Early Modern Europe* (Farnham and Burlington VT: Ashgate, 2011); Bernard Guenée, *La Folie de Charles VI: roi bien-aimé* (Paris: Perrin, 2004); Margaret McGlynn, 'Idiots, Lunatics, and the Royal Prerogative in Early Tudor England', *Journal of Legal History*, 26 (2005), 1–20; Pfau, 'Protecting or Restraining?'; David Roffe, 'Perceptions of Insanity in Medieval England' (publ. online by author, 2000) www.roffe.freeserve.co.uk/keel.htm, accessed 18 June, 2003; Andrew T. Scull, *The Insanity of Place, the Place of Insanity: Essays on the History of Psychiatry* (London: Routledge, 2006); Turner and Vandeventer Pearman eds., *The Treatment of Disabled Persons*; Turner, ed., *Madness in Medieval Law and Custom*; Turner, *Care and Custody*.

36 This was the common arrangement throughout the Middle Ages. See Roy Porter, *The Greatest Benefit to Mankind: A Medical History of Humanity* (New York, London: W. W. Norton, 1997), 177 and *passim* 65–77.

37 Bartholomaeus Anglicus, *De proprietatibus rerum*, edited by John de Trevisa (London: Berthelet, 1535), I. 10 (p. 13r); 'Of the commune or inner sence', Cap. x (translation by the author).

38 There were variations on how the functions were arranged, though all of the theo-
    ries agreed that the memory was in the back. They often included the functions of
    the five senses and common sense, fantasy, cogitation, estimation, and memory.
    One example of an illustration of the brain is in Nancy G. Siraisi, *Medieval and
    Early Renaissance Medicine: An Introduction to Knowledge and Practice* (Chicago,
    London: University of Chicago Press, 1990), 82–83: figure 13. For more on the
    medieval brain see: Roger Frugard, *Chirurgia* [c.1180], in *Anglo-Norman Medicine*,
    edited by Tony Hunt in 2 vols. (Cambridge: D. S. Brewer, 1994), 53, I. XXVI.
39 For more on this topic, see Turner, *Care and Custody*, 63–90.
40 *CIPM* v. 8, no 284 (p. 209) and no 340 (p. 236).
41 Emma Beston's case is quite interesting. For more information, see: David
    Roffe and Christine Roffe, 'Madness and Care in the Community: A Medieval
    Perspective', *BMJ* 311 (1995), 1708–1712, accessed 18 June, 2003 at BMJ.
    com; Wendy J. Turner, 'Town and Country: A Comparison of the Treatment
    of the Mentally Disabled in Late Medieval English Common Law and Chartered
    Boroughs', in *Madness in Medieval Law and Custom*, 31–33; and Turner, *Care and
    Custody*, 63–65, 87–88, and 154.
42 *Calendar of Inquisitions Miscellaneous (Chancery), Henry III–Henry V*, 8 vols.
    (London: HMSO, 1916–2003), hereafter *CIM*, v. 4, no 227 (pp. 125–128).
43 *CIM* v. 4, no 227 (pp. 125–128).
44 The *Prerogativa Regis* was probably not intended as a statute. It was, though, his-
    torically treated as one. Since common law was mostly oral, the *Prerogativa Regis*
    represented actual legal policy and may have been distributed as a writ in the
    Middle Ages (which is rather how it reads). The *Prerogativa Regis* can be found
    in *The Statutes of the Realm* Vol. I (London: Dawsons of Pall Mall, reprint 1963
    of 1810 edn). The chapters relevant to mental health are 11 and 12. Chapter 11
    deals with – as I read it – the intellectually disabled, which is about 'born fools'.
    This chapter was at least in part active in English law until 1961; it was repealed
    in the Crown Estate Act of Elizabeth II. The Inquiries Act (2005) finally changed
    'next heir' to 'nearest relative'. (See: Trevor Turner, Mark Salter and Martin Deahl,
    'Mental Health Reform Act', *Psychiatric Bulletin* 23 (1999): 578–581.) Chapter 12
    of the *Prerogativa Regis* deals with 'lunatics', which I take to mean those persons
    suffering with neurotic or psychotic disorders; it was repealed in 1959 in chapter
    72 of the Mental Health Act, which was amended by the Inquiries Act of 2005.
45 The most important for understanding the intellectually disabled are: Glanville,
    Bracton, Britton, the *Fleta*, the *Mirror of Justices* and the *Year Books of Edward
    II*. See: Ranulf Glanville, *De Legibus et Consuetudinibus Regni Angliae* [1187–89],
    edited by George E. Woodbine (New Haven: Yale University Press, 1932); Henry
    de Bracton, *Bracton's Noetbook*, edited by Frederic W. Maitland, 3 vols. (London:
    Clay, 1887) and *De legibus et consuetudinibus Angliae: On the Laws and Customs
    of England* [c.1220–50], edited by George E. Woodbine, translated by Samuel
    E. Thorne, 4 vols. (Cambridge, MA: Harvard University Press, 1968–77); *Britton*,
    edited and translated by Francis M. Nichols, 2 vols. (Oxford: Clarendon Press,

1865); *Fleta* [c.1290], edited and translated by Henry G. Richardson and George O. Sayles, 4 vols, Selden Society Publications 72, 79, 99 (London, 1955, 1972, 1984); *The Mirror of Justices*, edited by W. J. Whittaker with introduction by F. W. Maitland, Selden Society Publications 7 (London, 1893); *Year Books of Edward II*, edited by Frederic W. Maitland et al., Selden Society, 29 vols. (London: Selden Society, 1903–88). See also: Ralph V. Turner, *The English Judiciary in the Age of Glanvill and Bracton, c.1176–1239* (Cambridge: Cambridge University Press, 1985).

46   On memory in the Middle Ages, see: Mary Carruthers, *The Book of Memory: A Study of Memory in Medieval Culture*, Cambridge Studies in Medieval Literature (Cambridge and New York: Cambridge University Press, 2008), and *Medieval Craft of Memory: An Anthology of Texts and Pictures* (Philadelphia: University of Pennsylvania Press, 2002); Shulamith Shahar, *Growing Old in the Middle Ages: 'Winter Clothes us in Shadow and Pain'*, translated by Yael Lotan, 1995 (London, New York: Routledge, 2004), 72, 82; Patrick J. Geary, *Phantoms of Remembrance: Memory and Oblivion at the End of the First Millennium* (Princeton, NJ: Princeton University Press, 1994); Timothy J. Reiss, *Mirages of the Selfe: Patterns of Personhood in Ancient and Early Modern Europe* (Stanford, CA: Stanford University Press, 2003), 243–297.

47   TNA: PRO C 66/235, m 1d and *Calendar of the Patent Rolls Preserved in the Public Record Office: Edward III*, 16 vols. (London: HMSO, 1893–1916), hereafter *CPR*, 1350–1354, p. 208 (23 January, 1352).

48   Officials holding lands about to be claimed by the crown often sold off all movable goods, including timber or buildings, in an effort either to get more money than originally agreed upon or to recoup losses if they had invested in the property. See: Turner, *Care and Custody*, 201–209.

49   Gilbertus Anglicus, 16–20; and Bartholomeus Anglicus, 87v.

50   *The Roll and Writ File of the Berkshire Eyre of 1248*, edited by M. T. Clanchy, Selden Society 90 (London: Selden Society Publications, 1973), no 440, 186–187.

51   TNA: PRO SC 9/1, m 3 and SC 9/2, m 6. *Rotuli Parliamentorum, ut et Petitiones, et Placita in Parliamento*, 6 vols. (London: Record Commission, 1783, reprint 1832), Vol. I, 23a and 60a. Paul Brand (ed.), 'Edward I: Parliament of 1290', Text and translation, in C. Given-Wilson et al. eds, *The Parliament Rolls of Medieval England*, CD-ROM (Leicester: Scholarly Digital Editions, 2005).

52   TNA: PRO KB 27/922 m 54 dorse.

53   TNA: PRO C 145/180, m 9 and *CIM* v. 3, no 365, p. 130.

54   *CIM*, v.4, no 283 (pp. 161–162).

55   *CFR* v. 7, p. 68.

56   *CIPM* v. 13, no 143 (p. 114).

57   *CIPM* v. 20, no 494 (p. 156).

58   *CIM* v. 4, no 227 (pp. 125–126).

59   TNA: PRO C 133/46, m 2; *CIPM* v. 2, no 611 (pp. 373–374); and *CFR* 1272–1307, p. 230.

60   TNA: PRO C 133/98, m 9 and *CIPM* v. 3, no 614 (p. 492).

61   *CIPM* v. 18, no 1186 (p. 409–410). See also: *CFR* v. 13, pp. 28 and 88.

62   TNA: PRO C 66/259, m 27d and *CPR* 1358–1361, p. 409.

63   *CPR* 1361–1364, p. 186.

64   TNA: PRO C 54/212, m 29 (top). See also: *Calendar of the Close Rolls Preserved in the Public Record Office: Edward III*, 14 vols. (London: HMSO, 1896–1913), hereafter *CCR*, 1374–1377, p. 4 (1 February, 1374).

65   *CPR* 1370–1374, p. 419.

66   *CIPM* v. 11, no 219 (p. 189).

67   *CIPM* v. 19, no 20 (p. 5).

68   *CIM* v. 3, no 747 (p. 283). See also: TNA: PRO C 145/197, m 19.

69   *CCR* 1369–1374, p. 526.

70   TNA: PRO C 54/126, m 17d cancelled; C 260/13, no 6; C 262/5, no 2; and *CCR* 1307–1313, p. 132 (3 Dec. 1308).

71   TNA: PRO C 135/125, m 25. See also *CPR* 1350–1354, p. 511 and 1354–1358, pp. 200–201.

72   *CIPM* v. 10, no 142 (pp. 132–133); TNA: PRO C 135/125, m 25. See also: TNA: PRO C 66/240, m 19d; C 66/245, m 13; *CPR* 1350–1354, p. 511; and *CPR* 1354–1358, pp. 200–201.

73   *CIM* v. 6, no 85, p. 40–41 and no 127 (p. 59–60); this reference covers all other quotes to the end of this paragraph.

74   *CIPM* v. 16, no 1039 (p. 421).

75   *CIPM* v. 17, no 987 (p. 363).

76   *CIPM* v. 7, no 181 (p. 148).

77   The National Archives have updated his name to Atwood in their databases, but in all archival records he is 'atte Wode'.

78   TNA: PRO C 138/44, no 10. See also C 139/108, no 6; and E 149/102, no 7; as well as *CIPM* v. 21, nos 396–399 (p. 119); and *CIPM* v. 20, no 275 (p. 90).

79   See previous note. Each number in the folder of documents is sewn together in the archives. This testimony is on the second leaf in the number 10 group of folder C 138/44 in The National Archive. The abbot is of St John's of Colchester.

80   TNA: PRO C 136/109, no 13 and no 2 respectively.

81   TNA: PRO C 260/125, m 11b. For more on Joan Jordan, see: Turner, 'Town and Country', 29–30.

82   See TNA: PRO C 138/6, m 6 where his is listed as ignorant in 1415. See also the rest of that file and C 139/121, m 10; E 149/66, no 12; E 149/105, no 8; *CIM* v. 6, no 167 (p. 79); and *CIPM* v. 20, no 147 (pp. 48–49).

83   TNA: PRO E 149/ 214, no 3.

84   TNA: PRO JUST 1/858, m 32 (org. 33).

3

'WILL-NOTS' AND 'CANNOTS': TRACING A TROPE IN MEDIEVAL THOUGHT

Irina Metzler

Commenting on the early modern distinction between natural and moral disability, Chris Goodey summarized that the 'distinction between "will nots" and "cannots" survives today, in exactly the same terminology, in education policy for pupils with emotional and behavioural difficulties'.[1] This chapter investigates how the trope of will-nots versus cannots runs from at least the Middle Ages, if not antiquity, through to modern times. Until the middle of the twentieth century, it was common practice amongst educational theorists and practitioners (e.g. teachers) to refer to those children who were not learning as ably as the 'norm' as either will-nots or cannots. Will-nots, as the name suggests, were those who were able but reluctant to learn, children deemed refuseniks, those obstreperous enough to willfully sabotage their learning objectives, while the cannots were the poor innocent incapables, those nowadays categorized as learning disabled, who are deemed unable to learn and therefore blameless for their underachievement. Conceptually separating one from the other, the fraudulent and the genuine, like the chaff from the wheat, was part of standard pedagogical training.

What at first sight appears to be a modern assessment of learning (in/dis) ability has in fact got much older roots. The Roman educationalist Quintilian (c.35–c.95 AD), in his handbook on the art of oratory and rhetoric, *Institutio Oratoria*, addressed the problem of children with learning disabilities in the wider sense and already suggested that there were different types of learners, some slower, some faster. Quintilian's art of rhetoric was not just an instruction for public speaking, but above and beyond such simple aims concerned itself with educational theories in general and also, like no comparable antique text, provides an insight into the entire Graeco-Roman educational system. His influence during the Middle Ages and the Renaissance was immense.

Quintilian supported the idea, promulgated by his Greek predecessors, of cutting down class sizes. He was also very direct about the varying capabilities of children (what twenty-first-century fashion calls 'diversity'). He compared children to vessels, whose variously constricted shapes meant various capabilities of containment and retention, saying 'that those with very narrow mouths could not hold all the liquid if one tried to pour too much into them'.[2] Also, consideration should be given to the amount of learning a child's mind could receive, since children were different from one another, some being 'slack', some 'impatient of control' and some requiring constant application to form the mind.[3] According to Quintilian there were very few children who genuinely could not learn, with this number of ineducables being so small that they could be regarded on a par with prodigious births or monstrosities. If children were unable to learn, the fault would be found not in their inborn talent but in the insufficiency of attention paid to them by others. His educational optimism was such that he was convinced that in principle the mental ability to be educated exists in all men. This he states at the very beginning of his text (Book I chapter 1,1–2):

> I would, therefore, have a father conceive the highest hopes of his son from the moment of his birth. ... For there is absolutely no foundation for the complaint that but few men have the power to take in the knowledge that is imparted to them, and that the majority are so slow of understanding that education is a waste of time and labour. On the contrary you will find that most are quick to reason and ready to learn. Reasoning comes as naturally to man as flying to birds, speed to horses and ferocity to beasts of prey: our minds are endowed by nature with such activity and sagacity that the soul is believed to proceed from heaven. Those who are dull and unteachable are as abnormal as prodigious births and monstrosities, and are but few in number. A proof of what I say is to be found in the fact that boys commonly show promise of many accomplishments, and when such promise dies away as they grow up, this is plainly due not to the failure of natural gifts, but to lack of the requisite care. But, it will be urged, there are degrees of talent. Undoubtedly, I reply, and there will be a corresponding variation in actual accomplishment: but that there are any who gain nothing from education, I absolutely deny.[4]

In *Institutio oratoria*, Book II.8, Quintilian looks at the different 'styles of learners', as modern parlance would have it, and argues that individual teaching styles need to be adopted for individual learners. He then states that those intellectually less gifted should be not be pushed beyond their boundaries: 'In the case of weaker understandings, however, some concession must be made and they should be directed merely to follow the call of their nature, since thus they will be more effective in doing the only thing that lies in their power'.[5]

Quintilian was almost modern in his educational theories, as well as in his emphasis that early childhood education (in modern parlance) for infants and younger children lays the most important foundations for subsequent 'higher' education. Quintilian argues that the earlier education commenced, the better.[6] He counters the ideas of some Roman educationalists – that children should not commence learning to read until they were seven years old – by stating that 'a child's mind should not be allowed to lie fallow'.[7] If children are capable of moral education, Quintilian argues, they surely are capable of literary (and other 'academic') education, and once able to speak the child is receptive to learning in general, even if this just lays the foundation for serious study in later years. In fact, the younger the child, the better such foundational learning is, due to the greater capacity for memory: 'Let us not therefore waste the earliest years: there is all the less excuse for this, since the elements of literary training are solely a question of memory, which not only exists even in small children, but is especially retentive at that age'.[8] He picks up this theme again in Book I chapter 12, 8–11, arguing that smaller children make better learners because they pick things up quickly and learning *per se* comes naturally to them: 'For the mind [literally: natural disposition] is all the easier to teach before it is set. This may be clearly proved by the fact that within two years after a child has begun to form words correctly, he can speak practically all without any pressure from outside'.[9]

With regard to the notion that imitation is insufficient to advance learning, Quintilian poses the question of how anything could have been invented. He looks back at earlier times and asked why we should not be allowed to invent something that did not exist previously, arguing that these 'primitive' – to use a modern way of describing it – ancestors of ours, who did not have the benefits of formal education, possessed an innate desire to invent and create: 'these rude [i.e. uneducated] men were prompted only by the nature of their mind that they created so much'.[10] By extrapolation, then, the creative urge that is innate to all humans is also innate to intellectually disabled humans, so that not being able to receive education in the formal sense does not preclude invention or creative abilities.

Education and schooling in antiquity were largely an oral matter, based on drill, imitation, and reading aloud. It is thus easy to imagine how blind or hearing-impaired children lapsed into a situation which made them appear similar to those who were intellectually disabled. Deaf people, who were functionally incommunicative and hence by implication akin to the mentally disabled, were not supposed to take legal action according to Roman law.[11] A similar attitude in Jewish law placed deaf-mutes, imbeciles, and minors in the same category.[12] The link between children as incomplete adults, and intellectually disabled persons (regardless of whether adult or children) as equally incomplete has often been made, in many different cultures across many different periods. Thus a sixth-century Byzantine letter (from Hermopolite in Egypt) written by a father to a teacher mentions that a pupil is foolish, childish, and without sense or intelligence.[13]

At the turn of the fourth to fifth century, Augustine highlighted logic and numbers as higher aspects of mental reasoning, as opposed to the baser knowledge gained by the senses, praising the faculty of 'reason', held to be uniquely human. But at the same time, Augustine could caution against the trickery that logic can be used for.

> There are many 'sophisms', as they are called, or invalid deductions, framed as a rule in the guise of valid ones, designed to trap not just dull people [*tardos*] but also clever ones who are less than consistently alert. The following proposition was put by X to Y: 'you are not what I am'. Y agreed; that was, after all, true up to a point, or else Y was just being simple-minded [*simplex*] because of X's deviousness. X added, 'I am a man', and when Y granted this too, he concluded 'therefore you are not a man'.[14]

The *Didascalion* of Hugh of St Victor

So much for a brief overview of Roman and late antique views on education and individual intellectual development. Medieval educational theories surface in the *Didascalion* of Hugh of St Victor, who in the early twelfth century had already drawn attention to the different abilities of learners, and also pointed out that these are not totally fixed, but malleable by the educator. Hugh certainly knew of Quintilian's earlier work, even if in an incomplete version, mentioning the Latin author in his own text.[15] In his *Didascalion*, composed at Paris in the 1120s, Hugh tries to describe and define all areas of human knowledge, advocating the necessity of *scientia* for the attainment of human perfection whilst considering varying ages and abilities of students. In the Preface, he wrote:

> There are many persons whose nature has left them so poor in ability that they can hardly grasp with their intellect[16] even easy things, and of these persons I believe there are two kinds. There are those who, while they are not unaware of their own dullness, nonetheless struggle after knowledge with all the effort they can put forth and who, by tirelessly keeping up with their pursuit, deserve to obtain as a result of their will power what they by no means possess as a result of their work. Others, however, because they know that they are in no way able to compass the highest things, neglect even the least, and, as it were, carelessly at rest in their own sluggishness, they all the more lose the light of truth in the greatest matters for their refusal to learn those smallest of which they are

capable. ... Not knowing and not wishing to know are far different things. Not knowing, to be sure, springs from weakness; but contempt of knowledge springs from a wicked will.[17]

Furthermore, Hugh distinguishes between ability and willingness to learn. 'And still it is one thing when one is not able, or to speak more truly, when one is not easily able to learn, and another when one is able but unwilling to learn'.[18] Hugh was thus one of the first people to make the distinction, so popular with later educational theorists, between what came to be called the will-nots and the cannots: that is, those who are able but reluctant to learn and those, such as people nowadays categorized as learning disabled, who are deemed unable and therefore not culpable with regard to low levels of educational attainment.

As G. R. Evans notes, Hugh 'recognises that there are differences of natural aptitude. But he also thinks that aptitude can be improved or blunted'.[19] So nature may be a pre-given, but it is not immutable or unchanging. It can be malleable and, like a musical instrument, can be finely tuned or played badly. Aptitude, Hugh said, 'arises from nature, is improved by use, is blunted by excessive work, and is sharpened by temperate practice'.[20] In the *Didascalion*, there are different types of students, or in modern terms different types of learners. There are some 'who are naturally dull and slow in understanding things',[21] but there are also extraneous forces which impede learning, namely carelessness (*negligentia*), imprudence (*imprudentia*) and bad luck (*fortuna*).[22] Carelessness is caused by omission or negligence, in which case the student needs to be admonished, and imprudence by unsuitable order or method of learning, in which case the student needs to be instructed. But *fortuna* is more illuminating as far as Hugh's attitude is concerned:

> Bad luck shows up in a development, a chance happening, or a natural occurrence, when we are kept back from our objective either by poverty, or by illness, or by some non-natural slowness, or even by a scarcity of professors, because either none can be found to teach us, or none can be found to teach us well.[23]

Prefiguring yet more modern educationalists' theories, Hugh suggests that in such cases the student needs to be assisted (*adiuvandus*). Extrapolating from what Hugh wrote nearly nine centuries ago we may say that there may be slow learners but there are no such things as non-learners.

Modern education praises the quick learner. Speed has not always been valued, however. Quick-witted ripostes were not always valued above slow, cautious or considered thought. Here it is worth citing a few more excerpts from the *Didascalion*. According to Hugh, a slower learning pace may be better: 'Consider, rather, what your powers will at present permit: the man who proceeds stage by stage moves along best'.[24] Hugh must have regarded this as a good maxim, as he repeats this advice: 'the man who moves along step by step is the one who moves along best, not like some who fall head over heels when they wish to make a great leap ahead'.[25] One may compare this with the statement by Quintilian, undoubtedly a great influence on Hugh, in which he argues that precocious intellects who learn quickly but use that learning to raise a laugh only acquire small learning achievements, whereas the ideal learner will follow rather than anticipate the teacher: 'I regard slowness of intellect [literally: disposition] as preferable to actual badness. But a good boy will be quite unlike the dullard and the sloth'.[26] (One may also compare this with Isidore of Seville's *Sententiarum libri* for a similar discussion of quick and slow students.)[27] It has been suggested that Hugh added the passages on types of learners as a riposte against the temporarily influential Cornificians, a rival group of medieval educational theorists 'who preached that study was futile for those lacking natural ability, superfluous for those possessing it'.[28]

Hugh also made observations concerning the contents of learning and social status, noting, for instance, that different groups of people learnt different topics. He distinguishes technical or mechanical from liberal arts, stating the liberal arts are so called

> because they require minds which are liberal, that is, liberated and practiced (for these sciences pursue subtle inquiries into the causes of things), or because in antiquity only free and noble men were accustomed to study them, while the populace and the sons of men not free sought operative skill in things mechanical.[29]

Overall, developments in medieval educational institutions and systems between the twelfth and fourteenth centuries shaped the process of learning and the expectations placed on the learners. The rise of the universities is only the most familiar and best known strand of this story.[30] More importantly for my argument, these developments included such elements as examinations and standardisations in the shape of 'degrees' that were accepted all over western Christendom. 'This all tended to make the pursuit of knowledge a systematic and formal business', writes Evans.[31] However, as medieval commentators themselves were already aware, just because the educational institutions and the formalized structures of learning were new and under construction during the high Middle Ages does not mean that the activities they pursued were in themselves novel. Hugh points this out in a passage no doubt harking back to what Quintilian had already said on the subject:

> Before there was grammar, men both wrote and spoke; before there was dialectic, they distinguished the true from the false by reasoning; before there was rhetoric, they discoursed upon civil laws; before there was arithmetic, there was

knowledge of counting; before there was an art of music, they sang; before there was geometry, they measured fields; before there was astronomy, they marked off periods of time from the courses of the stars.[32]

Cicero in *De oratore* had already made a similar observation: 'Almost all things now comprehended in the arts were once scattered and disordered. So in music, ... in geometry, ... in astronomy, ... in grammar, all these things seemed unknown and without order'.[33] Hugh, like Cicero and Quintilian before him, advocated a theory of education that placed on an equal footing not only different learners but also different subjects of learning. 'Hugh had virtually abolished the stigmatic division between the manual and the cerebral arts within classification-schemes', observes B. B. Price. 'He fully recognized the traditional distinctions between the divisions of the arts, insisting, however, that these differences were not based on an inherent relative value of the studies (or the student)'.[34] One may speculate that, if Hugh were alive today, he would have been an advocate not just of inclusive schooling but also of comprehensive schools. Hugh furthermore writes: 'Indeed, man's reason shines forth much more brilliantly in inventing these very things than ever it would have had man naturally possessed them'.[35] When discussing human inventiveness as part and parcel of the 'lowly' mechanical arts, he also adds that without some measure of abstract thinking invention could never lead to practical, applicable results, since simple imitation may reproduce things but will not produce new and improved things. Thus even the lower orders of society, the peasants and artisans who made things, could be credited with the capacity for abstract thinking. As Price notes, 'Hugh was insisting that the populace at work in the kitchens, workshops, construction sites, markets, fields, forests, and village squares might well be contributing to the body of medieval thought'.[36]

Furthermore, Hugh of St Victor was aware of the possibility of a kind of inbuilt notion of rational thought, which may, however, not always manifest itself due to extraneous forces. In the Preface to his *Didascalion* he suggests:

This, then, is the dignity of our nature which all naturally possess in equal measure, but which all do not equally understand. For the mind, stupefied by bodily sensations and enticed out of itself by sensuous forms, has forgotten what it was.[37]

Hugh had in the same chapter stated that the soul is composed of all things, a notion that forms the psychological basis for the return of the human mind to the divine wisdom. The importance of this is that soul *qua* soul is alike in all people, similar to the notion expressed a century later by John Blund in *Tractatus de anima* that the soul of an idiot, as pure soul, is the same as the soul of a philosopher. Hugh realized that some of his students 'would never progress much beyond the beginning stages of the pursuit of knowledge'[38] but was not, it seems, particularly worried by that.

Beyond the *Didascalion*: medieval intellectual disability in natural philosophy

One may compare the concept of an innate capacity for rational thought, as found in the work of Hugh of St Victor, with the idea that knowledge of actions and objects (such as reading, writing, measuring) was possible before the formal invention of the arts. This concept, expressed by Quintilian and Cicero, is also found in the work of an Arabic scholar, Alhazen (Ibn al-Haytham, c.965–c.1040). Here the undeveloped state of children is used to point out that one may have knowledge of something even if one cannot rationalize or theorize about it in so many words.

> Children, Alhazen argues, comprehend many things that grown men comprehend; they distinguish and perform many operations *per distinctionem*. If two apples are shown to a boy, one more beautiful than the other, he will choose the more beautiful. This is only possible through comparison and distinction, and through a 'universal proposition' that what is more beautiful is better, and more worthy of being chosen. The child in effect makes use of such a proposition; he argues and distinguishes, but does not know it, nor does he know that he argues, or even what an argument is.[39]

Children, and the intellectually disabled, who have so often been compared to children, may then be capable of making 'innate' distinctions, possessing a kind of proto-rationality, but overall their defect is their mental weakness. Children are gullible and have 'ignorance of deceit' [*doli non capax*].[40] This statement relates to the so-called Children's Crusade (1212), where a number of chronicles describe the children's actions as done foolishly (*stulte*) and without discretion, and the adults who follow them are behaving equally so.[41] Among early educational theorists, therefore, Hugh may have been the exception rather than the rule. Most medieval authorities emphasized the need for education as a form of training. As Evans points out, 'In the thirteenth century Gilbert of Tournai outlines in his *De modo addiscendi* procedures for inculcating good habits of learning into children. These include the right use of faculties'.[42] Reason is adulterated by too much *imaginatio* and then develops vice, which in turn leads to wrong judgements, since often imagination is considered to be *bestialis* by Gilbert, thus lowering the human mind to the lower level of animals. In pre-modern thought, children start off at this level, but intellectually disabled persons never rise above it.

With regard to learning disabilities, an interesting concept is the medieval version of the 'rust metaphor'. Rust was used, since the thirteenth-century encyclopedists, as a mechanical metaphor for mental decline, as in the modern saying 'my mind's gone rusty'. This metaphor commonly referred to mental or cognitive impairment, not necessarily from birth but more often from lack of use, and especially due to the deteriorations of age. However, Vincent of Beauvais associated rust with lack of use in a developing mind. In chapter V, 'De tribus necessariis addiscenti' of his *De eruditione filiorum nobilium*, a tract on pedagogy written in the middle years of the thirteenth century and inspired by Hugh of St Victor but quoting numerous classical and patristic authorities (such as Quintilian, St Augustine, and, on girls' education, St Jerome), Vincent mentions 'rusting' of the mind (*rubiginem ocii*) through idleness: 'Just as iron that is not used becomes blunt and rusty, while use sharpens it and preserves it from rust, so the human mind is blunted by lack of use'.[43] Slow learners are rusty learners. Chapter X, 'De beniuolencia eiusdem ad retinendum', has passages on the stupidity of rustics and *fatui*, a word often equated with 'fools', who if they find a precious stone, since they are ignorant of its worth, throw it away;[44] a little later in the same passage the *rustici* and *fatui* who throw away the stone are now called imbeciles and ignoramuses, although in children this is not imbecility but weakness.[45] From the time of Vincent onwards, late medieval tracts amalgamated melancholy with mental slowness: for example, in early fifteenth-century French vernacular texts, intellectual slowness can arise also from over-use (too many external impacts and influences) that overstimulates the mind, while literary metaphoric mentions of 'sharp intellect' are found in French vernacular texts written just after the mid-fifteenth century, where intellect is like a tool sharpened on a whet stone.[46]

In general, learning disabilities are comparatively neglected in medieval medical and philosophical discourse, in contrast to modern psychology, where learning 'has generally been regarded as important'.[47]

> Some interest was shown by Aquinas, and his account of dispositions ... considers a few of the issues raised by modern accounts of learning. Psychological dispositions, such as the tendency to behave courageously or the ability to speak and understand a foreign language, are, according to Aquinas, acquired by acts of will.[48] Like modern behavioral repertoires they are generally acquired gradually and strengthened by repeated actions as the passive potentialities are acted on by active elements, and may be lost or extinguished through lack of use.[49]

The key concept for pre-modern notions of intellectual disability is, of course, passive potentialities, since if these are not fully present or fully developed, then no amount of active elements can influence the dispositions.

Far more concern was shown by medieval commentators both over the quality of the teacher (rather than the qualities of the students), and physical 'defects' over mental ones. William Wheteley, a schoolmaster at Stamford and Lincoln, may illustrate this point. William composed a commentary on the Pseudo-Boethian treatise *De Disciplina Scolarium* as a series of lectures in 1309, believing that his source text was indeed the work of Boethius – in fact, it had been written at Paris only about five decades earlier. His attitudes towards disability include material on deformity and education, namely that the physically deformed (such as lepers, the hunchbacked, the monstrous or those with otherwise defective members) should not be teachers (*doctrine mancipari*, literally those who hand over doctrine).[50] However, these strictures are all in relation to physical integrity, with not a word about mental deficiencies. Madness, folly, and what we would now term intellectual disability were not bounded as categorically in the medieval period as they are now. Although words like *fatuus* or *stultus* often indicate something approaching mental disability, this was not an exclusive meaning, and medieval usage of such terms could oscillate between sometimes bewildering varieties that can only be interpreted through context. More forthcoming was Nicholas Oresme (d.1382), who discussed 'fools' as part of his discourse on mental afflictions. In his *Quodlibeta*, Oresme included a section on psychology with some discussion of fools, asking the rhetorical question of why we do not get fool horses and fool cows as well as human fools.[51] And in *De causis mirabilium*, composed in the 1340s, Oresme looked at natural and reasoned explanations for miraculous phenomena, amongst other things treating the question whether madmen can prophesy. Oresme here regarded madness as the inability to censor or control oneself, as a lack of interactive control between thought and speech. He suggested that mad people were simply saying and doing things that sane people were prevented from saying or doing by their socialisation, education, or behavioural constraints, thus putting a very modern slant on the causality. The mad are in this way alike to the foolish; both are unrestrained. Therefore, mad people are not saying and doing things that are totally inexplicable: there's a method in the madness. Understanding a mad person's talk would be as difficult (or easy) as understanding the random rambling thoughts of a sane person.[52] 'Look inside yourself: if you were saying all the things which occur to you now on this, now on that, then no matter what or how much you said, people would surely call you a fool'.[53]

That saying 'silly' or 'stupid' things is the hallmark of the fool is also a theme in an anecdote related by Albertus Magnus. Albertus commented that the claim of a nun during the Swabian Ries heresy investigations (1270–73) to have suckled Jesus was not a heresy that one must refute by words, but a silliness that needs to be corrected by physical chastisement.[54] Apart from what was to Albert probably an amusing pun (*verberibus*, 'by whippings'; *verbis*, 'by words'), this citation provides an example of a deeper notion, namely that 'silliness' or folly (*fatuitas*) is not something that can be corrected by words. As fatuity is illogical and not malleable by reason, words must fail, hence physical action is the only effective influence. This is reminiscent of the beatings children must of necessity receive when they are too young or too recalcitrant to be reasoned with verbally, a practice unfortunately not just relegated to medieval times – although the many representations of the allegorical Grammar brandishing a birch rod, ready to beat pupils, betrays something of the general attitude of the Middle Ages toward the physical punishment of (small) children. Thinking of the nun cited above, one must also recall that women were thought to be especially prone to fatuity, as countless medieval moralistic tracts made clear. Medievalist scholarship has 'charted a complex topography, in which the female is associated with weakness, irrationality, impressionability, the sinful senses, porosity, and the demonic; and the male with strength, reason, self-independence, moral understanding, impermeability, the angelic, and the image of God'.[55]

Conclusions: universal schooling and numbers

Arguably it is only with the widespread advent of schooling for all children, of all backgrounds and abilities, that 'mental deficiency' becomes something that is recognized as not only a problem, but also as widespread:

> In the long term, perhaps the most important trigger in the development of the problem of mental deficiency was the introduction of universal elementary education in 1870. Mass education revealed that there was a hitherto largely unrecognized section of the population, who were not handicapped to the extent that they would be diagnosed as idiots, but who were not normal either and who needed special training if they were to be educated.[56]

The Enlightenment had set the course with regard to the future treatment of intellectually disabled persons, so that first the fool became an object for medical attention, and then at the end of the eighteenth and beginning of the nineteenth century an object for special education and rehabilitation.[57] The year 1861 saw the publication by Jan Daniel Georgens and Heinrich Marianus Deinhardt of what would remain to this day an important contribution to special education in Germany, namely their twelve lectures on 'idiocy' and 'idiot' asylums.[58] The main contribution by Georgens and Deinhardt is the analysis and definition of cognitive difference, distinguishing between endemic and sporadic idiotism ['endemischer und sporadischer Idiotismus'].[59]

> Sporadic idiotism is divided into four categories that are influenced by earlier concepts, both from the discourse of wonder and psychiatric ideas of temperament. Therefore sporadic idiotism is either: boredom (*Stumpfsinn*), melancholic idiocy (*melancholischer Idiotismus*), dullness (*Beschränktheit*) or foolish idiocy (*narrenhafter Idiotismus*). In doing so, Georgens and Deinhardt refer to older concepts of mental difference while modifying and transferring them into their concept of orthopedagogy.[60]

Orthopedagogy (*Heilpädagogik*) is a topic still writ large in Germany, perhaps due to the lasting influence of Georgens and Deinhardt, and so is the history of special education, a subject that seems especially dear to the hearts of German academics (perhaps because mainstreaming of children with mental and physical disabilities is still not practised as widely in Germany as in the UK or North America).[61]

The philosophical, religious, and legal problem has therefore been, for at least the medieval thinkers, how to distinguish between the will-not and the cannot. Amassing medieval evidence for the characterisation of the 'type' of the will-not and the cannot, this chapter has considered the tension between people regarded as not wanting to do something and people incapable of doing something despite perhaps wanting to. The 'genuine fool' was accorded preferential treatment in all these realms, but the 'pretend fool', regarded with suspicion, was morally dubious, or even dangerous (cf. Psalm 52 on the atheist 'fool'). Fools are not invariably people with intellectual disability in medieval philosophy: 'The wise man might be contrasted not only with the fool but also with those who are handicapped in their "knowing" by immaturity, mental defect, mental disturbance'.[62] Thus it seems that, according to Evans' reading at least, the difference between the medieval 'fool' and whatever label they attached to intellectual disability is similar to modern educationalists' differentiation between will-nots and cannots: the fool will not learn, understand, listen, while the person with intellectual disability cannot do so. As Goodey reminds us, this categorical distinction was already used by the Puritan preacher William Fenner in the seventeenth century: 'not because they cannot (though they cannot) but because they will not'.[63] This is reminiscent of Thomas Aquinas' distinction between stupidity (*stultitia*) and idiocy (*fatuitas*), respectively the will-not and the cannot, in his key text, the *Summa Theologiae*.[64] It is perhaps speculation on my part, but somewhere along the linguistic line in philosophical texts of the Middle Ages a semantic difference between *stultus* and *fatuus* began, with *stultus* meaning stupidity but also implying philosophical stupidity – that is, doing something stupid despite having the capacity not to do so – as opposed to the *fatuus*, the natural fool, who is foolish because he cannot help himself.

Precisely because intellectual disability, or 'folly', is not something writ large on the body, like a crippled limb, medieval commentators were worried by it, just as they were worried by deafness (equally invisible and fakeable, and also causing communication and moral issues). One fourteenth-century German medieval author, Konrad of Megenburg, linked physical physiognomy with intellectual disability, but he seems to be the exception among medieval writers. In general, it is the behaviour rather than the physique that is highlighted as being different from the 'norm'. So perhaps it is a sign of more modern times that physical appearance comes to be more strongly linked to intellectual disability. In general, medieval children appear to have been categorized by their learning ability as expressed through behaviour, not physiognomy.

One may conclude with a little glance at the numbers game: educationalists like Quintilian and Hugh of St Victor could only believe in the potential educability of everyone because they were only ever dealing with small numbers of pupils. Quintilian wrote for an audience who would have expected one-to-one tutorials for their children. Even in Hugh's schools at St Victor, class sizes would have been nowhere near what they are in a modern British school. It goes without saying that individual attention given to each learner helps an awful lot. The modern schooling system, since the nineteenth-century advent of universal schooling, is akin to the factory system – only those who conform to a norm can be successfully turned off the educational conveyor belt. This is not a new argument, of course; this critique has been made by various educational reformers since the late nineteenth century. However, with increasing pressure of numbers, it remains a valid one. A factory system, whether educational or material, is about standards, norms, and targets, which is exactly the language of contemporary education administrators. Learners who do not fit the category of 'normal' are too resource-intensive in this system, since they require just the kind of individual attention that Quintilian and Hugh could provide. The optimism of Quintilian and Hugh was borne out by their educational success, in that it seems their writings reflect their practice, rather than their texts being just empty theories.

Notes

1   C. F. Goodey, 'The Psychopolitics of Learning and Disability in Seventeenth-Century Thought', in *From Idiocy to Mental Deficiency: Historical Perspectives*

on People with Learning Disabilities, edited by David Wright and Anne Digby (London: Routledge, 1996), 115n8; see also C. F. Goodey, *A History of Intelligence and 'Intellectual Disability': The Shaping of Psychology in Early Modern Europe* (Farnham and Burlington VT: Ashgate, 2011), 190.

2 Book I chapter 2, 28, *The Institutio oratoria of Quintilian* [c.95], translated by H. E. Butler (Loeb Classical Library 124) (Cambridge, MA and London: Harvard University Press/Heinemann, 1980), Vol. I, 53.

3 Book I chapter 3, 6, *Institutio oratoria*, Vol. I, 57.

4 *Institutio oratoria*, Vol. I, 18–20/19–21. 'Igitur nato filio pater spem de illo primum quam optimam capiat ... Falsa enim est querela, paucissimis hominibus vim percipiendi, quae tradantur, esse concessam, plerosque vero laborem ac tempora tarditate ingenii perdere. Nam contra plures reperias et faciles in excogitando et ad discendum promptos. Quippe id est homini naturale; ac sicut aves ad volatum, equi ad cursum, ad saevitiam ferae gignuntur; ita nobis propria est mentis agitatio atque sollertia, unde origo animi caelestis creditur. Hebetes vero et indociles non magis secundum naturam homines eduntur quam prodigiosa corpora et monstris insignia, sed hi pauci admodum fuerunt. Argumentum quod in pueris elucet spes plurimorum, quae cum emoritur aetate, manifestum est, non naturam defecisse sed curam. Praestat tamen ingenio alius alium. Concedo; sed plus efficiet aut minus; nemo reperitur, qui sit studio nihil consecutus'.

5 *Institutio oratoria*, Vol. I, 268/269. 'Imbecillis tamen ingeniis sane sic obsequendum sit, ut tantum in id, quo vocat natura, ducantur; ita enim, quod solum possunt, melius efficient'.

6 *Institutio oratoria*, I.1, Vol. I, 15–19.

7 *Institutio oratoria*, I.1, 16, Vol. I, 26/27. 'nullum tempus vacare cura volunt'.

8 *Institutio oratoria*, I.1, 19, Vol. I, 28/29. 'Non ergo perdamus primum statim tempus, atque eo minus, quod initia litterarum sola memoria constant, quae non modo iam est in parvis sed tum etiam tenacissima est'.

9 *Institutio oratoria*, I.12, 9, Vol. I, 194/195. 'Nam et dociliora sunt ingenia, priusquam obduruerunt. Id vel hoc argumento patet, quod intra biennium, quam verba recte formare potuerunt, quamvis nullo instante, omnia fere loquuntur'. *Ingenium* meant an innate quality or temperament, a character or inclination, in which sense Cicero used the term (thanks to Chris Goodey for drawing this to my attention). Hugh of St Victor, below, also uses *ingenium* in this fashion.

10 *Institutio oratoria*, Book X 2, 5. 'an illi rudes sola mentis natura ducti sunt in hoc, ut tam multa generarent'.

11 See e.g. *Cod. Iust.* 6, 22, 10 pr.; also A. Küster, *Blinde und Taubstumme im römischen Recht* (Cologne: Böhlau Verlag, 1991).

12 See *Mishnah*: Menahoth 9, 8 (concerning sacrifice); *Mishnah*: Hullin 1, 1 (on slaughter); *Mishnah*: Rosh Hashanah 3, 8 (on respresenting the community). On these texts, see W. Cotter, *Miracles in Greco-Roman Antiquity: A Sourcebook for the Study of New Testament Miracle Stories* (Abingdon and New York: Routledge, 1999).

13 Papyrus SB V 7655, lines 22 and 25, online at http://perseus.mpiwg-berlin.mpg.
de/cgi-bin/ptext?doc=Perseus:text:1999.05.0239&query=line%3D%2316026,
accessed 29 January, 2013; also cited in Edgar Kellenberger, *Der Schutz der
Einfältigen. Menschen mit einer geistigen Behinderung in der Bibel und in weiteren
Quellen* (Zurich: Theologischer Verlag Zürich, 2011), 142n253. The original reads
'môros kai paidion kai anoêtos ... kai epeidê paidion estin kai môros'.

14 Augustine, *On Christian Teaching* [397/426], translated and introduced by R. P. H.
Green (Oxford: Oxford University Press, 1997), 58, paragraphs 117–118.
'Sunt enim multa quae appellantur sophismata, falsae conclusiones rationum et
plerumque ita veras imitantes, ut non solum tardos, sed ingeniosos etiam minus dili-
genter attentos decipiant. Proposuit enim quidam, dicens ei cum quo loquebatur:
Quod ego sum, tu non es. At ille consensit. Verum enim erat ex parte, vel eo ipso
quod iste insidiosus, ille simplex erat. Tum iste addidit: Ego autem homo sum. Hoc
quoque cum ab illo accepisset, conclusit dicens: Tu igitur non es homo'. [Latin:
R. P. H. Green (ed.), *Augustine: De Doctrina Christiana* [397/426], Book II, 31.48
(Oxford Early Christian Texts) (Oxford: Oxford University Press, 1995).]

15 *The Didascalion of Hugh of St. Victor* [c.1130]. III.ii, translated and introduced by
Jerome Taylor (New York: Columbia University Press, 1991), 86. On the ques-
tion to which extent the full text of Quintilian's *Institutio* was known throughout
the Middle Ages, see the overview given by Nancy van Deusen, 'Cicero through
Quintilian's Eyes in the Middle Ages', 47–64, at 48n2, in *Cicero Refused to Die:
Ciceronian Influence Through the Centuries*, edited by Nancy van Deusen (Leiden:
Brill, 2013).

16 What is translated using the modern psychological term 'intellect' in classical and medieval Latin generally meant 'understanding', 'comprehension', or
'discernment'.

17 *Didascalion* III.vii, 43; 'Multi sunt quos ipsa adeo natura ingenio destitutos reliquit
ut ea etiam quae facilia sunt intellectu vix capere possint, et horum duo genera mihi
esse videntur. Nam sunt quidam, qui, licet suam hebetudinem non ignorent, eo
tamen quo valent conanime ad scientiam anhelant, et indesinenter studio insist-
entes, quod minus habent effectu operis, obtinere merentur effectu voluntatis. Ast
alii quoniam summa se comprehendere nequaquam posse sentiunt, minima etiam
negligunt, et quasi in suo torpore securi quiescentes eo amplius in maximis lumen
veritatis perdunt, quo minima quae intelligere possent discere fugiunt. ... Longe
enim aliud est nescire atque aliud nolle scire. Nescire siquidem infirmitatis est,
scientiam vero detestari, pravae voluntatis'. [Original Latin text: Hugo von Sankt
Viktor, *Didascalion de studio legendi* [c.1130] (Fontes Christiani 27) (Freiburg:
Herder, 1997), 104.]

18 *Didascalion* III.vii, 44, Preface; Et tamen aliud est cum non possis, aut ut verius
dicam, facile non possis discere, atque aliud posse et nolle scire. Latin: Hugo von
Sankt Viktor, *Didascalion*, 106.

19 G. R. Evans, *Getting It Wrong: The Medieval Epistemology of Error* (Studien und
Texte zur Geistesgeschichte des Mittelalters 63) (Leiden: Brill, 1998), 101.

20 *Didascalion* III.vii, 91; 'Ingenium a natura proficiscitur, usu iuvatur, immoderato
    labore retunditur, et temperato acuitur exercitio'. Latin: Hugo von Sankt Viktor,
    Didascalion, 240.

21 Hugo von Sankt Viktor, *Didascalion*, Book V.v, 334. 'qui naturaliter sunt hebetes et
    tardi ad intelligendum'.

22 *Didascalion* III.vii, 126.

23 Ibid., 127; 'Fortuna est in eventu, casu, sive naturaliter contingente, quando vel
    paupertate vel infirmitate vel non naturali tarditate, sive etiam doctorum raritate,
    quia aut non inveniuntur qui doceant, aut qui bene doceant, a proposito nostro
    retrahimur'. Latin: Hugo von Sankt Viktor, *Didascalion*, 336.

24 *Didascalion* III.xiii, 95; 'Considera potius quid vires tuae ferre valeant. Aptissime
    incedit, qui incedit ordinate.' Latin: Hugo von Sankt Viktor, *Didascalion*, 254.

25 *Didascalion* VI.iii, 137; 'illum incedere aptissime qui incedit ordinate, neque ut
    quidam, dum magnum saltum facere volunt, praecipitium incidunt'. Latin: Hugo
    von Sankt Viktor, *Didascalion*, 364.

26 *Institutio oratoria* I.2, 2, Vol. I, 54/55. 'alioqui non peius duxerim tardi esse ingenii
    quam mali. Probus autem ab illo segni et iacente plurimum aberit'.

27 Isidore of Seville, *Sententiarum libri* III.ix. 5–8, *PL*, Vol. 83, cols 681B–82A.

28 *Didascalion* III.vii, 174n3. On the Cornificians, see Rosemary Barton Tobin, 'The
    Cornifician Motif in John of Salisbury's *Metalogicon*', *History of Education* 13:1
    (1984), 1–6.

29 *Didascalion* II.xx, 75; Latin: Hugo von Sankt Viktor, *Didascalion*, 192–194; also
    discussed by B. B. Price, *Medieval Thought: An Introduction* (Oxford: Blackwell,
    1992), 173. 'Sicut aliae septem liberales appellatae sunt, vel quia liberos, id est,
    expeditos et exercitatos animos requirunt, quia subtiliter de rerum causis dispu-
    tant, vel quia liberi tantum antiquitus, id est, nobiles, in eis studere consueverant,
    plebei vero et ignobilium filii in mechanicis propter peritiam operandi'.

30 Cf. Stephen C. Ferruolo, *The Origins of the University* (Stanford University Press:
    Stanford, 1985).

31 Evans, *Getting It Wrong*, 90.

32 *Didascalion* I.xi, 59–60; 'Priusquam esset grammatica et scribebant et loqueban-
    tur homines. Priusquam esset dialectica, ratiocinando verum a falso discernebant.
    Priusquam esset rhetorica, iura civilia tractabant. Priusquam esset arithmetica,
    scientiam numerandi habebant. Priusquam esset geometria, agros mensurabant.
    Priusquam esset astronomia, per cursus stellarum discretiones temporum capie-
    bant'. Latin: Hugo von Sankt Viktor, *Didascalion*, 150–152; summarised in Evans,
    Getting It Wrong, 95.

33 *De oratore*, I.xlii.187–188, cited in *Didascalion*, 95.

34 Price, *Medieval Thought*, 173; cf. J. A. Weisheipl, 'Classification of the Sciences in
    Medieval Thought', *Medieval Studies* 27 (1965), 75–78.

35 *Didascalion* I.ix, 56; 'Multo enim nunc magis enitet ratio hominis haec eadem
    inveniendo quam habendo claruisset'. Latin: Hugo von Sankt Viktor, *Didascalion*,
    142.

36 Price, *Medieval Thought*, 175.

37 *Didascalion* I.i, 47. 'haec est illa naturae nostrae dignitas quam omnes aeque naturaliter habent, sed non omnes aeque noverunt. Animus enim, corporeis passionibus consopitus et per sensibiles formas extra semetipsum abductus, oblitus est quid fuerit'. Latin: Hugo von Sankt Viktor, *Didascalion*, 116.

38 Evans, *Getting It Wrong*, 207.

39 David Summers, *The Judgment of Sense: Renaissance Naturalism and the Rise of Aesthetics* (Cambridge: Cambridge University Press, 1987), 155; cf. Alhazen, *Opticae thesaurus. Alhazen Arabis libri septem nuncprimum editi ...*, edited by F. Risner (Basel, 1572) (facs. New York, 1972, edited by D. C. Lindberg), II, 13. Alhazen's text known in Latin as *Perspectiva* was probably translated in the late twelfth or early thirteenth century, cf. D. C. Lindberg, 'Alhazen's Theory of Vision and Its Reception in the West', *Isis* 58 (1967), 321–341.

40 William F. MacLehose, *'A Tender Age': Cultural Anxieties Over the Child in the Twelfth and Thirteenth Centuries* (New York: Columbia University Press, 2008), 188.

41 MacLehose, *'A Tender Age'*, 193–196.

42 Evans, *Getting It Wrong*, 60; cf. Gilbert of Tournai, *De modo addiscendi*, edited by E. Bonifacio (Turin: Società editrice internazionale, 1953), IV.xx.

43 Arpad Steiner, ed., Vincent of Beauvais, *De eruditione filiorum nobilium*, chapter V, 'De tribus necessariis addiscenti' (Wisconsin: Medieval Academy of America, 1938), 22. 'Ubi ferrum uocatur humanum ingenium siue mens propter perspicacitatis accumen. Et sicut ociositas ferrum obtundit ac denigrat, rubiginat et consumit, Econtra uero usus illud exacuit, dealbat, elimat et a corrupcione rubiginis conseruat, Sic humanam mentem ocium uel desidia obtundit ac cetera predicta in ea facit'.

44 Steiner, ed., *De eruditione filiorum nobilium*, 39: 'sicut rustici, fatui sc., lapidem preciosum inuenerint, non reputant, quia uirtutem eius ac preciositatem ignorant, et ob hoc illum quasi vile quid proiciunt'.

45 Steiner, ed., *De eruditione filiorum nobilium*, 39. The original passage reads 'sicut imbecilles et ignaui cito proiciunt lapidem'.

46 Julie Singer, '"Une enroullure de sapience": The Mechanics of Melancholy and Intellectual Disability' (paper presented at Medieval Academy of America meeting, St Louis University, St Louis, Missouri, 22 March, 2012).

47 Simon Kemp, *Medieval Psychology* (New York: Greenwood Press, 1990), 157.

48 St Thomas Aquinas, *Summa theologiae*, 1.2.54.4; 1.2.51.4.

49 Kemp, *Medieval Psychology*, 157–158, with *Summa theologiae*, 1.2.50–53.

50 'Nota quod leprosi, gibbosi, monstuosi et in ceteris membris officialibus defectuosi no debent doctrine mancipari propter multa. Leprosi non, quia lepra est morbus contagious et sic leprosus sanos lepra posset inficere ... Item, nec gibbosus seu in aliis menbris defectuosus, quia istius non accidunt nisi propter debilitatem nature vel propter inobedienciam materie. Si propter debilitatem nature, cum natura sit fundamentum in corpora et debile fundamentum semper minetur ruinam et

statum deteriorem, ex tali defectu in principio posset oriri magnus error in fine, nam modicus error in principilis facit maximum in principiatis. Et ideo cavendum est ne tales doctrine mancipetur'. Michael Johnson, ed., *A Critical Edition of the Commentary by William of Wheteley on the Pseudo-Boethian Treatise De Disciplina Scolarium* (PhD thesis, State University of New York at Buffalo, 1982), 46. There are also some observations on the same theme a little earlier: 'Ostendit cuius disposicionis menbrorum pueri debent esse qui debent doctrine mancipari … id est illorum menbrorum ex quibus integratur homo principalitur; et similiter illorum menbrorum que maxime deserviunt arti et discipline, cuiusmodi sunt oculi et aures; et similiter illorum menbrorum que maxime deserviunt operibus clericatum consequentibus, ut sunt manus et digiti et brachia que deserviunt scripture et operibus divinis in altari' (42). I am grateful to Ben Parsons at the University of Leicester for supplying me with this reference.

51 Lynn Thorndike, *A History of Magic and Experimental Science*, Vol. 3 (New York: Columbia University Press, 1934), 465.

52 Bert Hansen, *Nicole Oresme and the Marvels of Nature: A Study of his* De causis mirabilium *with Critical Edition, Translation, and Commentary* (Toronto: Pontifical Institute of Medieval Studies, 1985), 3–16.

53 Hansen, *Nicole Oresme*, 252–253. 'Vide in te: si loquereris omnia que tibi occurrunt modo de uno modo de alio, que et quot tu diceres, certe homines dicerent te fatuum'.

54 Cited in Herbert Grundmann, *Religiöse Bewegungen im Mittelalter* (Hildesheim: Georg Olms, 2nd edn. 1961), 414 n128, and mentioned by Caroline Walker Bynum, *Holy Feast and Holy Fast: The Religious Significance of Food to Medieval Women* (Berkeley, Los Angeles, and London: University of California Press, 1987), 85 and 337 n87, who translates Grundmann's note (above; he referred to the nun's Albernheit, literally: 'foolishness, silliness') as 'idiocy'. The original Latin reads 'Dicere quod aliqua lactet puerum Jesum cum matre usque ad lassitudinem et defectum, fatuitas est verberibus potius quam verbis corrigenda'. The source is a collection of notes regarding nearly one hundred statements by heretics collected by Albertus Magnus in the bishopric of Augsburg, which under the title *Determinatio magistri Alberti Magni de novo spiritu* was added to a collection of the so-called Passau Anonymous, modern edition by Alexander Patschovsky, *Der Passauer Anonymus. Ein Sammelwerk über Ketzer, Juden, Antichrist aus der Mitte des 13. Jahrhunderts*, MGH Schriften 22 (1968).

55 Nancy Caciola, *Discerning Spirits: Divine and Demonic Possession in the Middle Ages* (Ithaca and London: Cornell University Press, 2003), 175.

56 Mathew Thomson, *The Problem of Mental Deficiency: Eugenics, Democracy, and Social Policy in Britain, c.1870–1959* (Oxford: Oxford University Press, 1998), 13–14.

57 Ruth von Bernuth, 'From Marvels of Nature to Inmates of Asylums: Imaginations of Natural Folly', *Disability Studies Quarterly* 26.2 (2006), no pagination, online publication at www.dsq-sds.org, accessed 1 August, 2014.

58 Jan Daniel Georgens and Heinrich Marianus Deinhardt, *Die Heilpaedagogik: Mit besonderer Berücksichtigung der Idiotie und der Idiotenanstalten. Bd. 1: Zwölf Vorträge zur Einleitung und Begründung einer heilpädagogischen Gesammtwissenschaft* (original 1861, reprint Giessen: Institut für Heil- und Sonderpädagogik, 1979). For the impact of this work, see Anne Waldschmidt, 'Paradoxien des Normalismus: Normalitätsvorstellungen im heilpädagogischen Diskurs', in *Zeichen und Gesten: Heilpädagogik als Kulturthema*, edited by H. Greving, C. Murner and P. Rödler (Gießen: Psychosozial-Verlag, 2004), 98–112.

59 von Bernuth, 'From Marvels of Nature to Inmates of Asylums'.

60 Ibid.

61 See for instance Sieglind Ellger-Rüttgardt, *Geschichte der Sonderpädagogik. Eine Einführung* (Stuttgart: Reinhardt/UTB, 2008), an introductory textbook to the subject aimed at university courses, which of course only starts with the Enlightenment.

62 Evans, *Getting It Wrong*, 159.

63 William Fenner, *Wilfull Impenitency the Grossest Selfe-Murder* (London, 1656), 4, cited by Goodey, *History of Intelligence*, 190.

64 *Summa Theologiae*, II pars 2, quaestio 46 in 3 articles *De stultitia*. 'And folly differs from fatuity, … in that folly implies apathy in the heart and dullness in the senses, while fatuity denotes entire privation of the spiritual sense. Therefore folly is fittingly opposed to wisdom'. [Et differt stultitia a fatuitate, … quia stultitia importat hebetudinem cordis et obtusionem sensuum; fatuitas autem importat totaliter spiritualis sensus privationem. Et ideo convenienter stultitia sapientiae opponitur.]

4

'SOME HAVE IT FROM BIRTH, SOME BY DISPOSITION':[1] FOOLISHNESS IN MEDIEVAL GERMAN LITERATURE

Janina Dillig

The fool is a prominent character in medieval German literature, and often serves not only a comic but also a didactic purpose. To the contemporary reader this seems like a potential contradiction, but the logic underlying this contradiction can be found in the Christian idea of foolishness as something typically human that can be overcome by reason – an idea likely generated by depictions of foolishness, idiocy, or stupidity in the fifteenth and sixteenth centuries. Indeed, the German author Sebastian Brant uses this concept in his *Narrenschiff* [*Ship of Fools*], first printed in 1494. He explicitly names the fostering of reason and wisdom as the objective of his collection of fools:

> This collection was gathered through the effort and work of Sebastian Brant for the good, for sanatory instruction, for admonition and for the propagation of wisdom, reason and public decency as well as for the contempt and punishment of foolishness, blindness, madness and stupidity in all places and humankind.[2] [All translations are by the author unless otherwise indicated.]

Brant's text is a prominent example of the popularity of the contrast of reason and foolishness in the sixteenth century, since it is one of the most successful German books of that period. Scholars have frequently identified the reason/ folly opposition expressed in this work, combined with the increasing importance of the individual in philosophical discourse, as a signpost on the route to modern concepts of (intellectual) disability:

> Significantly, as the individual and his reason re-emerge as the central focus of social and political discourse, so too does the disabled subject, reason's Other. [...] The drive to define categories of reason and unreason, and the explicit formulation of disability as a state in opposition to the rule of reason, emerge simultaneously.[3]

Following this argument, scholars have argued that the modern image of the natural fool develops after the Christian – and medieval – idea of the universal fool becomes individualized. However, the medieval idea of foolishness is not that simple, as Stainton notes, because several discourses are interleaved in the medieval conception of the fool.[4] It is the aim of this chapter to add to this discussion with a reading of earlier medieval texts that present medieval folly as something more complex and diverse than a simple opposition to reason. This study focuses on Middle High German texts (roughly encompassing the period from 1050–1350) that feature foolish characters and thus invoke forms of foolishness or stupidity which may not only be described as folly but also as medieval precursors of a concept of intellectual disability.[5]

I understand literature as a symbolic institution of the imaginary, in the sense that the Greco-French philosopher Cornelius Castoriadis uses this term in *The Imaginary Institution of Society*. According to Castoriadis, literature can be understood as a form of expression not only of the individual imaginary, but also as a symbolic expression of society. It reflects the discourse of society while also influencing it.[6] Defining literature as a symbolic institution in this way allows us to understand texts not only as the products of cultural discourse, but also as performative elements within it. Any depiction of foolishness or stupidity in literature can thus be conceived as an active part of the discourse on foolishness or stupidity pertaining to the particular society in which the work was written.

When one uses the terms 'intellectual disability' or 'learning disability' in a historical-literary analysis, one has to be careful to avoid anachronisms. While recent studies have established that disability is not a natural category but an unstable concept which each historical society defines differently,[7] most historical studies on disability concentrate on either physical disability or mental illness in the form of madness. And while mental illness is commonly accepted as a relative concept, and madness often seen as a consequence of or associated with extreme intelligence, scholarship has tended to ignore intellectual disability because it is still often seen as something that is self-explanatory and 'natural'.[8] One can assume that there are and have always been people in every society who cannot (or do not) act in a way perceived as intelligent. However, the kinds of behaviours and actions that are considered signs of a lack of intelligence differ from society to society:

> Of course there are always people around who seem unable to grasp certain complex everyday activities. What changes, though, is the content of those activities and their centrality to the life which the rest of us in any one era expect to lead. At any given historical moment, the people thus excluded seem to be a

separate and permanent natural kind, but in fact their psychological profile alters radically in the long term along with the social context feeding it.[9]

As Goodey suggests, identifying someone as intellectually disabled in a historical context is quite difficult, if not impossible, since sources are not fully reliable as to what signs indicate intellectual disability at a given point in time. This is especially difficult for medieval concepts of foolishness and their relation to intellectual disability.

In order to identify different kinds of disability I use Susan Wendell's definition of 'disability as a form of difference from what is considered normal or usual or paradigmatic in a society'.[10] Following Wendell's concept of disability, we can establish how societal reactions to the foolish character determine whether the fool is considered to be disabled or whether he is an integrated part of society. Not every type of folly that is described as different equates to a form of intellectual disability, especially because the fool is a very multidimensional character in medieval culture: 'He was the wild man and the one who plays the wild man; the idiot or the maniac and the one who plays the idiot or the maniac; the dreamer and the breaker of dreams; Harlequin the aggressor and Pierrot the victim'.[11]

What complicates the discussion around folly, foolishness, and intellectual disability in the Middle Ages is the fact that foolishness was also institutionalized through the character of the court jester. The behaviour of the jester seems to lie outside the norm of intellectual behaviour and as such seems to imply intellectual disability in most depictions. Thus, for a long time, scholarship considered the court jester to be an example of some precursor of intellectual disability. However, more recent critical historical research shows that there is no proof that court jesters were commonly intellectually different; on the contrary, there are university records and iconographic illustrations of court jesters with bodily impairments, which do not imply an intellectual impairment as well. Thus the historical institution of the court jester does not account for the conception of a form of intellectual disability in the European Middle Ages.[12] This example demonstrates that depictions of foolishness do not always imply natural foolishness. And so natural fools have to be separated from so-called 'will fools' or 'artificial fools' (*wille tôre* in Middle High German[13]).

In addition, while will fools usually imitate the behaviour of so-called natural fools (for example, in the role of court jester), the behaviour of will fools may also be copied by natural fools. Hence, the concepts of will fool and natural fool are not independent of each other. Especially after 1500, '"natural idiocy" and "artificial folly" are engaged in a deep exchange of meaning and value'.[14]

These diverse meanings of the term 'fool' demonstrate why references to foolishness can only be the starting-point for an investigation of intellectual disability in medieval literature. In what follows, the Middle High German words for fool (e.g. *tôre, narre, gief*) will be used as markers for a wide range of possible forms of disabilities. Only by being able to understand the range of foolishness depicted as lying outside of societal norms will it be possible to tentatively describe the function of precursor notions of intellectual disability.

The fool in the medieval medical discourse

To understand further how some medieval precursor of the idea of intellectual disability might have been imagined in medieval society, it is helpful to turn to historical discourses on the natural fool, especially medical ones. However, simply taking the Latin medical discourse as the background for vernacular literary texts is problematic because they not only differ in terms of language but also in terms of their target audience. This is why I focus on a vernacular text of the fourteenth century: *Buch der Natur*, one of the first German encyclopaedic sources on nature, by Konrad von Megenberg. This German scholar wrote his compendium around 1350, and his systematic collection of all things in nature can be seen as a benchmark in modern natural sciences.[15] Its popularity is demonstrated by the eighty manuscripts and six incunabula which have survived.[16]

As a medieval scholar, Konrad did not write as a modern scientist would; instead he was transcribing what Augustine referred to as the *Liber Naturae* ('The Book of Nature'), God's addition to the *Liber Scripturae* (the Bible). Medieval scholars understood nature as the manifestation of God's power in the world and thus as something that could be theologically interpreted.

> Thus Konrad of Megenberg did not write a book on nature but a *liber de natura rerum*, a book on the special properties of things, which was meant to clarify the meaning of natural things and their different significances in medieval printed texts. Often the descriptions of creatures are followed by moral and allegorical interpretations.[17]

Konrad's text contains a chapter entitled *Von der wunder menschen*,[18] on 'wondrous things', including one article in which he tells the reader about two types of wondrous humans: 'Some [who] have a deficit of the body, some of the soul'. [*Etleich habent geprechen an dem leib und etleich an der sel werk*].[19] According to Konrad, bodily deficient humans include people who are either missing body parts or have too many. In other words, *geprechen an dem leib* describes different kinds of physical disability. Impairments other than bodily ones, by contrast, can be associated with *geprechen an der sel*.

Translating *sel* as 'soul', however, does not do full justice to what Konrad means here, especially as he is writing in German rather than Latin, which had two words, *animus* and *anima*. Strictly speaking, the former describes the persona of individuals, while the latter, derived from the Greek *psyche* but adapted to Christian religious usage, denotes in a more abstract sense the animating principle of the body. By Konrad's time the terms were beginning to be interchanged, albeit not necessarily legitimately in the eyes of contemporaries. Be that as it may, the medieval idea of the soul (*anima*) also often includes what we would today call the mind. For example, in the ninth century Johannes Scotus describes the soul as the animating principle of the body, encompassing life, intellect, ratio, mind, cognition, and memory as its essential parts. This later became a standard description.[20] Only later still did the intellect or mind sometimes become described as an accidental property – as opposed to an essential property – of the soul.[21] Yet even the Aristotelian philosopher Thomas Aquinas admits that if mind and intellect were accidental properties of the soul, the soul could still not be separable from its possibilities. Therefore, he understands mind and intellect as possibilities which are immortal just like the soul itself.[22] Other medieval thinkers, such as Albertus Magnus, maintain that, despite the Aristotelian influence on Christian scholars, the intellect is an essential part of the soul.[23] I specifically mention Albert Magnus in this context because Konrad von Megenberg himself asserts that his *Buch der Natur* is a vernacular adaptation of a compendium written by Albertus Magnus: 'Thus I translate from Latin into the German language a book that Albert collected in a masterly fashion from the forefathers'.[24]

If we read Konrad's *Buch der Natur* in the light of Albertus Magnus's theory of the intellect as an essential property of the soul, the expression *geprechen an der sel* describes something wrong with the whole functioning of the soul, including not only the intellect and the mind but also its other essential parts. This 'wrongness', however, is described not as a disease but explicitly as a deficit, the precise sense given by *gebrechen*.[25]

In another passage from Konrad's text, the deficit of the soul is described as something which 'Some have ... from birth, some by disposition'.[26]

Konrad first discusses 'natural fools', that is, those fools who have their deficit from birth. He explains their deficit through what in the Middle Ages was called the soul's powers: 'Those who have a deficit from birth on, those are the natural fools. They do not have the cells of their soul's powers correctly situated in their head'.[27]

The doctrine of the soul's powers was common in medieval philosophical, theological, and medical discourses. However, each discourse describes these powers in different ways, with different numbers and different ways of understanding them.[28] For the purpose of this chapter, I focus on the medical version, where perception and cognition are considered to occur through three 'cells' or ventricles that process everything first recognized by the senses. The first ventricle contains the power of the imaginative faculty, or *imaginatio*, which processes all sensual impressions; these impressions are then transferred to the reasoning faculty, and are finally saved by the *memoria*. In some formulations of this structure, however, the reasoning faculty is sub-divided into *ratio* and *intellectus*. While *ratio* differentiates all impressions, it is the *intellectus* that allows the human mind to process these impressions into an understanding of divine reason.[29] Finally, in order for the soul to act, humans must also have a will. Even if the will is not considered to be a power of the soul, it is nevertheless defined by Albertus Magnus as something that moves *ratio* and the other soul's powers.[30]

In accordance with the logic of the soul's powers, Konrad does not define natural fools by their lack of intellect. Instead, he understands foolishness to be the result of an incorrect and misordered process of perception and cognition; that is, the soul's powers are not working in the way that is considered normal. This incorrect ordering may also manifest itself physically: 'One may verify [the deficit of the soul] by the fact that they have malformed heads, either too big or too small'.[31]

Notably, since natural fools do not have anything missing from their souls, they are considered complete humans. Their souls nevertheless work differently from those of normal adults and that is why they can be compared to the souls of children: 'They do not work like other human souls, but have human souls in the sense that children do'.[32] In the European Middle Ages, children were considered to have souls, but it was often believed that their souls were not as fully developed as those of adults.[33]

With this in mind it is clear that what marks natural fools as different from birth is the way the soul's different components process sensory impressions. As a consequence of this 'wrong' processing, natural fools act and look differently and are thus recognized as 'disabled' in the sense that they are limited in their adult mental capabilities; but their souls are not incomplete or partial. As such, these precurser forms of intellectual disability were not considered to be a consequence of sin, at least in the academic vernacular discourse.

In contrast to natural fools, fools by disposition do not show any physical signs of difference. Instead they can be considered disabled because they live outside of human society, as animals do: 'Those who have the deficit through disposition are those raised in the wild, far away from reasonable people, and live like cattle'.[34]

Konrad makes a clear distinction between those he considers natural fools and those he labels fools by disposition. Still, as the following examples will show, the distinction between the natural fool and fool by disposition is not always as explicit, just as the distinction between the natural fool and the will fool is often hazy. And it becomes even more complicated when we bring into the picture questions of the social standing of the 'deficient' people in medieval society.

The will fool in Middle High German literature

To understand the social standing of fools, I will use the example of a character who disguises himself as a fool, a situation occurring in several medieval stories.[35] One such character can be found in the Middle High German story 'Die Halbe Birne', recorded around 1300,[36] about the knight Arnold who participates in a joust to prove his worth as a potential husband for a princess. The princess appreciates Arnold's knightly deeds on the first day of the joust, and she is pleased when her father invites him to dine with them.[37] However, when Arnold shares a pear with the princess, employing non-courtly table manners, she is outraged.[38] His mistake is not to peel it, and he thus earns the enmity of the princess. She reacts to this breach of 'exaggerated courtliness'[39] by insulting the knight in public, thus diminishing his reputation and honour (êre).

To seek revenge, Arnold disguises himself as a fool. In this guise he is allowed into the court and even into the bedchamber of the princess because she wants to be entertained by him – thus he is accepted as a court jester. When Arnold exposes himself by lifting his tunic we are told that 'she became very aroused at the sight of the oafish fool's swollen eleventh finger'.[40]

The princess takes the fool into her bed, where he in turn refuses to participate in any kind of sexual activity. She prods and strikes him, but he does not perform and is consequently thrown out of the bedchamber. Now, however, the fool holds a higher moral standing than the princess, because of his ability to show sexual self-control.

The next morning, Arnold returns as a knight to fight again in the joust. When the princess again insults him publicly, he repeats the words she had used the night before, which is when she realizes that 'The fool who left us unsatisfied was the courtly knight'.[41]

The situation is reversed and the princess knows it. It is no longer he who is disgraced, it is she. Afraid he might expose her, she marries him and he wins her kingdom, so that 'Both the people and the land came under his power'.[42]

Arnold's performance as a fool reveals two important factors in terms of how people thought about foolish behaviour in the courtly society of this story. Firstly, the fool not only wears different clothes from the knight, he also wears his hair short and his skin is sunburned and dark. Furthermore, Arnold carries a club as a signifier of his status as a fool.[43] Once thus equipped, Arnold becomes the perfect fool: 'His hair was cut short like a fool's, and he was dressed as a fool. He was painted black like a moor. His tunic ended at his knees. He took a club in his hand, and that was how he left. Women and men alike took him for a fool'.[44]

As a fool, Arnold has possibilities for manoeuvre within the court that he does not have as a knight. He cannot act against the princess as a knight, but he can get his revenge by disguising himself as a fool. As a knight, Arnold has entrance to the Arthurian-type court, but only as a fool does he gain entrance to the inner sphere of the princess's life, her bedchamber. This additional room for manoeuvre allows him to prove himself superior to the 'exaggerated courtliness'[45] of the princess. As Müller points out, '[Through the] figure of the (alleged) fool – feeble-minded, deaf-mute, dirty, ragged, ugly and brutal – he negates point by point the norms on which the self-conception of courtliness is based'.[46]

In considering the function which his disguise fulfils in the story, one can say that by playing a fool and acting outside of the norms of knightly behaviour Arnold uses the social status of someone whose behaviour is considered to be different, and thus disabled, as an auxiliary means to gain what he wants. This 'disabled' behaviour is largely accepted because of the social standing of a court jester. As nobody recognizes the fool as a knight, the disguise allows him to re-establish his honour (êre) and win the hand of the princess. According to this logic, the fool is clearly an accepted part of courtly society. Foolishness adorned with the appropriate status symbols, such as specific clothing, haircut, and skin tone, as well as a club, implies integration in courtly society. However, if anyone had recognized Arnold in his 'fool' disguise, it would surely have led to negative consequences, because in so disguising himself he transgressed social boundaries.

The natural fool in Middle High German literature

Not every knight in Middle High German literature who wears the clothes of a fool is a will fool like Arnold. Let us consider the example of Parzival, the eponymous hero of the epic *Parzival*, one of the most popular stories in the Middle Ages, written by Wolfram von Eschenbach some time before 1210.[47] Parzival's father dies before his son is born, and the grieving mother removes her child from any kind of civilization. Parzival is then raised without formal education of any kind; he learns neither of God nor of his royal heritage.[48] One day, the child sees four knights and wishes to become one. To prevent this, his mother dresses him as a fool before he leaves her: 'The queen then thought, People are really quick to mock. My child will wear fool's clothes on his royal body. When he is fought with and beaten he will come back to me'.[49]

However, the text suggests that, after leaving his mother, his clothes are not alone in making Parzival a fool. He also misinterprets social behaviour several times. For example, his mother tells him that he should accept a ring and the kiss of a lady; but when he sees a lady, he steals her ring and forces her to kiss him, leading the narrator to refer to him as 'Parzival, the foolish one'.[50]

On several occasions, Parzival's behaviour is considered to lie outside of normal societal expectations. The act of stealing the kiss, and his generally foolish behaviour, can be understood as signs of an intellectual disability because he makes no conscious decision to act in this way. However, Parzival finds teachers who not only inform him of his identity but also teach him what it means to be a knight, and even about his heritage concerning the Holy Grail. In the end, after several quests and duels, Parzival becomes the Grail King.

Clearly the narrator uses Parzival's intellectual disability as a means to show how much he has to overcome in order to reach his status as the Grail King. We can therefore use the concept of 'narrative prosthesis' to describe how this disability functions in Wolfram's text. 'Narrative prosthesis', a term coined by David T. Mitchell and Sharon L. Snyder, describes how disability is commonly used as a narrative device. They point out that in modern literature, the paradox of disability lies in the fact that it is on the one hand inherently marginalized and on the other hand a prevailing characteristic of narrative discourse;[51] this paradox is possible because disability is used as a 'crutch upon which artistic discourse and cultural narratives have leaned to ensure the novelty of their subject matter'.[52] Only when something is not normal can it form the basis of a story worth telling. Consequently, disability is often used as an 'other' that produces and supports an illusion of normativity and thus affirms discursive power structures.

While the concept of narrative prosthesis is used by these authors mostly in the context of physical disability, it can be applied to cognitive disability as well.[53] Parzival's disability is used not only to emphasize the hero's 'development' from the fool in the wild to the Grail King, foregrounding how he overcomes his lack of education, but also to demonstrate his innocence, since the behavioural mistakes he makes are merely the result of his intellectual disability, or stupidity. As thus, Parzival's disability is not only in contrast to reason but also to sin, when his intellectual disability is used as prosthesis to demonstrate his childlike disposition, which includes innocence. However, at first glance his disability seems to be curable; he is able to rectify his deficit through the right teachings. Therefore, Parzival seems to be a fool by disposition, as Konrad von Megenberg describes it, and not a natural fool. Not only is he literally raised in the wild, he also has no physical markings for his intellectual disability. On the contrary, his beauty and strength are underlined several times in the text.[54]

Yet Parzival's foolishness is not that easily remedied. Bumke argues that Parzival never fully overcomes it, because it is not a result of his lack of education but rather a deficit in his *ratio*.[55] After Parzival leaves his teacher Gurnemanz, who instructs him in what it means to be a knight, the narrator comments that 'the worthy Gurnemanz freed him from his foolishness'.[56] In speaking to Gurnemanz, however, Parzival does not seem to be of the same opinion: 'He then said: Sir, I am not wise'.[57]

It cannot therefore be said that Parzival, having arrived at Gurnemanz's place as a fool, leaves as a fully educated knight, because the protagonist himself has his doubts.[58] These doubts are given credit by the later progress of the story, when Gurnemanz's teachings lead in fact to Parzival's biggest mistake. Arriving at the Grail Castle for the first time, Parzival remembers Gurnemanz's advice and does not ask his host about his wound. By not asking, Parzival keeps his host in agony and has to fight for a second chance to ask his question before he can release his host from his pain.[59]

Nor does Parzival's other teacher, Trevrizent, who teaches him about his heritage, remove his foolishness.[60] Even after Trevrizent tells him that the killing of family in a duel is a sin, Parzival keeps fighting duels, including one against his own brother. Bumke further points out Parzival's continuing and key characteristic, established by the narrator at the beginning of Wolfram's epic as 'He, the brave but not wise one'.[61]

In conclusion, Bumke argues that Parzival does not overcome his stupidity until the end: 'The Parzival plot does not show the way to wisdom. It is the stupid Parzival who is appointed by God, not the wise one. Parzival's stupidity is not a deficit to overcome but his *habitus*'.[62]

Following Bumke's interpretation, Parzival is not just a fool by disposition, but also by birth. He is a natural fool, which becomes especially obvious when his behaviour leads to comical situations which mark him as different. His disability, though, does not have negative connotations, and is not only used to emphasize his innocence but even to represent a form of purity, akin to the idea of holy stupidity (*sancta simplicitas*).[63] Consequently, a natural fool like Parzival is eventually able to become the Grail King.

Not every story of a natural fool has such a happy ending. Another example of foolishness in Middle High German literature is found in the story 'Des Mönches Not', probably written at the end of the thirteenth century.[64] Again, the story is about a young man who lacks education, just as Parzival does. The young man is raised in a monastery in the wilderness, in a clerical setting: 'A little child was given to a monk to live a pure life. It did not know the world. The monk sends the child to a monastery in the woods'.[65] The child studies his books dutifully. However, all his bookish wisdom does not help the young man when he reads about courtly love, or *minne*. To learn more about the practice of *minne*, he asks a male servant for an explanation. Instead of explaining the courtly virtue, the servant leads the boy to a prostitute, who in turn gets angry with the astonished boy, because he does not move at all while lying in bed with her. She starts hitting the boy who, as a result, deems *minne* very painful. This is when the narrator calls the young monk a *tôre*.[66] By contrast with Parzival, the young monk is a fool because he gathers the wrong information from the wrong sources and thus comes to a wrong conclusion.

Nevertheless, the young monk's wrong deductions do not have any immediate consequences, apart from creating humour for the reader. On the way back to the monastery, he asks his servant whether it is possible to become pregnant from *minne* and if so, who the pregnant party will be: 'This I can tell you, says the servant, the one who lies underneath'.[67]

As a result, the young monk panics: 'As it was me who lay underneath, I am going to give birth to a child. I have entirely lost my honour'.[68]

The monk's lack of knowledge of female anatomy and human reproduction leads to foolish behaviour. He seeks an abortion. He hears of a cow that lost her calf after being hit by a peasant. He seeks the same solution, and pays the peasant to hit him; while being beaten up, the monk sees a rabbit running away and believes it to be it his 'child'. The young monk follows the rabbit into the woods but cannot catch it, and concludes that his child is lost. While searching for his 'child', he is found by the other monks and consequently diagnosed as being a fool: 'They all would have sworn that he was out of his mind'.[69]

First, the other monks try to exorcise the young fool. But this does not help; he still mourns for his unbaptized child. There seems to be no remedy, so the other monks react to him as if he were a natural fool and isolate him. However, when he finally gets a chance to recount his incorrect deductions to his abbot, the latter is able to clarify why the monk might have thought he was pregnant. However, the young man still does not know that he never actually experienced sexual intercourse, nor that he never came close to learning about *minne*. Consequently, he accepts punishment for a sin he never committed. The original deficit of the monk is never corrected, as can be seen in the last words of the abbot to him: 'You shall go to the choir to sing and read and you shall be a good child'.[70]

The monk's folly persists, therefore, even after his confession, and his abbot continues to treat him like a child.[71] He does not learn about *minne* and thus stays a fool by disposition, as Konrad describes it. While the narrative uses this foolishness to underline his innocence in a manner similar to that employed in the story of Parzival, his foolish behaviour is primarily employed as a way of provoking laughter in the reader. Contrary to Parzival's disability, the monk's disability is depicted as something negative and used as a narrative prosthesis to indirectly critique clerical education because it leads to foolishness. As a consequence, 'Des Mönches Not' is one of the earlier examples of a fool character rendered as a tool for clerical satire, a genre which becomes even more popular in the following centuries. The fool therefore gains a didactic purpose in literary discourse, similar to the fools in Brants' *Narrenschiff*.

Conclusion

In summary, we have seen that in Middle High German literature foolishness is described in different forms. While these few examples of fools in Middle High German literature by no means form a complete list, they exhibit a variety of representational possibilities available even before foolishness became a popular theme in the fifteenth and sixteenth centuries. All examples use foolishness – in both forms as 'natural' fools and 'will' fools – as narrative prosthetics; however, they do not confine themselves to contrasting folly with reason. On the contrary, the young monk and Parzival appear as fools whose foolishness indicates innocence or even sainthood. As such, foolishness is not only depicted as part of the discourse of reason, but also of sin. This innocence may form a basis for comical situations, which relates them to the court jester, the socially accepted form of the will fool, and also leads to the sixteenth-century use of foolishness for didactic purposes. Parzival, however, is a different example. His innocence leads to salvation and serves no comic purpose. As such, the history of foolishness and its link to intellectual disability is more diverse in the Middle Ages than suggested by the early modern discourse of folly serving a comical and didactic purpose.

Notes

1   Original text: 'Etleich habent daz von geburt und etleich habent das von gewonhait.' Konrad von Megenberg, *Buch der Natur* [c.1349–50], edited by Robert Luff and George Steer (Tübingen: Max Niemeyer Verlag, 2003), 524.
2   Original text: 'So zů nutz / heilsamer ler / ermanung / vnd ervolgung / der / wißheit / vernunfft / vnd gůter sytten / Ouch zů verachtung / vnd straff der narrheyt / blindheit / Irrsal vnd dorheit / allerstadt / vnd geschlecht / der menschen /

mit besunderm fliß / mueg / vnd / arbet / gesamlet ist / durch Sebastianum Brant.'
Sebastian Brant, *Das Narrenschiff* (Tübingen: Max Niemeyer Verlag, 1986), 3.

3 Stainton, 'Reason's Other: The Emergence of the Disabled Subject in the Northern
   Renaissance', *Disability and Society* 19.3 (2004), 241.

4 Ibid., 241.

5 Hilkert Weddige, *Mittelhochdeutsch* (München: Beck, 2001), 7.

6 Jan-Dirk Müller, *Höfische Kompromisse. Acht Kapitel zur höfischen Epik* (Tübingen:
   Max Niemeyer, 2007), 9–17.

7 Lennard Davis, 'Constructing Normalcy: The Bell Curve, the Novel and the
   Invention of the Disabled Body in the Nineteenth Century', in *Disability Studies
   Reader*, 2nd edn, edited by Lennard J. Davis (New York: Routledge, 2006), 3–16;
   Susan Wendell, *The Rejected Body: Feminist Philosophical Reflections on Disability*
   (New York: Psychology Press, 1996), 35–56.

8 C. F. Goodey, 'What is Developmental Disability? The Origin and Nature of Our
   Conceptual Models', *Journal on Developmental Disabilities* 8.2 (2001), 4 and 8;
   Patrick McDonagh and Tim Stainton, 'Editorial: Chasing Shadows: The Historical
   Construction of Developmental Disability', *Journal on Developmental Disabilities*
   8.2 (2001), ix.

9 C. F. Goodey, *A History of Intelligence and 'Intellectual Disability': The Shaping of
   Psychology in Early Modern Europe* (Farnham and Burlington VT: Ashgate, 2011),
   1.

10 Wendell, *The Rejected Body*, 66.

11 Lucy Perry and Alexander Schwarz, 'Introduction', in *Behaving Like Fools: Voice,
   Gesture, and Laughter in Texts, Manuscripts, and Early Books*, edited by Lucy Perry
   and Alexander Schwarz (Turnhout: Brepols, 2010), 2.

12 Ruth von Bernuth, 'Aus den Wunderkammern in die Irrenanstalten – Natürliche
   Hofnarren in Mittelalter und früher Neuzeit', in *Kulturwissenschaftliche Perspektive
   der Disability Studies*, edited by Anne Waldschmidt (Kassel: Bifos, 2003).

13 See Heinrich von Freiberg's *Tristan: der willetôre Tristan* [c.1290], edited by Karl
   Bartsch (Amsterdam: RODOPI, 1966, v. 5192).

14 Patrick McDonagh, *Idiocy: A Cultural History* (Liverpool: Liverpool University
   Press, 2008), 142 and 146–149.

15 Ulrike Spyra, *Das 'Buch der Natur' Konrads von Megenberg. Die illustrierten
   Handschriften und Inkunablen* (Köln: Böhlau Verlag, 2005), 3.

16 Werner Chrobak, 'Die Schriften Konrads von Megenberg', in *Konrad von
   Megenberg. Regensburger Domherr, Dompfarrer und Gelehrter (1309–1374) zum
   700. Geburtstag. Ausstellung in der Bischöflichen Zentralbibliothek Regensburg 27.
   August bis 25. September 2009*, edited by Paul Mai (Regensburg: Schnell & Steiner,
   2009), 58.

17 Original text: 'So schrieb auch Konrad von Megenberg kein Buch der Natur,
   sondern einen Liber de natura rerum, ein puoch von der eigenchait der ding,
   mit dessen Hilfe erst der Sinngehalt der Naturdinge und ihre unterschiedlichen
   Bedeutungen innerhalb der mittelalterlichen Typologie klar werden sollten. An

die Beschreibung der Kreaturen schließen sich häufig moralisch-allegorische.' Interpretationen an. Spyra, *Das 'Buch der Natur' Konrads von Megenberg*, 5.

18 Konrad von Megenberg, *Buch der Natur* [c.1349–50], edited by Robert Luff and George Steer (Tübingen: Max Niemeyer Verlag, 2003), 522.

19 Ibid., 523.

20 Burkhard Mojsisch, 'Seele', in *Lexikon des Mittelalters 7* (Darmstadt: Brepols, 2000), 1675–1677.

21 Burkhard Mojsisch et al., 'Seele', in *Historisches Wörterbuch der Philosophie*, edited by Joachim Ritter et al. (Darmstadt: Schwabe Verlag, 1995), 13. Aristotle differentiates between essential and accidental properties of everything. For example, a stone wall has the essential property of stone but its colour is accidental, since the colour changing would not change the wall by itself.

22 Mojsisch, 'Seele', 1675–1677.

23 Ibid.

24 Original text: 'Also trag ich ein puoch / von latein in dauetscheu wort / daz hat Albertus maisterleich gesamnet von den alten.' Konrad von Megenberg, *Buch der Natur*, 26.

25 Matthias Lexer, *Mittelhochdeutsches Handwörterbuch. Erster Band A–M* (Stuttgart: Hirzel, 1979), 760.

26 Original text: 'Etleich habent daz von geburt und etleich habent das von gewonhait.' Konrad von Megenberg, *Buch der Natur*, 524.

27 Original text: 'Di den geprechen habent von gepurt, das sint di naturleichen torn, [...] die habent ir cell der sel chreft niht recht geschicht in dem haubt.' Ibid.

28 Nikolaus Haase, 'Das Lehrstück von den vier Intellekten in der Scholastik: von den arabischen Quellen bis zu Albertus Magnus', *Recherches de Théologie et Philosophie Médiévales* 66 (1999), 21.

29 Armin Schulz, *Erzähltheorie in mediävistischer Perspektive*, edited by Manuel Braun, Alexandra Dunkel, and Jan-Dirk Müller (Berlin: De Gruyter 2012), 39.

30 Rolf Schönberger, 'Rationale Spontanität. Die Theorie des Willes bei Albertus Magnus', in *Albertus Magnus. Zum Gedenken nach 800 Jahren: Neue Zugänge, Aspekte und Perspektiven*, edited by Walter Senner et al. (Berlin: Akademie Verlag 2001), 229.

31 Original text: 'Daz prueft man dar an, daz si ungeschickteu haubt habent, aintweder ze groz oder ze clain.' Konrad von Megenberg, *Buch der Natur*, 524.

32 Original text: 'Di wuorkent nicht nach den werchen menschleicher sel und habent doch menschen sel sam di chint.' Ibid.

33 Joachim Bumke, *Blutstropfen im Schnee. Über Wahrnehmung und Erkenntnis im 'Parzival' Wolframs von Eschenbach* (Tübingen: Niemeyer, 2001), 78; Michael Goodich, *From Birth to Old Age: The Human Life Cycle in Medieval Thought, 1250–1350* (Lanham: University Press of America 1989), 85ff.

34 Original text: 'Di aber den geprechen habent von gewonhait, das sint di in den waelden erzogen warden, verr von den vernunftigen laeuten, und lebent sam daz vih.' Konrad von Megenberg, *Buch der Natur*, 524.

35   See, for example, the tradition of the Tristan stories as well.

36   Older studies mention Konrad von Würzburg as the author of 'Die Halbe Birne', but there is no conclusive proof of his authorship. See Klaus Grubmüller, 'Kommentar', *Novellistik des Mittelalters* (Frankfurt a.m.: Bibliothek des Mittelalters, 2011), 1084.

37   The narrator explains that Arnold is invited 'durch sînen manlichen muot' [because of his knightly attitude]. 'Die Halbe Birne', in *Novellistik des Mittelalters. Märendichtung*, edited by Klaus Grubmüller (Frankfurt a.m.: Bibliothek des Mittelalters, 2011), V. 68.

38   Arnold is described as acting 'nach gebiureschlîcher art' [in a discourteous fashion] ('Die Halbe Birne' V. 86).

39   Stephen L. Wailes, 'Konrad of Würzburg and Pseudo-Konrad: Varieties of Humour in the "Märe"', *The Modern Language Review* 69.1 (1974), 114.

40   Original text: 'si enbran als ein zunder / von der angesihte, / daz dem tumben wihte / der elfte vinger was ersworn.' 'Die Halbe Birne' V. 286–289.

41   Original text: 'der tore, der uns hât betrogen, / daz was der ritter wolgezogen.' Ibid., V. 458f.

42   Original text: 'beide liute unde lant / wart im untertænic.' Ibid., V. 479f.

43   See William McDonald, 'The Fool-Stick: Concerning Tristan's Club in the German Eilhart-Tradition', *Euphorion* 82 (1988), 127–149.

44   Original text: 'daz hâr wart im abe gesniten / nach tœrlîchen siten, / und gekleidet als ein tôr. / er wart geswerzet als ein môr. / daz kleit im an dem knie erwant. / einen kolben nam er in die hant, / dâ mite huop er sich von dan. / beide wîp unde man / ersâhen in für einen gief.' 'Die Halbe Birne', V. 177–183.

45   Wailes, 'Konrad of Würzburg and Pseudo-Konrad', 114.

46   Original text: '[Durch die] Figur des (angeblichen) Narren: schwachsinnig, taub-stumm, schmutzig, zerlumpt, hässlich, brutal, negiert er Punkt für Punkt die Werte, auf denen das höfische Selbstverständnis beruht.' Jan-Dirk Müller, 'Die hovezuht und ihr Preis. Zum Problem höfischer Verhaltensregulierung in PS-Konrads "Halber Birne"', in *Mediävistische Kulturwissenschaften*, edited by Jan-Dirk Müller (Berlin: Schwabe Verlag, 2010), 212.

47   Joachim Bumke, 'Wolfram von Eschenbach', in *Die deutsche Literatur des Mittelalters. Verfasserlexikon Band 10*, edited by Burkhart Wachinger et al. (Berlin: De Gruyter, 1999), 1378.

48   Bumke, *Blutstropfen im Schnee*, 77. The narrator tells us that Parzival was 'küne-clîche vuore betrogen' [cheated out of his royal education] and later Parzival has to ask 'what is God?': 'ôwê muoter, waz ist got?' (Wolfram von Eschenbach, *Parzival*, 2 vols., edited by Karl Lachmann (Stuttgart: Reclam, 1981), 118, 2 and 119, 17.

49   Original text: 'do gedâhte mêr diu künegîn / der liute vil bî spotte sint. / tôren cleider sol mîn kint / ob sîme liehten lîbe tragen. / wirt er geroufet unt geslagen, / sô kumt er mir her wider wol.' Wolfram, *Parzival*, 126, 24–29.

50   Original text: 'Parzivâl der tumbe.' Wolfram, *Parzival* V. 155, 19.

51 David T. Mitchell and Sharon L. Snyder, *Narrative Prosthesis: Disability and the Dependencies of Discourse* (Ann Arbor: University of Michigan Press, 2000), 47.

52 David T. Mitchell and Sharon L. Snyder, 'Introduction: Disability Studies and the Double Bind of Representation', in *The Body and Physical Difference: Discourses of Disability*, edited by Mitchell and Snyder (Ann Arbor: University of Michigan Press, 1997), 13.

53 McDonagh, *Idiocy*, 16.

54 Bumke, *Blutstropfen im Schnee*, 83.

55 Ibid., 103.

56 Original text: 'der werde Gurnamanz / von sîner tumpheit geschiet.' Wolfram, *Parzival*, 188, 16f.

57 Original text: 'dô sprach er 'hêrre, ichn bin niht wîs.' Ibid., 178, 29.

58 However, other scholars argue this point: see, for instance, Thomas Strässle, *Vom Unverstand zum Verstand durchs Feuer. Studien zu Grimmelshausens 'Simplicissimus Teutsch'* (Bern: Peter Lang, 2001), 383.

59 Bumke, *Blutstropfen im Schnee*, 87.

60 Ibid., 101.

61 Original text: 'er [Parzival] küene, traeclîche wîs.' Wolfram, *Parzival*, 4, 18.

62 Original text: 'Die Parzivalhandlung zeigt keinen Weg zur Weisheit. Es ist der tumbe Parzival, der von Gott zu Gral berufen wird, nicht der wîse. Parzivals tumpheit ist kein zu überwindender Makel, sondern sein Habitus.' Bumke, *Blutstropfen im Schnee*, 105.

63 Ibid., 108.

64 Grubmüller, 'Kommentar', 1221.

65 Original text: 'Ein kleinez kint wart gegeben / zu einem münch in ein reinez leben. / im waz diu werlt unbekant. / do wart ez anderswa gesant / zu einem kloster in einen walt.' 'Des Mönches Not' [c.1290], in *Novellistik des Mittelalters. Märendichtung*, edited by Klaus Grubmüller (Frankfurt a. M.: Bibliothek des Mittelalters, 2011), V. 9–13.

66 Ibid., V. 145.

67 Original text: '"daz wil ich rehte sagen", / sprach der kneht; "der under leit"'. Ibid., V. 262f.

68 Original text: 'nu bin ich armer under gelegen, / nu wirt ein kint von mir geborn. / so hab ich min ere gar verlorn.' Ibid., V. 268–270.

69 Original text: 'si hetten des alle gesworn, / daz er unsinnic wære.' Ibid., V. 508f.

70 Original text: 'du solt gen zu kore / singen unde lesen / und solt ein gut kint wesen.' Ibid., V. 532–535.

71 André Schnyer, '"Des Mönches Not" Mit Michel Foucault neu gelesen', *Wirkendes Wort* 37 (1987), 271.

5

EXCLUSION FROM THE EUCHARIST: THE RE-SHAPING OF IDIOCY IN THE SEVENTEENTH-CENTURY CHURCH

C. F. Goodey

Under the microscope of history of ideas, we can observe concepts of 'intellectual disability' by this or any other name being born, forming, re-forming, and completely metamorphosing. It is thus a historical and a cultural category. As such it contrasts with the underlying, seemingly cross-cultural persistence of the pathology that has given rise to such concepts over the centuries. Currently known to psychiatry as specific phobia, it occurs in individuals but also expresses itself socially, often as a fear of contamination.[1] Key works in anthropology, psychiatry, sociology, and psychology have built influential theories of social out-group formation more or less explicitly around this phobia. Its importance is evident not only because of their authors' well-known and seminal influence in their own disciplines, but because it transcends the range of those disciplines and emanates moreover from an equally disparate range of approaches: conservative and marxist, visionary and commonsense.[2] It must be said that none of them uses intellectual disability to illustrate their theories. Nevertheless, the highly specific case I analyse below – the radical creation of a particular type of idiocy – fits just such a framework.

In its acutest social form, a paranoid anxiety is projected on to the categorisation of some particular group supposed to be only quasi-human and thereby not just unequal, not just untouchable, but requiring physical elimination. And while the phobia itself seems to remain a historical constant, the essential characteristics of the 'extreme', albeit notional out-group undergo an almost one hundred percent blood transfusion from one era to the next. The mind sciences, once the preserve of theology, are implicated in this. The same scientific psychiatry that might see its ancestors' categorisation and elimination of twelfth-century heretics as a phobic reinforcement of the era's religious dogmas is also responsible for the categorisation and elimination of twenty-first century 'intellectual' disability as a reinforcement of our own era's cognitive dogmas.

Psychology and the formalisation of gossip

Whatever the shifting nature of the out-groups thus projected, 'intellectual' or otherwise, a core symptom of the phobic disorder in its social form is its obsession (suggested particularly by Gabel) with the formal, codified assessment of human types.

One example of this from the early modern period, specifically the mid-seventeenth century, is the diagnostic manuals which priests used to assess the understanding and hence the possible religious status of the individuals in their flocks. These were among the direct precursors of a modern science of the mind.

Throughout the English revolution of the mid-seventeenth century, churchmen disagreed about whom to exclude from taking holy communion, who should do the excluding, and how this exclusion was to be practised. The dispute had kept resurfacing from the early church fathers onwards, but this was a key moment which, more than any other, determined the eventual course of English Puritanism.[3] The constant reclassifications of potential contaminants of church ritual – hypocrites, the unregenerate, the lustful, drunk or willfully ignorant, the merely uneducated, children, the 'distracted' and the mad – fluctuated in tandem with larger socio-political processes. The ferocity of the debate in the 1650s reflects that decade's social revolutionary chaos. Near the end of it, the label 'idiot' – whatever that may mean – arrives on the list. It emerges from a dialectic of disputes which acknowledge the socio-political context, even if they do not directly match its competing ideologies. In that particular deployment of the label we start to see an outline of the modern psychological definition into which we have talked ourselves.

The psychology of intelligence and the emotions is a formalisation of gossip. As human beings continually group and regroup and, in so doing, observe each other, the behaviour of one group is first whispered about by others, then recorded, then classified, then becomes a matter of social anxiety, public policy, and professional authority, and finally, in the modern era, of science. What started off raising an eyebrow ends up, for a group that has achieved dominance, as a pathological fact of nature. So we must first ask what phobic classificatory urges would have formed the gossip of the mid-seventeenth-century social and religious elite, of the pastor or magistrate (often the same person) who had power to formulate judgements on the outward and inward states of others.

What did words like 'nature' and 'intellect' evoke for this elite? Rather than seeing people's inner states in terms of nature versus nurture, they would have grown up with a three-way doctrine: nature, nurture, and necessity. Determinism lay not in nature but in God's necessary preordination of people's status. In social terms this meant high or lowly. In terms of (Calvinist) religion it meant elect or reprobate: God had chosen the elect pre-natally for salvation, the reprobate for damnation. 'Nature', by contrast, standing in the middle, was dispositional: a deep but acquired habit. It also meant fleshly corruption: 'natural man'. On the medieval 'ladder of nature', reason was not specifically human but part-overlapped with the divine intellect, to which humans could only aspire. The *merely* human bit of it was mundane and, like nature itself, corrupting: a hindrance to faith.

Elements of modern intellectual disability's 'cognitive' profile, particularly the inability to abstract or generalize, reason logically, process information or maintain attention, are recognisable from late medieval texts onwards. However, they characterized lower social classes, and in a sense all females: that is, the majority. No analogy was being drawn here between these large groups and some small, separate 'intellectually disabled' group as we now define it, since none such was yet conceptualized beyond the legal sphere of property inheritance (and then somewhat hazily).[4] The same goes for the terminology. 'Idiot' could describe the labourers on the magistrate's estate and possibly his own womenfolk. Every pastor possessed a Vulgate (Latin) Bible describing the disciples, without irony, as *idiotae* – 'laymen', by contrast with the church's learned *doctores*; in the early medieval church, the word indicated a novitiate on his way to ordination.

True, there were also 'natural fools'. 'Natural' meant they were born that way. But they were not incurable; the idea of lifelong intellectual disability was not yet available, because 'natural' conditions were not 'necessary' in the sense of preordained. They could be cured by divine providence. For the most part, natural foolishness, for which the criteria scarcely resemble modern ones, was simply the organic aspect of some bodily disposition such as imbalance of the humours; their 'rational soul' had been infused by God and thus could hold no imperfection.

Contamination and communion

Something like this mind-set, by now somewhat fragmented, was still in place on the eve of the mid-century debate about 'free' (open) admission to the eucharist that was triggered by a 1651 book of sermons. Typically for religious publishing, it went through three editions within a few months, with published responses to it coming rapidly, like a blog. Its author, John Humfrey, ordained in the Presbyterian church with its largely Calvinist doctrine, nevertheless disliked its practice of continuously assessing and barring from holy communion people it deemed ignorant or lacking grace. Like his friend, the hugely influential Richard Baxter, he thought that interrogating people on their catechism should be voluntary: he advocated freedom *to* receive eucharist but also *from* formal examination by church elders. No one, not even the pastor, could really know the heart of a 'true believer', only God. Humfrey's stricter Presbyterian opponents objected that free admission would 'take away the use of the keys ... and leave us no discipline in the church'. But, says Humfrey, these opponents work the keys 'in so far, that being unable to work them out again ... they have both shut out the sacrament from the church and the church from the sacrament'.[5] In short, to assume the right to exclude people is not only hubristic, it also damages the church as an institution.

Humfrey does make exceptions. In addition to those already excommunicate, children and madpeople ('the distracted') should be kept away. Many Protestant congregants were perceived as 'deficient' in their understanding of the ritual of bread and wine, especially as they had to work out its metaphorical significance (by contrast with Catholics who accepted transubstantiation as an act of faith). Catechisms correspondingly tended to demand proper thought-out answers. However, this should not prevent people participating. Their deficiency was the sign of an internal (and thus indiscernible) 'unworthiness', which was in turn an indicator of the 'obliquity' of 'natural man' that affects everyone else too. He does not discriminate between those lacking understanding and those possessing it. The one justifiable exclusion is if 'the *outward* work itself be amiss' (my emphasis). Lack of 'Christian deportment at the table' was presupposed in children and small numbers of distracted, mad adults.[6] Such behaviour was obvious, so their exclusion needed no formal assessment.

The theological question – whether outward behaviour might be a proven sign of people's inner elect or reprobate status or whether that is a secret known only to God – was also a political one. Presbyterians anxious about the presence of reprobates corrupting the purity of ritual genuinely thought they could guess people's inner religious identity; but they were equally anxious about the usurpation of their own powers by others among the social elite (known as 'Erastians') who sought to put the church under state control. However, in 1649 the state was in dire jeopardy. Not just the monarch but the Church of England had gone to the executioner's block. What was to replace it: a wary religious pluralism – Cromwell's existing policy – or a uniform church administration? The Presbyterians, hoping for the latter, sought to replace Charles at its head. In asserting their right to assess sane adult congregants, and ban some of them, they were pursuing ecclesiastical authority as well as social order, an order that could be re-established only if they themselves were in charge.

Humfrey's initial text was prompted by scepticism about these grandiose pretensions. He claimed that his policy of free admission was a superior, less coercive variant of orthodox Presbyterian discipline. He presented himself as defending a uniform church against the Cromwellian Independents' view that admission to communion was for each individual congregation to decide by itself. Presbyterian practices of formal assessment might drive the excluded into separate doctrinal groupings ('even as in the peeling of an onion'[7]), thus undermining authority; as Locke pointed out some years later when justifying religious tolerance, one had to be cautious about laying down the law to communicants whom political events had liberated into a newfound confidence in their own faith. Humfrey, the orthodox Presbyterians, and the Independents all had a common goal: the post-revolutionary unification of religious and political authority, and hence the preservation of religion, gentry, and tithes. What they were split about was how to cure splits.

It was from the debates following publication of Humfrey's text that more precisely defined 'idiots' would eventually emerge. As we shall see, by the time of his *Second Vindication* in 1656, the list of exclusions now did contain this category. And he would end up drawing a precise distinction not only (a) between idiots and children/madpeople, but also (b) between idiocy and the intellectual defiencies of the general population. What exactly 'idiots' meant is another matter, but for the moment let us note that they will contribute to the modern definition.

Rationales for exclusion

The first opposition to Humfrey came from orthodox Presbyterian Roger Drake. Both Humfrey and Drake stand on the verge of that momentous shift across late seventeenth-century doctrines, Protestant and Catholic alike, over the place of reason in religion. A positive and specifically human reason, no longer corrupted automatically by the flesh, starts to be inserted within the substructure of a person's faith, thus starting to influence what defines an 'idiot'. Drake, while claiming that scripture is against Humfrey (on the one hand it forbids us 'to admit all pell mell', on the other hand it does not 'forbid children and distracted persons'), disingenuously concedes to his opponent's intellectually oriented stance.[8] He will advance his own case not 'scripturally', as he normally ought, but 'with reason', engaging with Humfrey's philosophical contradictions, slippery-slope arguments, and absurd consequences.

The contradiction is as follows. If, as Humfrey claims, the communicant's inner state cannot be discerned, there is no reason to exclude children and mad, distracted people. They may sometimes 'by their ... unseemly gestures ... prove troublesome to the congregation', but not always. So how can Humfrey say they are incapable 'by nature'? What is this nature? Humfrey appears to say that children and madpeople suffer from some discrete condition over and above the general corruptions of 'natural man'. He *is*, therefore, implicitly claiming to know about their internal states. And since the idea of internal states covers reprobates, who commune and receive in secret hypocrisy and thereby contaminate the sacraments, Humfrey should be trying to screen these out too. Moreover, even if, as he says, we do not know who is regenerate, 'Who knows how God may work at the Word, though not by the Word?' Eucharistic rite may require the recipient to understand the Word as an 'active instrument' of conversion, but the Word may also be its 'passive occasion', working by sheer providence. In that case it may be effective for anyone, even for children and madpeople – or indeed for 'innocents'.

Humfrey's slippery slope argument is that infants can receive baptism but not the eucharist. Since that is 'because they cannot examine themselves ... , then I answer: no more can grossly [generally] ignorant persons, who therefore ... upon Mr Humfrey's principles ... must be kept away'. These, a majority, may easily be taught to parrot outward professions of faith, no less than 'a child of three years old or a madman'. Drake challenges Humfrey to find a clear distinction between this type of deficiency and the sheer 'uncapability' he sees in children and madpeople. Drake agrees that 'outward profession is ... the ultimate reason of admission', but it has to be 'accompanied with suitable knowledge and conversation', and the latter requires pastoral assessment: a 'verbal' profession as opposed to an assumed or 'virtual' one. People 'cannot ... be discerned unless tried'. Humfrey is condoning the laxity of the old church regime 'if ... he think their very coming ... be sufficient'. He might find himself giving communion to 'brutes and swine', plague victims, the 'stark staring drunk', and complete strangers displaced by the social upheavals, who may well be excommunicate.[9]

Humfrey's absurd consequence, finally, is that in practice he might exclude more people than a strict Presbyterian would. First, says Drake, a madman may be 'better many times than sundry of those for whom he opens the door', since many of the latter may be hypocritical fakers. Secondly, 'all grossly ignorant persons ... need instruction. And is not this previous trial before the eldership used of purpose, that ignorant persons might be put upon enquiry after knowledge?' Hence Drake's strict assessments may 'permit a freer admission than Mr Humfrey', because they are educational. 'Nor is the proper end

... exclusion from, but preparation of all sorts [of people] for the sacrament for which in a few months (by God's grace) we dare undertake to fit the meanest'.[10]

This 'few months' is key to the debate: a practical deadline. The task is to prepare *all* the generally ignorant, *especially* the meanest of them, for the expected rule of the saints. This quasi-millenarian hope was shared at some level by Humfrey as well as Drake (and Cromwell). They were simply at odds over how to prepare. What kinds of people would hinder its arrival? For Drake the 'willfully' ignorant are the obstacle. They 'are much more uncapable' than the generally ignorant but educable, or children and madpeople whom providence may suddenly grant an understanding.[11] Assessment should allow for 'children, distracted and excommunicated persons [to] attend the sacrament' but not actually receive it till they become as 'capable as persons visibly worthy'. This is 'positive suspension', contrasting with Humfrey's merely 'negative suspension (which is a bare non-admission)'. Lifting their suspension will then depend on their ability to provide 'evidence' of their receptivity to grace, through 'trials and attempts at edification'.[12]

Humfrey's choice of children and madpeople as his exclusions diverts attention from the real, dangerous polluters of sacred ritual: reprobate hypocrites, who conceal their willful ignorance. Drake likens Humfrey simultaneously to a reactionary Papist and a radical democrat or Leveller. In the first respect, free admission 'lays the axe to the root of Reformation', leading to 'a chaos of darkness and ignorance'. Decoded, this means he is an 'Arminian', following the quasi-Romanist ecclesiastical policies of Charles I and his Archbishop, William Laud. True, these men's heads had recently been removed. However, the papal Antichrist might easily grow new heads on new bodies. It was the policy of openness in Laud's Church of England that had let in amongst the godly a 'sinful mixture' of reprobates and recusants. Drake is warning against a return to the old regime. But in the second respect he is also warning against letting the revolution run too far: Humfrey's open admission policy was 'mere church-levelling', which 'lays all common' – therefore 'the more careful had we need be of our property and enclosures'.[13] As for most writers in this dispute, the uppity labourer and the reprobate are two faces, one social, the other religious, of a single social contaminant, threatening in-group and hierarchical rule.

A natural disability of the intellect

Charles I's 1649 execution replaced an unchallengeable fount of authority with a chasm. Some of Cromwell's colleagues proposed filling it with a republican, semi-democratic written formula. But Cromwell banked on another kind of 'election' instead: political rule by God's elect, to prepare for the kingdom of heaven on earth. In July 1653, not long after the first exchange between Humfrey and Drake, he had a new parliament appointed to enact this. The collapse of the Barebones Parliament or Parliament of Saints (as it was variously known) after a mere six months – the saints found it hard to agree on anything, let alone be moderately pleasant to each other – marked the end of that policy, by which time the moment for a constitutional solution had passed too. Cromwell was now cornered into a quasi-monarchical role. With hindsight, restoration of the monarchy was from this point inevitable. Religious optimism receded in step with political downturn. While the kingdom of the saints remained inevitable, its postponement gave more time for preparing the mass of congregants with the appropriate frame of mind and behaviour, and also for greater awareness of the size of that task.

Against this political background, in 1654, Humfrey replied to Drake. Humfrey's *Rejoynder* deals with Drake's obsessive attacks on his own initially casual remark about reason being temporarily absent in children and madpeople. Answering the charge that if one cannot know an inner condition like reprobation, then nor can one know the inner incapability of children and madpeople, Humfrey replies,

> I explain [that children and madpeople] *are uncapable* in the first sense, in saying, *by nature*, and, *that can discern no meaning* [in the eucharist] ..., which I do clearly to distinguish infants, the distracted and natural fools from the barely ignorant of age, who are capable to learn ... First, because this very discerning cannot be the duty of the former, who are *naturally* uncapable ... And secondly, because signs cannot work upon the unintelligent (which they wholly are) to receive any *real* effect by them.[14] (emphasis in original)

Humfrey had not mentioned natural fools in his first text. Their arrival here, perhaps picking up on Drake's stray reference to 'innocents' above, helps support Humfrey's argument that children and madpeople are incapable 'by nature'. Natural fools seem an even firmer example of the same type.

We must beware of hindsight, however. The 'nature' of these fools was not deterministic like our modern, genetic 'nature', nor inevitably lifelong. True, Humfrey sounds sceptical about providential cure. Drake, he says with irony, 'speaks miraculously well' of what the deaf (and, implicitly, fools, among whom the deaf were often still numbered) might gain from a passive, unhearing receipt of the Word. Nevertheless, if fools are incapable by nature of understanding eucharistic ritual, the 'nature' in their case is still the softer-edged early seventeenth-century concept. Sixteenth- and seventeenth-century determinism ('necessity') was divine, the cause of election and reprobation and categorically *not* a cause of human ability or disability.

Nevertheless, Drake's attack forced Humfrey into highlighting the role of active understanding in grasping the metaphorical character of the eucharist (by contrast with the idolatrous belief in transubstantiation). This began to suggest that human nature may have some neutral intellectual aspect free from the corrupting 'natural man'. By 1654 Humfrey would have encountered the theory of a permanent 'natural disability of the intellect', devised by the French Protestant Moise Amyraut in the 1640s and endorsed by Baxter. This would become the thin end of the wedge for an entirely new way of classifying human types.[15] Its novelty was the clear separation of intellectual disability from failures of the will; it excused people in the former case from fulfilling their covenant with God. In a shocking reversal of accepted psychological causality, Amyraut and Baxter posit a type of people who *will* not because they *cannot*. Most church leaders of a Calvinist persuasion resisted this separation, because it seemed to imply (a) space for a positive natural intellectual *ability* as well as disability, and similarly uncorrupt and free from religious obligation; and (b) a primordial distinction between intellectually able and disabled which might subvert that between elect and reprobate. If such creatures existed, naturally and permanently lacking reason, their place in the hierarchical scale of nature would surely have to be reclassified as non-human. Orthodox opponents offered this argument as a *reductio ad absurdum*, but we shall see how Humfrey started to take the possibility seriously.

He corresponded at this point with Baxter.[16] How should he respond to Drake? Baxter simply advised Humfrey against admitting known scandalizers to communion; his own book on the right to the sacraments, two years later, does not mention idiots or fools.[17] But we know that Baxter agreed with Amyraut on the possibility of a natural, incurable intellectual disability.[18] This concept somehow pushed children and the mad closer to the intellectually able; though 'unintelligent' (Humfrey's phrase), they have a potential ability to understand eucharistic symbolism at some point in their lives. It merely fails to operate during their childhood or distractedness. This now *contrasts* them with fools, since the latter, without providence, will *never* be able. Humfrey broaches this hypothesis just once in the *Rejoynder*, when he says that eucharist is for everyone, 'let members of a church be never so grossly ignorant (and not idiots)' – his first use of the latter term in this dispute.[19]

Discerning Christ's body in the bread and wine by analogy requires what Humfrey calls 'intelligence'. In theology, *intelligentia* was the actualisation of *intellectus* within the individual. Protestants promoted it as favouring a narrative understanding of the Word, over the idolatrous adoration of images and the 'darkness and ignorance' of Romanist transubstantiation. Free admission evoked the old, quasi-Catholic state church, which had elided the elect-reprobate division in favour of perseverance (and obedience) for all. Humfrey accuses Drake of advancing a divine-right claim of his own: 'A power of discriminating the guests ... is a power ... even over God's ordinance'. And 'when a power must be established, clothed with a divine right ... [it is] no wonder if tender Christians ... rise up for their precious liberty', as they had done a decade earlier.[20] Drake, not he, was risking a return to chaos.

In arguing over natural categories of intelligence and unintelligence, the disputants to begin with had been indulging in a rhetorical and trivial diversion, both sides still believing the essential demarcation to be that between God's elect and the reprobate. Within a few decades a whole new social order would begin to be built on the foundations of just such trivia. They helped launch the historical process whereby the impending religious utopia of rule by a saintly elect would become today's meritocratic utopia of rule by rational exam-passers (the difference between the two being not so great in the long historical view).

Who is truly human?

Meanwhile, others joined in. Humfrey was supported by John Timson, himself a labouring *idiota* fallen among *doctores* (he was 'a husbandman, who ... follows the plough all day and studies [contemplates] and then writes down his thoughts and reads at night').[21] Although one's own means, says Timson, are 'ordinarily successful' to benefit from the eucharist, they are not sufficient; one needs the additional element of grace, which is only 'given according to ... God's own will'.[22] So far, so conventionally Calvinist. However, 'means' here no longer signifies, as it had done for early Calvinists, the individual's passive ability to receive a faith unilaterally implanted by God. Faith now consists of certain 'abilities' which 'all men stand bound to employ'. And it is the reasoning element among them that dominates, because it is something the pastor can directly observe and assess. These abilities, merging mundane 'natural graces' with God-given, divine grace, together comprise what he calls 'intelligence'. One needs reason, not just sober deportment, at the altar rail: 'and this I think is [not] Pelagianism, but the tenor and scope of the covenant of grace to man'. The pastor did not ask himself, does this person have the intellectual ability to examine his conscience or understand the analogy in the bread and wine, and leave it at that. Such would indeed have been a 'Pelagian' style of assessment, i.e. it would have assumed, heretically, that the communicant could achieve grace purely by his own means. What the pastor wanted to know was: would the communicant *by-pass* his intellect? People who did that might swerve into an idolatrous belief in transubstantiation. And that, not mere *absence* of intellect in a modern sense, is what would have defined them as foolish.

In support of Drake, John Collinges responded to both Timson and Humfrey. He accuses the latter of an Erastian desire to put 'the government of the church ... into the hands of the civil magistrate'. This tarred Humfrey with the late monarchist regime, whose policy this had been too.[23] Humfrey and Timson heretically posit a 'mere natural capacity to exercise reason', a morally neutral intellectual nature, as the basis of 'full right to the sacrament'. Just as Drake's passing gibes about infants and madpeople expanded into a central point of debate, so Collinges adopts a playful rhetoric about natural species and the scale of nature – who is truly human? – that will eventually seep into the core of the dispute. It is 'incumbent upon the officers of the church to keep the fellowship of the church pure' from pollution. It is no good being against pastoral assessment in the name of being humble, before an impenetrable God. Surely there must be *some* people disqualified from attendance. (As the long history of contamination phobia shows us, a category of the excluded exists *a priori*, before one has decided on the actual characteristics of the group that is to fill the slot.) All who are 'not visible church members' – unknown people turning up for the first time, those already known as ungodly, or refusing instruction – are 'dogs and swine'. If Humfrey will admit anybody without due edification, says Collinges, including people 'appearing notoriously unfit for it and unable to it', and still insist that it 'is a pure communion, he hath proved that ... a communion made up of a saint, a hog, a dog, a madman and a fool is a pure communion'.[24] Animal insults were a normal part of many sermons, but in these years the language of natural kinds was becoming more than just rhetoric and was starting to be used to challenge the real species membership of certain human-looking creatures on intellectual grounds; hints are there in Baxter, in the political Leveller Richard Overton, and certainly in Locke's founding text of modern psychology, *An Essay Concerning Human Understanding*.

Species difference, says Collinges, consists in the inability to hear or obey 'reproofs'. That is why some people are like animals. Assessment is possible because, however limited the merely human capacities of the elders doing the examining, those capacities are attuned to the congregant's *moral* inner nature, to which his intellectual inner nature is subordinate:

> Suppose one had committed incest ... immediately before a sacrament; such a wretch may be in a capacity to exercise reason, yet surely Mr Timson hath large principles if he thinks such wretches have a plenary right ... Something besides church membership must be added to give one a plenary right to the sacrament;

or else infants and distracted persons must have a plenary right. And something besides an ability to exercise reason.[25]

Collinges does occasionally recall the original, common aim behind the diversionary rhetoric: 'And for the point of examination (so much boggled at), it is only in order to the settling of our churches', in other words, to ensure the unity of the church as it prepares for godly rule and the second coming.[26] But he is sidetracked by dogs and swine as much as Drake had been by infants and madpeople. These digressions would soon put down firm roots, helping to establish a modern 'idiot' type that occupies a distinct, abnormal biological niche and is therefore implicitly non-human.

Human nature, human reason, natural intelligence

Collinges, like Drake, thought the pastor should deny admission to those whose assessment revealed their moral unfitness – a sign they were not regenerate at that point and might never be. Humfrey and Timson said the sacrament should be withheld only because of inappropriate outward behaviour in church, which said nothing about elect or reprobate status. They had, so far, solved the contradiction between their policy of free admission and their exclusion of madpeople by identifying a 'natural reason' from which madpeople and children were disabled, and by separating this disability from the reprobate's (unknowable) inability to respond to God-given grace. Humfrey had not in fact (as Collinges tried to suggest) claimed also that natural intellectual ability should be the basis for rights – a truly modern thought. Timson, however, is pushed forward under his own momentum, by the cut-and-thrust of debate. He reaches for a more definite basis on which to categorize people: the law. Infants and madpeople, he says, are barred from eucharist because of 'their *natural and rational* incapacity actually to enjoy their right' to it (my emphasis).[27]

In a subsequent text, he adds that one must distinguish between 'a real right in point of title, and a right of actual [active] ... enjoyment'. A minor, for example, inherits but does not manage his dead father's estate.[28] Before the early modern period the concept of rights was not categorically linked to intellectual competence. The 'Aristotelian' convention was that one possessed reason simply *qua* human being, regardless of whether one could or did use it. Timson's legalistic reference, however, introduces a simple distinction, an explicitly natural-intellectual one, in which the individual either has reason or does not. There is 'a clear difference between infants [or] distracted, and the [generally] ignorant ... : the one not in a natural capacity as the other is, nor in a rational capacity as the other is'. There is now a sharper difference between childlike and mad intellects on the one hand and the general ignorance of the majority on the other. The outline of a new law of nature within human beings – expressed as the *immediate use* of a *specifically human* reason – is about to emerge from out of the old conventions. Humfrey and Timson, in reaching for the precision of positive law, start to create a modern-looking precision of natural differences among human types with intellectual ability as the criterion.

Legal references seemingly resolved the contradiction between their advocacy of free admission and their exclusion of infants and madpeople. But awkward questions remained. Infants may eventually acquire a rational nature and madpeople recover it; in *this* sense, there is no essential difference between them and the general population, the 'grossly ignorant'. While being 'in minority or under distraction is a bar to admission, it is not a bar to church membership ... A difference in the degree alters not the kind ... We do not find a different rule to church members of the same kind'.[29] So even infants and madpeople have a latent 'right' to communion if not its actual use. Yet the primary symptom of contamination phobia is precisely its belief that some items are categorically dirty and must be excluded. If not children and knowable madpeople, and if not unknowable reprobates, then who?

When Amyraut and Baxter theorized a natural intellectual disability, they were merely defending the doctrine of predestined reprobation against Catholic attacks, by mollifying its harshness. People who scored zero on their catechism, they said, were surely excused responsibility for fulfilling their side of the covenant with God, and could not be damned. But those two writers still needed to avoid the accusation of being universalists, encouraging pollution of the eucharist as Catholics did by allowing unworthy individuals to participate. Humfrey and Timson were less concerned with mollification. They were answering critics who had asked how they could distinguish between the generally ignorant whom they admitted and the madpeople whom they barred, given their belief that no one can know the 'inner man' (who is elect or not) and that assessment was therefore inappropriate. Who could possibly not sense the necessary distinctions between a genuinely and a spuriously human kind? Only heretics believe in the universal possibility of salvation. In response, Humfrey and Timson avoided universalism and stuck with the harsh necessity of distinctions – but only by translating their assumptions about difference in the inner man to a new realm of 'natural intelligence' where human nature and human reason meet – or not.

Spiritual fools and natural fools

If this new division arose at the expense of election and reprobation, it was through the dialectics of dispute. Practical details of pastoral decision-making were involved too. Humfrey and Timson were under pressure to render their assumptions real: to identify the categories they were suggesting in the actual people that presented themselves for communion. For the orthodox Presbyterians, says Timson, natural qualifications such as reason and age are mere 'superadditions' to primordial predestination; this downplaying of nature is 'frivolous', even 'perverse', as reason and age are 'essentials to the more perfect being of a man', 'presupposed' elements of his nature. But he and Humfrey, championing open access and seeing the natural imperfections of madness and childhood as curable by time and education respectively, still needed to prove that they were as good gatekeepers as their opponents or better.

Orthodox Presbyterians constantly tried to provoke them into defining more clearly their (absurd) exclusions, especially the adult ones. This forced Humfrey and Timson to emphasize the numbers and range of 'grossly ignorant' adults who *can* be admitted – by inverse correlation with a small minority of them who are compacted into strangeness and pathology in order to yield a precise definition. Collinges has challenged Timson to say whether he would admit someone so ignorant that they did not even know if Christ were man or woman. Timson turns it back on his opponent: 'I am sorry that any should be so grossly ignorant. I thank God I never have known any such; if Mr Collinges have, I hope not in his parish'.[30] This last jibe signals Timson's belief that excluding the grossly ignorant from communion, as the Presbyterians did, only *encourages* ignorance, rather than being (as they claimed it to be) a wake-up call to the person concerned that he needed educating. If the Presbyterians insist on assessing the aspiring communicant, surely it is *their* job 'to determine of the lowest degree of what is necessary to receiving or excluding in respect of every member'.[31] The most fundamental categories of human difference may be merely nominal (only God knows the truth about whether someone is elect), but that does not relieve the Presbyterians of their duty to justify, precisely, the exclusions they nevertheless feel entitled to make.

Collinges concedes that 'Where the scriptures do not distinguish, we must not distinguish'. He simply thinks the presbytery's second-best practices will do. Timson, by contrast, tries to identify a natural distinction between human groups, one that is real and essential, enabling the pastor to be sure. Having noted how Collinges 'stretcheth the metaphor of dogs', Timson himself allows this human/animal model of difference (he calls it 'frivolous and improper', though it is actually in scripture) to turn into a serious one. The excluded thus become a separate and only quasi-human natural kind. Isaac La Peyrère's theory that Jews are of separate natural origins from Gentiles was in the head-lines in these months, as they began their return to England. But Jews, says Timson, are members of the same 'kind' or species as Christians 'by nature'.[32] Old and New Testament alike are 'fitted for reasonable man, as instrumental to convey a blessing of grace'; and the Passover ritual of the Paschal Lamb, symbolizing as it does the blood of a future Messiah, is equivalent to the eucharist. Thus there is no reason to think of Jews as any less deserving than children. Both groups are simply under a temporary incompetence, not being fully 'grown' in the covenant. Yet hovering around this explanation as to why Jews, like children or madpeople, are not actually 'a different subject' or natural kind is the now logically existing hypothesis of exactly some such group. If a group, whose claim to be human was questionable, *did* exist in nature, definable by an inner, natural difference, surely it would constitute as great a danger to church unity and a future kingdom of the saints as reprobates do.

When Drake and Collinges said a line could not be drawn between children/madpeople and the grossly ignorant, they were not really arguing for the admission of either group, they were just ironically trying to expose the weakness in their opponents' argument. Another orthodox disputant, Humphrey Saunders, is more direct. When 'ministers and godly people assert ... the lawfulness of their administering the Lord's Supper in select company', they must beware the real danger: hypocrites, offering a 'dead and contradic-tory profession'.[33] Such tricksters may superficially present as intelligent, but in fact their incapability is one which subsumes that *faux* intelligence. The latter is the real disability:

> Folly and madness can never be denied to be, wherever sin reigns ... That which we examine ... is whether people can examine themselves, which we are assured many cannot ... Upon this ground infants, fools and madmen are not admitted, because unable to examine themselves. Now such as be wicked men cannot be (rationally) supposed either able or willing to try, or judge themselves, they are spiritually fools ... A natural man ... may play the ape, and do (as to outward works) what he sees others do, but as for discerning in the ordinance, or search-ing his own heart before, these are things far above him.[34]

Humfrey's insistence on the positive status of nature, says Saunders, might lead him to conclude that reprobates – who are in fact '*spiritual* fools and madmen' (emphasis added) – are merely products of nature, not of a deter-ministic, predestinate decision by God. This conclusion, however, would be heretical. Conversely, if natural disability really does 'keep back others', these latter must be 'other [than] *spiritual* fools and madmen'.[35] Clearly, if – good Christian that Humfrey surely is – he wants to carry on recognizing the existence of 'spiritual death', then he needs to associate natural disability with some other category than children (since they will at some point develop reason) or madpeople (since they will at some point regain it): in other words, he must identify a category lacking even a latent right of admission.

Legal idiocy and providence

These nuances are then drawn out further by Thomas Blake, a less partisan writer who maintains some distance on the dispute. Blake stresses that '*present* inaptitude and capacity' are the bar to admission; conversely, '*present* aptitude and capacity' are things any communicant could lose. Just like excommunicates, madpeople are 'member[s] under cure'.[36] As we noted above, a conceptual space that was not apparent before thus arises for *permanent*, lifelong incapacity. Blake subdivides this as follows: '1. Such that through inabilities cannot make any improvement ... 2. Such that ... obstinately will not'. Who, more precisely, are that first group? They break down further: people weakwilled in their quest for 'spiritual improvement' (by contrast with the 'obstinate' in group 2, whose will is strong but disobedient); 'those that by reason of minority and nonage are not yet ripe for the use of reason', such as children; those who have been 'bereft of it, as distracted persons [or] aged persons grown children', and who can be admitted 'upon recovery or upon their [lucid] intervals' after 'prudent' assessment – and 'those that by providence are denied it, as natural idiots'. This last group, though 'natural', is curable too, since the providence or 'hand of God' that denied them reason from birth can also instil it. Thus, although this new 'idiot' terminology suggests to us a sharper definition than those stray mentions of 'innocents' and 'natural fools' in earlier texts, it still brackets them with madpeople and 'the same with infants': they all have a latent right, even if they cannot use it at present.

However, the word 'idiot' had other connotations, of a fiscal character. By the seventeenth century these afforded no role for providence. In theological texts the word had rarely meant anything other than 'layman'. With the gradual intrusion of its fiscal significance into theology, marking a permanent absence of reason, came resonances of a more mundane discriminatory motivation. The Tudor monarchy, invoking obscure medieval jurisprudence, had established a Court of Wards which distinguished between the limited rights of the lunatic to his estate (limited only outside his lucid intervals) and the permanent lack of rights of the born, incurable idiot.[37] A legal idiot was precisely *incurable*; unlike a madman's estate, an idiot's could be sequestered under permanent guardianship. Until 1646, when the Court was abolished, profits could be used to finance the state. Blake seems obsessed with juridical metaphors for man's relationship with God. Was he associating ability to understand the symbolism of eucharist with ability to understand the administration of one's estate? There was as yet no underlying concept of a general intelligence as a firm common denominator for both. Nor did the characteristics of 'idiots' brought before the Court of Wards correspond closely with those of modern 'intellectual disability'. But reason was becoming increasingly important to faith.

To repeat: the fiscal construction of idiocy was not based on some prior psychological one which scarcely existed at the time. If Blake replaces the 'fools' and 'innocents' of previous texts with the more definitive 'natural idiot' of the courts, it is not because he is a proto-psychologist feeling his way towards a precise, quasi-scientific definition. True, he defines 'cannots' as 'ignorant by negation', while 'willnots' are merely 'ignorant by disposition'. But this makes the latter *more*, not less, disabled than the former. Their obduracy hides a popish, idolatrous approach to the sacrament, which to them is like 'the painted frontispieces that we see in many books ... The ignorant beholder sees nothing but an outside ... Such an [*sic*] one sees bread and wine, but what they mean, he knows nothing'.[38] The beholder's blind unintellectual devotion is not incompatible with an intelligently calculated hypocrisy. For Blake the ultimate pathology is to be unwilling. If the unwilling are also unable, it is because God has predetermined their reprobation, not because they lack everyday intellectual ability. They cannot because, necessarily, they will not. And people who by contrast do lack intellectual ability, by 'nature' (i.e. from birth), remain capable of providential cure.

From grace to reason

In his next response Humfrey repeats his opposition to formal assessment, on the grounds of divine inscrutability about communicants' religious status.[39] As we have seen, his argument should in theory lead towards greater inclusivity. To sum up so far: if we cannot know people's destiny in the afterlife, then here on earth they must be given the benefit of doubt. In the early 1650s, any such standpoint had to be hedged around with clear signals that one was not assuming the quasi-Catholic hints at a universal possibility of salvation. This provoked Humfrey and Timson into claiming to know *some sort* of distinction among aspiring communicants, but one that necessarily ran along some other line than that of election and reprobation. Humfrey saw this line as a 'natural' one, existing in the real physical universe.

By now, he has forgotten that the original point about madpeople and infants had been a playful diversion. It has become the centrepiece of his argument. He juxtaposes an initially secondary, natural-intellectual distinction alongside the elective one. The unwitting result is the promotion of the former, by osmosis. The natural distinction, as Timson had already noted, resembles the legal one between the use of a right and its mere possession: for example, between heirs 'of age and capacity' and those 'want[ing] the use of reason' because they lack it while young. And the elective distinction resembles the legal one between an 'active' and a 'passive' right; it is the elect alone who, being regenerate, can exercise an active right to 'the effectual benefits' of the Lord's supper (the unregenerate cannot benefit, even if they receive it passively). The eucharist, he says, marks a distinction in both senses at once: (1) the 'use of that right', i.e. a subjective, natural intellectual ability to understand eucharistic symbolism, and (2) the objective, predestined, unalterable facts of election. When Humfrey juxtaposes these two discourses (1) starts to swallow up (2). He spends many paragraphs on the first and just two sentences on the second – but these latter are enough to endow (1) with the status of an objective science. Thus he belongs in that seamless historical process, revealed later through Locke and many popular religious and educational writers of the eighteenth century such as Isaac Watts and Jonathan Edwards, whereby 'I am in grace' gradually became 'I am intelligent'.

In this text Humfrey's original formula, 'infants and distracted persons', becomes 'infants, idiots, distracted, with the like'. Thanks to Blake's intervention, positive, juridical idiots are now on his list of the excluded. However, they do not quite fit his original argument that his exclusions from the open admission system were not self-contradictory since they were temporary. When the fiscal needs of the state invented 'idiots' both incapable of managing their estates and incapable of recovery, the latter distinction became the whole point of the category, and according to Humfrey the same holds for the religious right to the sacraments. With hindsight, we can see how with the idea of birth-to-death incapacity the legal category helps to bring into view a previously unthinkable sub-species of creature who, as well as being not human for legal or ethical purposes (not having even latent rights), is perhaps not even human in essence.

Humfrey's intentions were largely benevolent: he thought idiots' condition excused them from their obligations to God. Furthermore, his *ad hoc* need for this new distinction within the realm of the excluded, between infancy and madness on the one hand and idiotism on the other, stems from his urge to demonstrate to Presbyterian colleagues that *ignorant* people, i.e. generally or 'grossly' ignorant, should be admitted, since their exclusion might lead them to split off into separate congregations. He purposely omits infants and madpeople here and instead uses only his 'idiots' to make the contrast. What emerges is a spectrum of innate intellectual nature, with its own cut-off point between the low end of normal and the downright pathological. For the first time in this debate we encounter a category that may be generally ignorant but, as Humfrey puts it, is simply 'ignorant *in the first place* ... such as are of age *and reason*' (emphasis added). Even these people should be admitted. Ministers should speak to them 'in as few plain words as they can'.[40] The result will be instruction, and with instruction, conviction. Despite their natural ignorance, such people are 'intelligent church members', educable by the eucharist which is itself a 'teaching sign'. Humfrey tries to anticipate his Presbyterian opponents' likely objection here: 'If ... some are so grossly ignorant that they are not capable for the present to learn, or be instructed by public teaching, then may you number them amongst idiots, and such as have not the use of reason?' Humfrey slips in 'for the present' in order to evade the objection: although some grossly ignorant people are virtually indistinguishable from madpeople and children, they are ultimately educable – but there is a separate category of people who are not, because they have never had the use of reason and never will.

Humfrey's construction of a category grossly ignorant 'in the first place', i.e. naturally of weak understanding but educable, helps throw into relief his contrasting concept of an absolute, permanent idiot; it is one of the early markers for the nineteenth century's distinction of its idiots from higher-level 'imbeciles'.[41] In this way he refutes opponents who assert that, by the logic of his novel criterion of natural intellect, he must believe a majority of the population to be 'in an utter incapacity to be edified'.[42] There *is* such a category, he says, but it is very small. Humfrey's 'idiotism' is a trench he has dug where he can safely sit out any further raids on the validity of open admission for everyone. If someone tries to blur the issue by insisting as before that even idiots are providentially curable, he will 'confess' to the truth of this merely 'upon a pinch ... to avoid intolerable cavil'.

Church unity (in which political unity is implicit) was best served by minimizing exclusions, said Humfrey. This demanded (a) maximizing the difference between people admitted and the residual hardcore of the excluded, but (b) doing so on grounds other than election and reprobation. It threatened to throw the baby out with the bathwater, since Humfrey was as concerned as everyone else about the eucharist being polluted by the presence of reprobates. His hints at a morally neutral intellectual nature were merely instrumental; they allowed him, as a pastor, to operate certain 'real' or 'necessary' exclusions without seeming to try and stand in for God. But his opponents saw this exclusion of 'idiots', by intellectual criteria drawn from nature, as

usurping and threatening the principle of predestined election and reprobation to which both sides subscribed. Perhaps they were right to be anxious. It is
certainly the case that after the dissolution of the Barebones Parliament came
a dramatic decline in public debate about election and a rapid rise in socially
calming sermons about reason's positive role in faith.

The triumph of incurability

Drake made a final contribution, replying to Humfrey's *Rejoynder* and *Second
Vindication*. Much of this just repeats his earlier performance. He opposes
Humfrey's idea that there can be a purely natural incapability which might
excuse someone from their religious obligations. There is 'only a *moral* instrument of conversion', not a natural one. As for Humfrey's exclusions, 'God's
operation upon infants and others naturally uncapable [is] secret', and 'arbitrary'. The religious value of the human individual is passive, not intellectually
active: 'The creature's work is to get in the way and road of grace, that the very
shadow of mercy passing by, may overshadow some of them'.[43] Any boundaries other than elective ones are inconceivable. (One could also infer here, as
others did, that some of those 'naturally incapable' by intellect may be elect.)
Culpability is moral and applies to everyone owing to the Fall – irrespective of
their natural capacity or incapacity, and irrespective of whether incapacity is
intellectual or physical (blindness, paralysis etc). Humfrey must 'either admit
all church members', including his idiot exceptions, 'or give us a better rule ...
His rule of visibility is natural intelligence, when church members have the use
of reason; our rule is spiritual intelligence'.[44] Terms that look ordinary enough
to us must be read carefully in their seventeenth-century context: 'natural
intelligence' is Drake's imputation to Humfrey of a self-evidently outrageous
concept.

Unlike reprobation, which God determines pre-natally and forever, intellectual incapacity is curable by the sacraments themselves: 'If an infant may
be bewitched by ... the Devil's ministers, and that witchery be removed by a
spell ... which the babe cannot understand ..., why may not the same babe
be regenerated by ... God's minister?' Baptism can have this effect. If so, a
'cure' can also 'heal ... when they come to riper years', i.e. by means of the
eucharist. Intelligence, on the other hand, 'might prove a bar, he being thereby
capable of an act of unbelief, which might hinder the cure'.[45] Although Drake
is simply restating old arguments, he now uses the term 'idiot', following its use
in Humfrey's *Second Vindication*. Consequently, permanence and incurability loom larger: 'Wherefore are idiots kept away [by Humfrey], but because
they are children in understanding, and cannot put forth those acts which are

necessary to worthy receiving? Are not all grossly ignorant persons children also in understanding? ... If yet he say ignorance may be cured, so may distraction and madness also'. In omitting idiotism from this latter phrase, Drake neatly sidesteps Humfrey's point, which was precisely that idiots (unlike madpeople) were incurable.

Conclusion

It was Blake, the most moderate of the disputants, who had unwittingly set up the taxonomic framework in which Humfrey could hone his distinction between the ineducably idiotic and the educably 'ignorant in the first place'. Blake and his orthodox colleagues were trying to reclaim the territory of fundamental ontological difference for election and reprobation as against human reason and its absence, and to halt the intrusion of reason into faith. But by 1655 the horse had bolted. Moreover, once Cromwell re-established a quasi-monarchical authority, the threat to church unity passed and so the dispute faded; a Royalist, Church of England account of the disputes in 1657 already has a historiographical tone.[46] The longer historical perspective shows the transition from election to intelligence to be more or less continuous, yet here is what looks like a turning-point. Locke, though himself embedded in Calvinist tradition, was only a few years later drawing his seminal distinction between the generic, species-defining, and educable 'moral man', a logical reasoner, and the pathologically idiotic 'changeling', prototype of the modern intellectually disabled person.[47]

Orthodox Presbyterians had stuck to the doctrine that ignorance is moral and willful, unable to countenance that of a natural, intellectual idiotism which might be as deeply ingrained and absolutely defined as reprobation was. But it was their own attack on Humfrey's originally hazy notions that had forced him into such a precise category. Simply by the way they engaged with him, they had raised demons rather than quelling them. Collinges belatedly grasped their mistake in 1658. Attacking the entitlement of 'gifted' lay brethren to preach, he could not resist complaining that among them were exceptional numbers of people advocating free admission. We have already noted Timson's dubious status as a layman and, worse, a peasant. 'As for Mr Humfrey', says Collinges, the Presbyterian hierarchy ought not to have risen to the bait; they should not have 'by an answer serve[d] him with a wind, which might tempt him to spread his sails'.[48] They had pressed him too hard with ironical arguments that did not truly reflect their own beliefs, thus unwittingly colluding with him in 'creating monsters.'

Monsters of this natural-intellectual, 'idiotic' type, in many respects novel for their time, were in embryo the exclusion necessary to the Enlightenment's ensuing unity of 'man'. To put it another way: the disputes were not some merely discursive stage in the abandonment of predestinarian theology for a secular science of the mind, but also a material shift in the way shamanistic knowledge elites maintain and reconstitute their phobic exclusions, and the zealous divisiveness they encourage.

These disputes about people's inner capabilities and inclinations were also central to anxieties, sometimes explicit ones as we have seen, about the maintenance of a unified political rule, the very existence of a whole social elite and perhaps, reflected through the latter's eyes, the status within nature of the human species itself. One practical feature of elite knowledge systems in both religion and psychology is their categorisation of certain people whose identity actually turns out in the long historical term to be arbitrary. The philosophy of science, like the authorities cited at the start of this article, tends to stress that knowledge elites are incapable of thinking beyond the preservation of their own closed systems from contamination.[49] So if, according to one of its classic case studies, there is no agreed scientific account of why aeroplanes stay up, can we expect to know why a merely conceptual entity like intellectual ability or disability stays up?

Yet we cannot leave the matter at that. History does not only teach us to doubt. As our case-study indicates, when an outgroup descriptor like intellectual disability is being shaped and re-shaped, it is for understandable socio-political and administrative reasons. It may belong in the history of ideas, but this is inextricable from histories of a more practical sort. Neither works without the other. In history from above, concepts assume a life of their own, whose purpose is to shore up elite defences against social contamination. In history from below, people may be liberated from discriminatory practices of elimination and segregation – but to be effective this requires a freeing-up of conceptual boundaries too. The episode examined here represents just one moment – a historically specific phase in the interrelationship between concept and practice – on a journey from elimination by excommunication to elimination by pre-natal testing, and from segregation by the catechism to segregation, via the church-school curriculum, by the cognitive ability test. The relationship between these phases is not that of some cross-historical identity, equivalence, or parallel. It is that of landmarks on a concrete historical path within a unitary conceptual landscape.

Notes

1 American Psychiatric Association, *Diagnostic and Statistical Manual of Mental Disorders* (2013), 5th edn.

2 See, in particular, Mary Douglas, *Purity and Danger: An Analysis of Concepts of Pollution and Taboo* (London: Routledge, 1966); Joseph Gabel, *False Consciousness: An Essay on Reification* (Oxford: Blackwell, 1975); René Girard, *The Scapegoat* (Baltimore: Johns Hopkins University Press, 1986); Henri Tajfel, *Human Groups and Social Categories* (Cambridge: Cambridge University Press, 1981). On the combined relevance of these texts, see C. F. Goodey, *Learning Disability and Inclusion Phobia: Past, Present, Future* (Abingdon: Routledge, 2016), pp. 15–25.

3 William Lamont, *Richard Baxter of the Millennium: Protestant Imperialism and the English Revolution* (London: Croom Helm, 1979), 157. For general background to these disputes, see E. Brooks Holifield, *The Covenant Sealed: The Development of Puritan Sacramental Theology in Old and New England 1570–1720* (New Haven CT: Yale University Press, 1974).

4 See in the present volume Introduction, n35, chapters 2 and 3.

5 John Humfrey, *An Humble Vindication of a Free Admission unto the Lord's Supper* (London: Edward Blackmore, 1651), 30.

6 Ibid., 72.

7 Ibid., 23.

8 Roger Drake, *A Boundary to the Holy Mount* (London: S. Bowtell, 1653), 13ff.

9 Ibid., 53.

10 Ibid., 57.

11 Ibid., 89.

12 Ibid., 105.

13 Ibid., Preface; A3.

14 Humfrey, *A Rejoynder to Mr Drake* (London: Edward Blackmore, 1654), 20.

15 See C. F. Goodey, *A History of Intelligence and 'Intellectual Disability'* (Farnham and Burlington VT: Ashgate, 2011), 189ff; for general background still see Brian Armstrong, *Calvin and the Amyraut Heresy: Protestantism and Scholasticism in Seventeenth-Century France* (Madison WI: University of Wisconsin Press, 1969).

16 Richard Baxter, *Certain Disputations of Right to Sacraments* (London: Thomas Johnson, 1657).

17 Ibid.

18 Baxter, *The Universal Redemption of Mankind* (London: John Salusbury, 1694, published posthumously).

19 Humfrey, *A Rejoynder to Mr Drake*, 24.

20 Ibid., A2.

21 Letters of Richard Baxter, 11 May, 1655, ms. Dr Williams Library, London.

22 John Timson, *The Bar to Free Admission to the Lord's Supper Removed* (London: Thomas Williams, 1654), 59ff.

23 John Collinges, *Responsaria Bipartita* (London: H. Hills, 1654), i.19, 24.

24 Ibid., ii.88.

25 Ibid., i.23.

26 Ibid., ii.174.

27 Timson, *The Bar to Free Admission*, 9.

28 Timson, *To Receive the Lord's Supper* (London: Thomas Williams, 1655), 4ff.

29 Ibid., 8.

30 Ibid., 17.

31 Ibid., 303.

32 Ibid., 322ff.

33 Humphrey Saunders, *An Anti-Diatribe* (London: Thomas Newberry, 1655), 217.

34 Ibid., 147.

35 Ibid., 180.

36 Thomas Blake, *The Covenant Sealed* (London: Roper, 1655), 225ff; see also Daniel Cawdrey, *A Sober Answer to a Serious Question* (London: Christopher Meredith, 1652), 13.

37 See chapters 2 and 9 in this volume.

38 Blake, *The Covenant Sealed*, 230.

39 Humfrey, *A Second Vindication of a Disciplinary, Anti-Erastian, Orthodox Free Admission to the Lord's Supper* (London: Edward Blackmore, 1656), 20ff.

40 Ibid., 29ff.

41 Goodey, *A History*, 199, 277.

42 Humfrey, *A Second Vindication*, 132.

43 Roger Drake, *The Bar Against Free Admission to the Lord's Supper Fixed* (London: Philip Chetwind, 1656), 25.

44 Ibid., 124.

45 Ibid., 421, 137.

46 William Morice, *The Common Right to the Lord's Supper Asserted* (London: Richard Roiston, 1657).

47 John Locke, *An Essay Concerning Human Understanding* [1689], edited by Peter Nidditch (Oxford: Clarendon Press, 1975). See also chapters 6 and 7 in this volume.

48 Collinges, *The Preacher (Pretendedly) Sent, Sent Back* (London: Livewell Chapman, 1658), preface.

49 David Bloor, *Knowledge and Social Imagery* (Chicago: University of Chicago Press, 1991), 2nd edn.

6

'A DEFECT IN THE MIND': COGNITIVE ABLEISM IN SWIFT'S *GULLIVER'S TRAVELS*

D. Christopher Gabbard

Modern conceptions of mental disability did not begin to take shape until the concept of intelligence came into formation. This development occurred at about the same time – roughly the later seventeenth century – that an individual's perceived possession of intelligence rose in value vis-à-vis more traditional status-bidding claims such as lineage (nobility) and election (being saved in the Christian sense). One's ability to think abstractly, regardless of birth, was privileged more and more by those seeking to curb the monarch's prerogatives and create a political order in which power devolved to individuals. Laying out the terms of this new order, John Locke invoked social contract theory, and argued that a society composed of freely associating individuals would be governed through reciprocal contracts. In making this argument, he maintained that the parties to these contracts would need to possess sufficient mental capability to understand the agreements into which they were entering. In sum, they would require intelligence, which Locke defined as the ability to engage in abstract thinking.

Locke's impact on Book Four of Jonathan Swift's *Gulliver's Travels* (1726)[1] is a well-worn topic of discussion among scholars. Most of the criticism rejects the idea that the philosopher exerted much influence. Rather, a substantial body of it takes its cue from Swift's letter of 29 September, 1725, to Alexander Pope in which he protests against the 'falsity of that definition *animal rationale*' and redefines the human as '*rationis capax*' (capable of reason).[2] With this letter in mind, most scholars have assumed that the targets of Swift's attack in the fourth book are the Stoics, the Deists, or the general cultural drift of Enlightenment thought. These positions are grounded in the thinking that Swift is exploring the age-old binary of reason versus the passions. However, a few scholars have diverged from this line of thought, most notably W. B. Carnochan, who argued that Gulliver's character satirizes Lockean epistemology.[3]

What has not been considered heretofore by Carnochan or others is a specific role Locke's *Essay Concerning Human Understanding* (1689)[4] may have played in regards to Book Four, one having to do with a distinction the philosopher draws between *person* and *man* (hereafter in most cases *human* or *non-person*). The categories of *person* and *human* provided Locke with a way to distinguish between offspring born of human parents and having human morphology who will grow up to become abstract thinkers (*persons*), versus those born with the same parentage and shape but who will never develop reasoning capabilities (*humans*). Locke's differentiation becomes explicit in those sections of the *Essay* discussing the changeling. When William and Mary signed the Bill of Rights in 1689 and England's subjects thereby entered into a contract with their king, not everyone, in Locke's view, could be party to this agreement. Those able to think abstractly could take part in the new public sphere, but those who could not do so could not participate. A novel political distinction thus arose à la Locke: *persons* (those with intelligence) qualified to be rights-bearing individuals and so could engage in public affairs, but *humans* (those lacking it) possessed a diminished set of rights (if any) and would be relegated to the private sphere, to the supervision of others. This distinction and Locke's invocation of the changeling figure underwrite what evolves into the modern concept of mental disability.[5]

In contemporary bioethics, one finds remnants of Locke's distinction expounded in the writings of Peter Singer[6] and Jeff McMahan,[7] who in turn are challenged by two other philosophers, Licia Carlson[8] and Eva Feder Kittay.[9] The latter accuse the former of practicing *cognitive ableism*, which Carlson defines as 'a prejudice or attitude of bias in favor of the interests of individuals who possess certain cognitive abilities (or the potential for them) against those who are believed not to actually or potentially possess them'.[10] Long before *cognitive ableism* was coined, however, Swift's Book Four critiqued this same bias, for its protagonist, Lemuel Gulliver, is a cognitive ableist *par excellence*. This chapter will argue that Gulliver epitomizes the attitude Carlson describes, that Locke's *person / human* binary broadly comes into play in the fourth book of the *Travels*, and that the character of Gulliver straddles the *person / human* divide, thereby vexing Locke's binary. Indeed, the characterization of Gulliver not only parodies Locke's distinction, but also exposes the Lockean notion of intelligence upon which it rests to be a fiction, one mainly useful for stoking self-esteem and self-deception that combine to form the cognitive ableist attitude of arrogance and complacency.

Jumping to conclusions

One of the most trodden paths in Swift criticism of Book Four is the meaning of Lemuel Gulliver's wholesale rejection of the Yahoos, his intense desire to 'distinguish myself, as much as possible, from that cursed race of *Yahoos*'.[11] And yet, the criticism curiously has avoided discussing the extreme lengths to which the narrator goes in rejecting them. To review, in Book Four Gulliver winds up on an island inhabited by rational horses, the Houyhnhnms, and irrational humans, the Yahoos, and comes to admire the former to such an extent he wishes to spend the rest of his life with them. However, in chapter nine their assembly expels him, and since he must leave, in chapter ten he builds a boat. Upon the completion of it, he makes what should be a remarkably troubling, even shocking, revelation:

> in six Weeks time with the Help of the Sorrel Nag, who performed the Parts that required most Labour, I finished a Sort of *Indian* Canoo, but much larger, covering it with the Skins of *Yahoos* well stitched together with hempen Threads of my own making. My Sail was likewise composed of the Skins of the same Animal; but I made use of the youngest I could get; the older being too tough and thick.[12]

This matter-of-fact, deadpan description seems designed to be overlooked. Does Gulliver capture, kill, and flay the young Yahoos himself? Or does he obtain the skins by some other means? The disclosure is provocative – even appalling. One of the few commentators to remark upon this passage is not a literary scholar but science fiction writer Isaac Asimov, who glosses the line 'the youngest I could get' in this way:

> How did Gulliver get the young Yahoo skins? Having but a limited time to complete his task, he could scarcely count on finding dead Yahoo infants. ... The conclusion is that he must have killed them for the purpose or had them killed.[13]

In this gloss, Asimov makes three rhetorical moves. First, he transforms 'youngest I could get' into 'dead Yahoo infants'. Second, he uses the word *infant*, which denotes, according to the *Oxford English Dictionary* (*OED*), either a 'child during the earliest period of life' or a 'person under (legal) age'.[14] And third, his phrasing, 'he must have killed them for the purpose or had them killed', leaves open the possibility that Gulliver commits, or is a party to committing, infanticide. However, outside of the narrator's phrase, 'the youngest *I could get*' (emphasis added), nothing in the text authorizes a reading that Gulliver engages in vicious and bloody infanticidal killing. No scene of slaughter and skinning appears, and even if one had appeared involving killing baby Yahoos, it would have been very odd, considering that a few chapters earlier Gulliver had noted that Yahoos 'are prodigiously nimble from their infancy'.[15]

Thus, Asimov's gloss begs the question: it assumes as true the two things in dispute, whether the Yahoos are human, and whether Gulliver commits or orders infanticide. On the other hand, with a few exceptions, critics have not much concerned themselves with figuring out how Gulliver obtained the skins. No one has asked if he found them or whether they were given to him. Gulliver does state, after all, that he '*made use of* the youngest I could get', with the 'made use of' suggesting he had no direct hand in the killing (emphasis added). However, the alternative explanations of the source generate many questions. Could these Yahoos have died from natural causes or internecine struggles, and he afterward stumbled upon the remains? And yet, do not bodies left in the sun quickly corrupt? And why would so many young ones have died? If they succumbed to disease, would Gulliver, a physician, have wanted to work with such material? Could the Sorrel Nag 'and another servant' have supplied him with the Yahoo skins?[16] Even conceding that they may have, why did they supply him with Yahoo skins rather than cowhide, which also is available?

To latch onto one of these alternatives as true would be to mistake a speculation for a conclusion. As to how Gulliver obtained the skins, the text will not yield an answer. One issue beyond dispute though is Gulliver's cavalier attitude: he registers neither objection nor hesitation. Most critics do not discuss Gulliver's nonchalance, and two mutually exclusive explanations can be produced for this reticence. Either his admission is so repellent that speaking about it proves difficult; or it invokes no ethical question worth discussing beyond whether killing animals and using their hides is morally justifiable. Toggling between these mutually exclusive explanations is Gulliver's own wording. On the one hand, throughout Book Four he uses phrases indicating he believes he is harvesting parts from animal carcasses: 'Springes made of *Yahoos* Hairs',[17] '*Yahoos* Tallow',[18] and 'hides of Yahoos'.[19] On the other, in chapter ten he uses the word *skin* three times: 'skins of *Yahoos*'[20] and, from the passage quoted above, 'Skins of the same Animal'. While the term *skin* can be applied interchangeably to animals and humans,[21] his back-to-back usage forces the reader to wonder why he prefers this word to the less equivocal *hide*. It would be a mistake to make too much of Gulliver's terminology, but his refraining from *hide* while repeating *skin* three times in succession at the moment in the text foregrounding Yahoo deaths does seem curious. In a way that *hide* does not, *skin* raises the question of whether the Yahoos may be considered human. Gulliver's preference for *skin* opens the door to the text taking a dramatic turn into the ethical realm, for, if the Yahoos have skin rather than hides, could they possibly be human? And if they may be human, one must choose an appropriate verb for the act of bringing about their demise. Regardless of who or what does this, are the Yahoos *killed*, as occurs with animals? Or are they *murdered*, as can only happen with humans?

No question seems to exist in Gulliver's mind as to this matter: in his eyes, the Yahoos are animals. However, one must ask whether he makes the same mistake as Asimov, but does so on the other side of the question, and from within the narrative itself. In other words, just as Asimov assumes as true the very question in dispute, namely, the humanity of the Yahoos – Gulliver similarly jumps to a conclusion, the difference between them being that in the latter's view they are not. What is the reader to think? As with the provenance of the skins, the text yields no definitive answer. This sort of indeterminacy forms a pattern in Book Four. Addressing a similar uncertainty (the derivation of the word *Yahoo* – more on this later), Carnochan writes of it that 'That would be a fairly characteristic Swiftian joke'.[22] The indeterminate species status of the Yahoos may be another such joke, but one perhaps told at the expense of the 'Gentle Reader'.[23] For if the text refuses to yield answers about acts so heinous – infanticide and murder – then it compels the reader to draw conclusions based on insufficient information. The joke, or serious point, of Book Four does not concern concluding one way or the other that the Yahoos are animal or human. Rather, the point may have to do with how one should act in such an ethically charged but uncertain situation.

Locke's changelings

It is not possible to speak about the beginnings of cognitive ableism as it bears on human status without talking about changelings and Locke. Thanks in great part to Locke, changelings exist at the fulcrum of the transition from a traditional way of determining human status to a more modern criterion. However, understanding this transition requires going back prior to Locke. The Aristotelian tradition's human essence and / or the presence of a soul – that is, human morphology and parentage – were all that mattered in determining whether an individual was to be considered human. In making such determinations, the governing binary was human versus animal. The soul was presumed to be present in a human form no matter how deficient the mind because '"soul" and "intellect" were notionally separate entities'.[24] Then, in the first half of the seventeenth century, René Descartes came along with the concept of mind-body dualism, and afterward it became possible to imagine a body without a working mind, with such a body representing 'a numerical subtraction from what makes us human'.[25]

Thus, it became conceivable to ask, are mindless humans *human*? Locke then enters the discussion. In the *Essay*, he debunks the concept of innate ideas and replaces it with a model in which humans are born with innate cognitive processes, or *abilities*. By doing so, he establishes a normative human mental standard that will bring about a paradigmatic shift in Western thinking. After Locke, shape and morphology alone no longer suffice to determine human status. Irvin Ehrenpreis makes the point that, by the Augustan period, 'it was a commonplace that the human body makes an insufficient mark of humanity; apes, monkeys, and monsters were invoked to prove this'.[26] In making the case for innate cognitive *abilities*, Locke summons examples in which the ability to reason and human birth/morphology do not align. He does so in order to point out that contradictions exist between those with human parentage and shape who grow up to think abstractly and those with the same prerequisites but who will never be able to reason. Definitions are important to Locke, and so he attempts to clarify matters by assigning the term *man* to the latter cases and *person* to the former. Locke specifically defines a *person* as a 'thinking, intelligent Being, that has reason and reflection, and can consider it self as it self, the same thinking thing in different times and places'.[27] In other words, a *person* is able to think abstractly, process information swiftly, and retain and quickly recall memories. Resemblance between parents and offspring now must be *intellectual resemblance.*[28] By making this distinction, Locke changes the focus as to what matters in such a way that to be a *man* no longer is enough: one must be a *person*. In this new person-human binary, *person* becomes the privileged term. Two things should be noted here: first, for Locke this is an all-or-nothing affair: either one is or one is not a person. He does not allow for gradations between one extreme and the other.[29] And second, the person-human binary supplants the former human-animal binary. Interestingly, to a considerable extent the former maps over the latter so that one must conclude that the human and the animal become equivalent when positioned vis-à-vis the new valorized term, *person*. In any case, the person/human distinction will have tremendous consequences, for it facilitates imagining a new social order in which those who believe themselves to be *persons* can assume prerogatives and power over those whom they deem to be merely *human*. Essentially, Locke's novel distinction facilitates restructuring society along the lines of *cognitive ableism*.

The chief example of a human birth in which there is physical but not intellectual resemblance to the parents is, according to Locke, the *changeling*. Locke needs the changeling to operationalize his argument about its opposite, the *person*, because, as C. F. Goodey notes, 'Pathology etches in the normal'.[30] *Changeling* was a holdover from folklore but also was much more. According to the *OED*, the first recorded usage appears in 1561 and refers to 'A person or thing (surreptitiously) put in exchange for another'.[31] The second, with a different meaning, appears two years later: 'One given to change; a fickle or inconstant person; a waverer, turncoat, renegade'.[32] The meaning most commonly attributed today did not appear until 1584: 'A child secretly substituted for another in infancy; esp. a child (usually stupid or ugly) supposed to have been left by fairies in exchange for one stolen'.[33] Then, in 1642, yet another meaning enters circulation: 'A half-witted person, idiot, imbecile'.[34] In the middle of the seventeenth-century, the four concepts – substitution, inconstancy, switching at birth, and imbecility – began to coalesce.[35] Thus, when Locke is writing the *Essay* in the 1670s and 1680s, he uses the word *changeling* – and uses it frequently – because it is common parlance, 'plain and "civil" (public) language'.[36]

'Changeling' also carried medical significance. Locke was a physician, and early modern doctors were still under the influence of *The Art of Medicine* by the second-century Roman Galen. In one part, this text describes the ancient concept of dispositional disabilities or mental weakness – the paradigm of problematic mental states.[37] While it is well known that Galen comments on the dispositional malady of melancholy, it is less well known that he discerned a related one: '"mobility" or "instability of opinion" (*mobilitas opinionum*)', which is to say, *changeableness*, the symptoms of which were thinking rashly or variably.[38] *Mobilitas opinionum* appears 'mainly in the (Latin) commentaries on Galen's *Art of Medicine*, which was the central component of the medical education curriculum – and this explains how it would have become a commonplace' even though it fell out of circulation when medical texts started to appear in the vernacular.[39] Those suffering from it were known as *changelings* on account of a propensity to change. Goodey describes how physicians would have understood the condition:

> Unstable opinion was a defect of the will. ... If a patient's opinion simply followed his appetites, it showed that his will was divorced from his reason. ... The paradigmatic mind changer was Eve, when she listened to the serpent. It went with her gullibility, a frequently cited medical symptom of unstable opinion. Instability undermined the patient's knowledge of what was true and (the same thing) what was good for him.[40]

Those with unstable opinions – those who were constantly changing, especially their religious beliefs – were known as *changelings*.[41] In Locke, the term undergoes further refining, coming to suggest an entity with human shape that is congenitally intellectually disabled. The *tabula rasa* of the changeling's mind will forever remain blank – nothing can be written there. A changeling thus is a mindless child who will grow up to become a perpetually irrational adult and so represents 'soulless bestiality'.[42]

Abstract thinking consists of reflecting on the process of thinking, and changelings are incapable of doing this.[43] Thus, they are equivocal men, existing in the interstices between species. At one point, Locke notes that *physically* monstrous births often are put to death without such killings being considered murder.[44] And yet, these physically monstrous births, if not killed, have been known to grow up and exhibit typical human consciousness.[45] Later, Locke points out a seeming contradiction – the killing of *physically* defective babies who grow up to be rational human beings, versus the saving of changeling babies that will grow up to be irrational beings.[46] Paul de Man notes that the changeling figure is 'powerfully coercive since it generates, for example, the ethical pressure of such questions as "to kill or not to kill"'. This question eventuates in that of 'what to do with the "changeling"'.[47] Locke suggests that readers engage in a thought experiment in which they distort the facial features of a newborn changeling just slightly, but enough, so that it no longer appears entirely human.[48] At what moment in this reconfiguring, he asks, does one stop calling the infant human, concede it is a soulless beast, and allow it to be destroyed? His implication is clear: changelings have transformed into an Other whose alterity is irreducible: 'the externally well-formed but mentally deficient changeling is in fact inhuman'.[49]

A Lockean thought experiment *in extremis*

With some justification, one can speculate that Swift some thirty years later in the 1720s took Locke up on his suggestion and engaged in his thought experiment. Could the result have been the Yahoo? How much Swift's Book Four distorts the Yahoos from the typical human form – if indeed it distorts them at all – depends on which chapter one is reading. If so, at what moment in Book Four does the reader concede that the Yahoos are soulless beasts, as Gulliver does, and allow them to be destroyed? Swift was familiar with Locke's *Essay*, and, according to Carnochan, his response 'ranges from ambivalent to critical'.[50] More recently, J. A. Downie comments that 'Locke's argument about real essences and complex ideas informs Swift's satire in Part Four'.[51] Locke's ideas indeed were circulating in the culture. While it may be going too far to assert that Swift was satirizing them, it can be argued that Book Four plays with them in tantalizing ways.

One can hardly read the entirety of the *Travels* without noticing, in addition to the numerous defects and distortions of body that Dennis Todd has pointed out,[52] the distortions in ways of thinking and the apparent defects in the minds of those the narrator encounters. These defects and distortions of mind reach a crescendo in Book Four vis-à-vis the Houyhnhnms and Yahoos. Hermann Real and Heinz Vienken point out that all that the reader knows about either of them derives entirely from Gulliver.[53] That said, for the purposes of this argument it is important to note that, within his admittedly limited and unreliable account, the Yahoos appear to utilize no language and do not seem to exhibit any ability to retain and recall memories. Because they seem to be unable to speak for themselves, readers 'have no recourse to' their minds, and they 'do not appear to have self-consciousness'.[54] If this indeed is the case, they can 'have no notion of a continuous identity. ... [Thus,] the Yahoos ... [do not] conform to the Lockean criteria of "person"'.[55] In other words, they answer to Locke's definition of *man*, not *person*. Most significantly, they instantiate changelings to the degree that they resemble changeling births who have grown up into adult form but who remain unable to think abstractly.

If the reader must mediate everything he or she knows about the Yahoos and Houyhnhnms through Gulliver, then who, or what, is *he*? Ian Higgins comments that from the book's beginning 'a faint hint of puritan zealotry attaches itself to Lemuel'.[56] In Book One's second sentence, Gulliver announces that he attended Emmanuel College, 'a Cambridge College of Puritan foundation'; the reader also learns he 'studied medicine at Leyden in the Netherlands, an educational destination abroad for Protestant dissenters'.[57] Moreover, Gulliver seems intent to impress the reader that he is a learnèd person. In fact, on page one he feels compelled to deliver a curriculum vitae of educational accomplishment to demonstrate his credentials as a narrator.

Furthermore, throughout the text he presents himself as one of the new, empirical men, someone who prides himself on his intelligence. And yet, does he live up to his own billing? Anthony Manousos describes him as a 'mechanical empiricist',[58] and, as Higgins points out, he is an empiricist to a fault: he outdoes everyone 'in over-particularity'.[59] Todd describes him as 'Literal-minded and superficial', someone who 'travels through the world like the stereotypical tourist, staring at everything and seeing nothing'.[60] As such, Gulliver becomes one of the satire's butts: he is 'a fully-fledged caricature of the "Modern"', a 'simplificateur of complex issues', and, at the end of the day, an '"enthusiast" or fanatic of ideal Reason'.[61] Most importantly, in the opening of Book One, Gulliver mentions that his formative years were spent under *Master Bates*, and this revelation allows the reader to connect his developing character with 'an unseemly self-absorption'.[62] Indeed, from the beginning, pride in his own intelligence is juxtaposed with a hint of mental masturbation. In sum, Gulliver manifests an intellectual narcissism that epitomizes cognitive ableism.

As a character priding himself on his intelligence, Gulliver sees in the Yahoos everything he wishes to define himself against. And yet, for a self-proclaimed intelligent person – as the epitome of cognitive ableism – he does not exhibit a high level of acuity. When he first comes to land in Book Four, he detects 'Tracks of human Feet' and, immediately after, spies 'these creatures', meaning the Yahoos.[63] However, while he does not refer to any other humans who could have made the tracks, he never ties the tracks to 'these creatures'. His failing to connect the two may be attributed to the visual impression made by 'these creatures', which causes him to be 'a little discomposed'.[64] His use of 'discomposed', which the *OED* defines as 'Disordered', reveals that his thoughts have deviated from their usual order on account of the Yahoos not meeting his expectation of a customary human form.[65] 'Their Shape', he states, is 'very singular, and deformed'.[66] The *OED* defines 'singular' to mean 'Different from or not complying with that which is customary',[67] and *deformed* as 'Marred in shape ... distorted'.[68] The Yahoos being 'marred ... distorted' and 'not complying with that which is customary' discloses that he recognizes traces of an original human form. In his perspective, then, the combination of these traces and deviations from them brings to the fore their monstrosity.

Monstrosity disorders Gulliver's mental processes, but not in the way one might think, for monstrosity itself is complex. David Williams demonstrates that *monster* has not held a consistent meaning through time. In Medieval theology, the concept served as a signifier of unintelligibility, while in post-Medieval thinking (scientific and aesthetic), it came to represent the exception, that which occupied the horizon of the human.[69] Both exceptionality and unintelligibility are forms of monstrosity, but with different valences. Dramatic irony consequently is created in the *Travels* when its naive narrator insistently views the Yahoos scientifically and aesthetically as exceptions, while the astute reader probes between the lines and realizes the Yahoos are unintelligible. Enhancing the irony is the reader's recognition that the narrator's prejudices in one direction bar him from looking in the other. Roger Lund notes that 'By the time we reach the early eighteenth-century, monstrosity had lost its power to shock or to amaze, and tended instead merely to annoy the observer because of its "unseemliness", inspiring mere repugnance at the violation of "conventions of beauty and decorum"'. In sum, Gulliver's animosity is aroused by the Yahoos' exceptional deviation from the '"conventions of beauty and decorum"'.[70] Their aesthetic deviance drives his behaviour and backfires on him a few lines later in the 'contact-zone' moment when he encounters one of them face to face.[71] In this scene he becomes the aggressor, giving the 'ugly monster' a 'Blow with the flat side' of his sword.[72] Of the approaching 'monster', David Nokes claims that it 'is a human being who approaches Gulliver, with his hand raised in greeting'.[73] While the text never authorizes Nokes' reading of the Yahoos as definitively human, Gulliver for his part hastily jumps to the opposite conclusion and so initiates the violence, to which the Yahoos respond by defecating on him. What the reader understands but Gulliver fails to grasp is that, if the new, empirical man persists in viewing the Yahoos as exceptions, he must come to terms with the fact that, on this island at least, he is the one who is the exception.

In Swift's Lockean thought experiment, the Yahoos differ just enough from the typical human form – the form as Gulliver has known it up until then – for him not to ask the question of whether they possibly may be human. Later, under the coaxing of his Houyhnhnm *master* (recalling the earlier 'Master Bates'), Gulliver acknowledges he has the same shape as the Yahoos,[74] and the young Yahoo female's sexual attack indeed confirms this species similarity. However, he deduces the wrong conclusion from his Houyhnhnm master and the female Yahoo, for, instead of accepting his and the Yahoos' shared humanity, he decides instead that he himself and they must be animals. Thus, he embraces 'the position of submissive servant to his Houyhnhnm 'master'',[75] the position of a faithful dog.

Why does Gulliver make the choice that he does? What are his criteria? Once he has encountered the Houyhnhnms, no entity with human shape in his estimation will ever be able to prove itself capable of being a person. Moreover, without discretion or moderation, he opts for reason as the marker of *person* to the extent that an entity with a human's shape is merely a human until he or she can demonstrate themselves to be a person. However, in the process of becoming enamored of the Houyhnhnms, Gulliver engages in a chiasmatic switching of the usual coordinates of shape and reason. Horses now possess reason; humans do not. Could this inversion constitute textual play regarding Locke's famous 'association of ideas'? Locke speculates that the mind can randomly associate unrelated ideas in such a way that they become irrevocably and permanently – but wrongly – linked together. Once one idea is invoked, 'the whole gang always inseparable shew themselves together'.[76] In this case, Gulliver detaches one idea, *ability to reason*, from another idea, *human shape*, then re-associates the former idea with *horse shape*: then, forever after, he cannot release himself from this new association. The Houyhnhnms now qualify as *persons* because, even though they do not have human shape, they do appear to him to possess the ability to reason. In fact, he frequently refers to them as *persons* and *people*. In one example, Gulliver states, 'I could with great Pleasure enlarge further upon the Manners and Virtues of this excellent people'.[77] Again, as with 'skins', it may be a mistake to make too much of Gulliver's word choice, but his diction does arouse curiosity. While it is possible *people* merely signifies *race,* as in *a people,*[78] *people* also signifies *person* in the plural.[79] In addition, while he does not restrict the term to the Houyhnhnms, he does use *persons* ten times and *people* six times to refer to them. His extensive usage of *person* and *people* to refer to the island's horses suggests that his mental wires have crossed so that, in his Lockean association of ideas, equine morphology becomes associated with rationality.

A further possible caricature of Lockean theory may be part of this textual play: Locke argues that names take on an importance and life of their own so that it becomes easy to forget *how* they became associated with the things they signify. Allen Michie draws attention to the fact that Gulliver first hears a horse neigh, which he transcribes as 'Yahoo'. He next learns to connect this name with negative connotations – brutishness, filth, and ignorance. Then he concludes he himself must be this thing he himself has named a Yahoo, so he not only links himself to the name, but he also assumes he must embody its bad attributes. In the final step, he undertakes an obsessive personal mission to divorce himself from every tincture of the name's connotations, all the while forgetting that he is the one who coined the term in the first place. As Michie sums it up, 'There is circularity to this argument'.[80]

In his self-constructed linguistic prison, Gulliver is caught in the middle, trapped in a Yahoo body but yearning to join the society of 'this excellent people'. The Houyhnhnms constitute an intelligence society – a regime in which those who display reason to competitive advantage become the elite and in which intelligence rather than honor (nobility) or election (being saved in the Christian sense) serves as the primary marker of social status. Gulliver wants to join the horses' intelligence society, but he has no way to enter into it except by occupying its fringe, becoming a marvelous oddity by playing the oxymoronic 'wonderful Yahoo' – a self-admitted freak on the outskirts. As Todd has demonstrated, this self-denigrating description recalls the kind of billing used in Augustan Britain to draw the public's attention to a freak show exhibit. Indeed, in Books One and Two, Gulliver's freakishly sized body already has been placed on display. Todd confirms that 'From the beginning, Gulliver has been driven by this desire for "Distinction"',[81] and in Book Four he once again earns a variety of it. Learning to speak Houyhnhnm and emulate their virtues, he attempts to carry through with his intention to become, in the worst possible way, a member of the island's intelligence society.

Blows to this aspiration come with the two meetings of the Houyhnhnm Assembly. In the session following the one in which they discuss 'Whether the Yahoos should be exterminated from the Face of the Earth',[82] the horses vote to deport him, a decision they base solely upon his Yahoo shape. For them, his shape serves as the primary indicator of his inability to reason. In so doing, they disregard the evidence of his rationality. Because he has the Yahoo shape he does, he cannot possibly be capable of abstract thought and, thereby, answer to their understanding of *person*. Gulliver now must build a boat, and it is in its construction that the killing, or murder, of Yahoos can be inferred. Obviously seduced by the Houyhnhnms' debate – not decision – about exterminating Yahoos, Gulliver takes his cue from the intelligence society he wishes to join: he too judges on the basis that Yahoo-shape indicates an inability to think abstractly.[83]

In terms of genre, Book Four moves back and forth between functioning as a beast fable and as a fictional narrative populated by humans. In a *mise en abyme*, the Yahoos replicate in miniature the generic oscillation between beast and human. This alternation should not stop readers from asking questions of Gulliver that they would not bother to ask of the beasts. In ethical terms, it would be one thing for beasts to kill Yahoos, and quite another for Gulliver to do the same or to have the killings carried out at his behest. In other words, the Houyhnhnms are horses confined to the beast-fable portion of the narrative, while Gulliver interacts with – as best as the reader can judge – creatures who may turn out to be of the same species as himself. Consequently, readers hold him – or at least should hold him – to a different standard.

As was noted at the beginning, when he informs the reader about the skins, he does so as a casual aside. In fact, his tone becomes so matter-of-fact that his obliviousness that anything morally may be at stake becomes the thing that most stands out. Is Gulliver's association with the killing of Yahoo babies for their skins a parodic version of Lockean thinking about changeling infants? After all, Locke strongly implies that if he could know *with certainty* at the time of birth that the changeling infant would grow up to be an irrational humanoid entity, he would endorse destroying that infant.[84] Additionally, as was noted earlier, de Man remarks that Locke's rhetorical moves in the unfolding of the *Essay* raise 'questions [such] as "to kill or not to kill"' and 'what to do with the "changeling"'.[85] In the *Travels*, the Yahoos as adult changelings confirm what Locke suspected them to be in their infancy. Gulliver then seemingly demonstrates what Locke would have done, or, at least, what Locke might have done with their skins.

Gulliver, the changeling

Gulliver appears neither to think about using the skins, nor even to know *how* to think about the moral implications the skins raise. And this inability brings to the foreground a central irony of Book Four, namely, that of the individual who aspires to join the intelligence society but who does not know how to think. And yet, thinking is only one of the things an intelligence society respects; it also values social hierarchy and order, which can only be achieved by an in-group defining itself in opposition to an out-group. Hence, the more Gulliver aspires to join the intelligence society, the greater grows his revulsion for its antithesis, the Yahoos. On one level, the Yahoos allude to human beings 'exemplified in nonreligious terms by [Thomas] Hobbes's portrait of life in a state of nature as "nasty, brutish, and short"'.[86] In *Leviathan* (1651), Hobbes describes a pre-social condition in which there prevails a 'war of every man against every man', where 'force and fraud are cardinal virtues', the strong prevail, and might makes right.[87] With Gulliver suddenly acting aggressively, or at least tolerating aggressive acts to be carried out for his advantage, the allusion's spotlight unexpectedly shifts, with readers experiencing whiplash, for now they must question whether it is Gulliver who is more brutish than the Yahoos. Is it Gulliver, the *strong* – in his own estimation the most intelligent – killing, or ordering the killing of, the *weak* – the least intelligent? Must the supposedly enlightened members of the intelligence society achieve social supremacy in the same way that every other group vying for dominance goes about attaining it, namely, by reverting to Hobbesian force? Enlightened intelligence resorting to brutishness to suppress those whom it considers brutish indeed presents the reader with a paradox.

Does any direct or indirect textual evidence suggest that the killing of Yahoos should be judged as immoral? In terms of indirect evidence, two pieces can be summoned. The first has to do with the *Yahoo* name. Herbert Zirker and Richard Crider have argued that Swift coined the word *Yahoo* from 'Yahu, variant of *Yahweh*, component of numerous names in the Hebrew Bible, including the Hebrew form of Swift's own first name, 'Yehonanian'.[88] As Crider explains, *Yahu* is a variant of the tetragrammaton, *YHWH*, and of Yahweh, 'the name agreed upon by scholars in the Christian era when they attempted to restore the vowel sounds of the tetragrammaton'.[89] YHWH is thought to be ineffable and to always be holy: its surrogates are assumed to be no less sacred. If this explanation has any truth in it, its point would be this: even if the Yahoos are fallen creatures, they are still made in Yahweh's image and bear his name. Most critics correctly contend that Book Four is not a religious book; however, Biblical allusions do enter into it. Claude Rawson concedes the veiled references to Adam and Eve and Noah's flood.[90] Once these exceptions are admitted, the allusion to *Yahu* must also come into consideration. What might be Swift's reason for alluding to the 'Yahuistic names'?[91] If *Yahoo* were a nonsense term Swift coined, the figures the word stands for would be equally nonsensical, and killing them would not rise to the definition of murder. If Gulliver kills animals, or has them killed, or benefits from their killing, that would provide the basis for a discussion of ethics having to do with the killing of animals; but if he murders, or is complicit in the murder of, humans, that becomes a foundation for an ethical debate directly relevant to this chapter. As has been said before, the text ultimately does not allow the reader to decide one way or the other; for, as with just about everything else connected with the Yahoos, the answer must be deferred. Consequently, the allusion to the Yahuistic' names is just one more piece of information to muddy the waters. Writes Carnochan, 'That would be a fairly characteristic Swiftian joke'.[92] Still, the joke would underscore what ultimately is at issue, namely, the Yahoos' uncertain species status: they are equivocal creatures, existing in the interstices between species. Final decisions as to their potential *personhood* must be endlessly deferred. At the very least, then, Gulliver lacks humility when faced with a complex ethical issue: he refuses to ask, or is incapable of asking, whether the Yahoos are human beings and whether killing them, or having them killed, or benefiting from their killing, amounts to murder or complicity in such acts. Most importantly, Gulliver's association with the killing provides an example of the individual with pretensions to being a 'person' assuming prerogatives over changeling-like creatures – humans in shape only – whom he considers to be non-persons.

While the indirect evidence of the word *Yahoo* does not provide anything definitive as to whether the killing of Yahoos should be deemed immoral, a second piece of indirect evidence, Gulliver's quoting of Virgil, may give some indication. After praising his 'noble Master, and the other illustrious Houyhnhnms', Gulliver recites the following line spoken about Sinon in the *Aeneid* (II: 79–80): '*Nec si miserum Fortuna Sinonem Finxit, vanum etiam, mendacemque improba finget* (Latin: 'Nor, if Fortune has made Sinon for misery, will she also in her spite make him false and a liar').[93] In Troy's last days, Sinon is the Greek who defends 'his veracity while attempting to persuade the Trojans to accept his gift of a giant wooden horse'.[94] The quote's proximity to the immediately preceding praise of the Houyhnhnms connects the Trojan Horse allusion to the intelligence society with which Gulliver has associated the horses. The vessel's surface appearance suggests the benefits of both Enlightenment reason and the tradition of rationality stemming back to the ancient Greeks. However, if the wooden horse's exterior is associated with the Houyhnhnms' seemingly benevolent intelligence society, then what threat lurks inside? Anne Barbeau Gardiner affirms that Book Four 'is about a new Trojan Horse', one that warrants the protagonist to do 'whatever cruel thing is useful to him'.[95] Penetrating the horse's outer shell to consider the hidden danger, one realizes that what looks like a benign gift turns out to be a vehicle for introducing a new social order that authorizes brutality in the name of reason. This returns to the paradox mentioned earlier. In Swift's time, the contours of the burgeoning order could be observed not just in the Augustan satirists' disdain for dunces, but also in the formation of the bourgeoisie, which pointed to its own increasing wealth as a sign of its superior intelligence. Furthermore, what lies concealed is not just brutality, but also the inauguration of rationally systematized violence: when they reach a consensus in their assembly, the horses' intelligence society will exterminate the unintelligent humanoid figures *en masse*. Thus, the allusion to the wooden horse seems to take a sharp turn into the ethical realm. And yet, it does not answer the question of whether the killings of Yahoo offspring in which Gulliver is implicated should be read as morally wrong. It raises the spectre of killing for reason's sake and of systemic killing, but on the question of whether the killing of Yahoo infants should be judged immoral it remains agnostic.

The strongest, direct evidence supporting a reading in which killing Yahoos can be understood to be unequivocally condemned appears in the intellectual resemblance Gulliver himself bears to the Yahoos. Like them, Gulliver too functions allegorically: as has been said, his empiricism marks him as someone with pretensions to membership in the new elite of the intelligence society. And yet, while he empirically *observes closely* in order to imitate the Houyhnhnms' speech and behaviour, this close observation leads to nothing more than earnest mimicry on the level of a parrot. Gulliver in effect demonstrates Goodey's point that the 'concepts of intelligence and intellectual disability are mutually reinforcing';[96] that is, the reader can observe in Gulliver both the affectation of possessing superior intelligence and the malady mentioned earlier, *mobilitas opinionum,* or instability of opinion. While it cannot be said that his character lives with an intellectual disability resembling any present-day diagnosis, he does answer to a dispositional disability that some physicians of his own time would have recognized. Because *gullibility* was 'a frequently cited medical symptom of unstable opinion',[97] the connection between the symptom and Lemuel's surname should be obvious. Does Gulliver suffer from *mobilitas opinionum?* So inconsistent is his character that critics debate whether he qualifies as one at all. Many assert that he really is just a figure supplying whatever Swift's satirical fancy requires in the moment.[98] However, a strong case can be made that Swift is not changing his protagonist from moment to moment to suit his own needs; rather, it is Gulliver the character who lacks stability. He is as protean as another seafarer, Odysseus, but without the cleverness. He can be considered changeable for five reasons of ascending importance.

First, from Book One to Book Four his chauvinistic British nationalism evaporates but without any explanation. For example, in Book Two he brags to the Brobdingnagian king about his nation's greatness, but by the end of Book Four he gleefully contemplates a fantasy of the Houyhnhnms overrunning an invading British force. Second, throughout the first three books and into the first chapters of Book Four, he has engaged in empirical thinking in the Baconian and Lockean traditions. However, midway through the last book, he switches to become a Cartesian rationalist, a way of thinking that had bewildered him in Book Three.[99] In other words, by the end he operates under an intellectual system that (at least to him) seems logical, and he has grown skeptical of the evidence of his senses. Indication of this change comes to light in his classification of the Portuguese sea captain, Pedro de Mendez, as a Yahoo. Gulliver's insistence on considering de Mendez to be a Yahoo despite all of the tangible evidence to the contrary found in the good captain's exceeding kindness illustrates just how much his mind is gripped by an *idée fixe*. Thus, he swings wildly from one system to its opposite without attempting to synthesize the two. Third, signals of *mobilitas opinionum* come to light in the shift in his attitude regarding brutality. Gardiner states that in 'Lilliput he was against persecution', refusing to use his tremendous bulk to subdue Blefuscu. However, in Book Four, after the Houyhnhnm Assembly debates genocide, he himself decides to join 'in on the persecution', at least to the extent that he employs the skins of dead young Yahoos.[100]

Fourth, a striking sign of instability of opinion occurs between the chapter in which he employs the skins of dead Yahoos, and the last,[101] in which he excoriates European colonizers for slaughtering natives. Gulliver is scathing in his denunciation, yet is unable to recognize that his own earlier behaviour with the skins intersects with the very thing he is criticizing. One must ask whether these other white colonizers similarly never stopped to consider whether their non-European victims might also be persons? The reader is supposed to glean that the ethical calculations – or lack of them – transpiring in the minds of these other Europeans engaged in slaughter similarly went on in Gulliver's mind but that he does not make the connection between himself and them. The disconnect inherent in killing natives, or ordering them to be killed, or at least using their skins, but then condemning those who kill natives, demonstrates an instance of 'thinking variably'. Thus, he answers to a dispositional disability that would have been recognized by some doctors of his own time. In sum, when he kills, or orders to be killed, beings who are the equivalent of Locke's *changelings*, he is bringing about the deaths of those whom he himself resembles intellectually, or at least semantically. Indeed, his dispositional disability – excessive changeability – is not controlled until the end (if even then), when, back at home in England, alone with his horses, he finally is 'stable-ized'.[102]

Lastly and most decisively in the matter of his changeability is the way he moves back and forth across the boundary separating *person* from *human*. After his rescue, Gulliver assesses everyone to be a *non-person*, including occasionally himself. Thus, within this narrative in which Gulliver appoints himself arbiter of everyone's personhood status, including his own, no *person* in the Lockean sense rises to the bar and meets the qualifications. In other words, no *person* exists within the story proper, except perhaps Gulliver himself. And even then, he qualifies as a *person* only sporadically; that is, he meets the requirements only during those moments when he is deeming everyone around him to be a Yahoo. But in this he does not remain consistent, for he toggles back and forth between being *person* when he is judging others to be Yahoos and being a *non-person* when he is excoriating himself for being a Yahoo. Prideful in one second, riddled with abject shame the next, he becomes the ultimate *changeling*, alternating between *person* and *non-person* in the blink of an eye, like a figure under a strobe light. By so doing, he becomes a parodic version of Locke's person/non-person binary, with the parody directing attention to the fundamental lack of viability and stability inherent in Locke's category of *personhood*. Gulliver's radical inconsistency in this matter calls attention to the fact that no individual – no matter how 'intelligent' – can think abstractly every second of every day for the duration of a lifetime. In other words, no individual can persist in the pure, whole, and lasting state of perpetual abstract thinking in the way Locke describes it. This realization may be behind what Swift intended in his letter mentioned earlier to Pope when he uses the phrase *rationis capax*. Human beings are *capable* of reason, but even the most intellectually gifted hardly practise it all of the time. Everyone lapses; everyone falls away for periods of time from being a perfect Lockean *person*.

As someone exhibiting extreme changeability in these five ways, Gulliver can be identified as a changeling. While Gulliver reluctantly but explicitly accepts his Yahoo bodily configuration, he is unable to perceive that he also resembles them intellectually. In fact, the more he attempts to emulate the Houyhnhnms, the more he thinks like a Yahoo. As a result, even as Gulliver bids for status based on what he deems to be his own flawless mental powers, he shares with the Yahoos what Locke terms 'a defect in the mind'.[103] Once resettled in England, he again asserts a kind of status bid based on intelligence, one appropriate for *that* island, when he announces in a 'Messianic tone' that he intends to teach his fellow, presumably unteachable Yahoos.[104] This tone goes to the issue of pride. Critics correctly note that the text attacks pride, but they do not go far enough because they speak of a vice along the lines of one of the seven deadly sins. Real and Vienken are more specific when they affirm that Gulliver, on account of 'his pride of reason', is '"mad" for reason'.[105] More precisely, Gulliver's pride – exhibited especially in the book's final lines – derives from his assumption that he is more intelligent than, and, therefore, superior to, others. Even more specifically, it is the pride of the new elite, one implicated 'in the rising faith of "progress", which assumed a perfecting of human behaviour in proportion to the increase of knowledge. All of these ideas, with their emphasis on men's completeness and self-sufficiency, would have seemed to ... Swift signs of an "age of pride"'.[106] Gulliver's pride is born of his believing neither that he is saved (one of the elect in the religious sense) nor that his ancestors were noble. Rather, his pride comes from a smug assumption of mental superiority. It becomes hubris when the reader begins to question whether this aspirant to the intelligence elite kills, or at least is implicated in the killing of, those whom he determines to be his mental inferiors.

Oddly, the reader may not notice these killings, for they occur *obscene* or off-stage, intimating they may have been designed to be easily overlooked. If they do register, the reader may excuse them, for Gulliver has so demonized the victims that the 'Gentle Reader' likely shares his antipathy and so believes they deserve whatever they get.[107] Overweening pride, therefore, may not be confined to Gulliver. Narrator and narratee together may become ensnared in a trap. As Laura Brown notes, 'Neither Gulliver nor Swift's reader can stand clear of this story. It is specifically structured to implicate its audience'.[108] Readers themselves are likely to aspire to join the intelligence society and perhaps themselves may be in the grip of cognitive ableist assumptions. The paradox resides in their being smart enough to understand the allegory's moral, namely, that those who fancy themselves intelligent should practise what Ralph Savarese terms 'an interpretive humility in the face of the cognitively "other"'.[109] However, in a further Swiftian 'joke', or irony, this lesson most likely will be lost on the Gentle Reader.

Ultimately, in addition to Gulliver, the arrogant and complacent readers of Book Four are the butt of Swift's satire. As Swift observes in the preface to *The Battel of the Books*, '*Satyr is a sort of* Glass, *wherein Beholders do generally discover every body's Face but their Own*'.[110] Readers are the butt because they pride themselves as much as Gulliver does on their own supposedly superior intelligence. Brown's insight that Book Four 'is specifically structured to implicate its audience' speaks to the issue of every reader's unperceived cognitive ableism, a prejudice resting on the assumption that intelligence and mental deficit are real things rooted in nature. Real they are for Locke, with the former serving as a punched ticket to personhood, the latter as a chute to changeling status.

An Essay Concerning Human Understanding so locks in a cognitive ableist bias that readers unwittingly influenced by Locke do not recognize how this bias limits understanding. This is the point of Book Four of *Gulliver's Travels*, with readers' general failure to concern themselves with the provenance of the skins attesting to the extent that Locke's views have prevailed. So insidious is the *person-man* binary that it stops consideration of ethics before it can begin. And yet, the skins' provenance provides a place to begin interrogating the way that Gulliver's rapid switching back and forth between person and man not only parodies Locke's *person-man* distinction, but also exposes the notion of intelligence upon which it rests to be a fiction. What may not be apparent to readers under Locke's sway – as it is not obvious to Gulliver – is the possibility that the trait he and they most pride themselves upon having – (intelligence) does not exist. And if it is not real, but a constructed concept, Locke's political legacy of liberal democracy should be reevaluated. These democracies operate on the assumption (or pretense) that almost all individuals have sufficient intelligence to enter into social contracts. The reality may be that few, if any, do. If intelligence is a fiction, these institutions' foundation has a catastrophic structural flaw.

Notes

1 Jonathan Swift, *Gulliver's Travels* [1726/1735], edited by Albert Rivero (New York: Norton, 2002).

2 Jonathan Swift, 'To Alexander Pope', in *The Correspondence of Jonathan Swift* [1725], edited by Harold Williams, 5 vols. (Oxford: Oxford University Press, 1963–65), iii, 103.

3 W. B. Carnochan, *Lemuel Gulliver's Mirror for Man* (Berkeley and Los Angeles: University of California Press, 1968).

4 John Locke, *An Essay Concerning Human Understanding* [1689], edited by Peter Nidditch (Oxford: Oxford University Press, 1975).

5 C. F. Goodey, *A History of Intelligence and 'Intellectual Disability': The Shaping of Psychology in Early Modern Europe* (Farnham and Burlington VT: Ashgate, 2011), 313–346.

6 Peter Singer, *Animal Liberation: A New Ethics for Our Treatment of Animals* (New York: Random House, 1975).

7 Jeff McMahan. *The Ethics of Killing: Problems at the Margins of Life* (New York: Oxford University Press, 2003).

8 Licia Carlson, *The Faces of Intellectual Disability: Philosophical Reflections.* (Bloomington: Indiana University Press, 2009).

9 Eva Feder Kittay, 'The Personal is Philosophical is Political: A Philosopher and Mother of a Cognitively Disabled Person Sends Notes from the Battlefield', in *Cognitive Disability and Its Challenge to Moral Philosophy*, edited by. Eva Feder Kittay and Licia Carlson (Malden MA: Wiley-Blackwell, 2010), 140.

10 Licia Carlson, 'Cognitive Ableism and Disability Studies: Feminist Reflections on the History of Mental Retardation', *Hypatia* 16.4 (2001), 124–145.

11 Swift, *Gulliver's Travels*, 200.
12 Ibid., 237.
13 Isaac Asimov, *The Annotated* Gulliver's Travels (New York: Clarkson Potter, 1980), 270.
14 'Infant, n.1–2', *Oxford English Dictionary* (Oxford: Oxford University Press, 2012), *OED Online*.
15 Swift, *Gulliver's Travels*, 224.
16 Ibid., 237.
17 Ibid., 197.
18 Ibid., 237.
19 Ibid., 200.
20 Ibid., 233, 237.
21 'Skin, n.8.a.', *Oxford English Dictionary*.
22 W. B. Carnochan, email to author, 28April, 2012.
23 Swift, *Gulliver's Travels*, 245.
24 Goodey, *History of Intelligence*, 308.
25 Ibid., 308.
26 Irvin Ehrenpreis, 'The Meaning of Gulliver's Last Voyage', *Review of English Literature* 3.3 (1962), 129.
27 Locke, *Essay* (2.27.9), 335.
28 Goodey, *History of Intelligence*, 275.
29 For more on the all-or-nothing nature of Locke's *person*, see D. Christopher Gabbard, '"What He Found Not Monsters, He Made So": The I-Word and the Bathos of Exclusion', *Journal of Literary and Cultural Disability Studies*, 2.1 (2008), 1–9.
30 Goodey, *History of Intelligence*, 333.
31 'Changeling, n.2', *Oxford English Dictionary*.
32 'Changeling, n.1', *Oxford English Dictionary*.
33 'Changeling, n.3', *Oxford English Dictionary*.
34 'Changeling, n.4', *Oxford English Dictionary*.
35 Goody, *History of Intelligence*, 229.
36 Ibid., 317.
37 Ibid., 180.
38 Ibid., 228.
39 C. F. Goodey, email message to the author, 8 September, 2014.
40 Goodey, *History of Intelligence*, 229.
41 'Changelings, n.1', *Oxford English Dictionary*.
42 Jonathan Andrews, 'Begging the Question of Idiocy: The Definition and Socio-Cultural Meaning of Idiocy in Early Modern Britain: Part 1', *History of Psychiatry* 9 (1998), 68.
43 Goodey, *History of Intelligence*, 289–290.
44 Locke, *Essay* (3.11.20), 519.
45 Ibid. (3.6.26), 454.

46 Ibid. (4.4.16), 571–572.

47 Paul de Man, 'The Epistemology of Metaphor', in *Aesthetic Ideology*, edited by Andrzez Warminski (Minneapolis and London: University of Minnesota Press, 1996), 40.

48 Locke, Essay (4.4.16), 572.

49 Lila V. Graves, 'Locke's changeling and the Shandy bull', *Philological Quarterly* 60.2 (1981), 258.

50 Carnochan, *Lemuel Gulliver's Mirror for Man*, 144.

51 J. A. Downie, 'Gulliver's Fourth Voyage and Locke's *Essay Concerning Human Understanding*', in *Reading Swift: Papers from the Fifth Münster Symposium on Jonathan Swift* (2008), 463.

52 Dennis Todd, *Imagining Monsters: Miscreations of the Self in Eighteenth-Century England* (Chicago: University of Chicago Press, 1995), 140–178.

53 Hermann Real and Heinz J. Vienken, 'The Structure of *Gulliver's Travels*', *Proceedings of the First Münster Symposium on Jonathan Swift* 1 (1985), 206.

54 Spencer Wertz and Linda Wertz, 'Some Correlations Between Swift's *Gulliver's Travels* and Locke on Personal Identity', *Journal of Thought* 10 (1975), 267.

55 Wertz and Wertz, 'Some Correlations', 268.

56 Ian Higgins, *Jonathan Swift* (Tavistock: Northcote House, 2004), 64.

57 Ibid., 64.

58 Anthony Manousos, 'Swiftian Scatology and Lockean Psychology', *The Gypsy Scholar* 7 (1980), 19.

59 Higgins, *Jonathan Swift*, 71.

60 Todd, *Imagining Monsters*, 150.

61 Herbert Zirker, 'Horse Sense and Sensibility: Some Issues concerning Utopian Understanding in *Gulliver's Travels*', *Swift Studies: The Annual of the Ehrenpreis Center* 12 (1997), 97, 89, 90.

62 Higgins, *Jonathan Swift*, 71.

63 Swift, *Gulliver's Travels*, 189.

64 Ibid., 189.

65 'Discomposed, adj.1', *Oxford English Dictionary*.

66 Swift, *Gulliver's Travels*, 189.

67 'Singular, adj.13', *Oxford English Dictionary*.

68 'Deformed, adj.2', *Oxford English Dictionary*.

69 David Williams, *Deformed Discourse: The Function of the Monster in Mediaeval Thought and Literature* (Montreal: McGill-Queen's University Press, 1996), 5, 324.

70 Roger Lund, 'Laughing at Cripples: Ridicule, Deformity and the Argument from Design', *Eighteenth-Century Studies* 39.1 (2005), 94.

71 Mary Louise Pratt, *Imperial Eyes: Travel Writing and Transculturation* (New York: Routledge, 1992), 6.

72 Swift, *Gulliver's Travels*, 190.

73 David Nokes, *Jonathan Swift, A Hypocrite Reversed: A Critical Biography* (New York and London: Oxford University Press, 1985), 326.

74 Swift, *Gulliver's Travels*, 200.

75 Liz Bellamy, *Jonathan Swift's* Gulliver's Travels (New York: St. Martin's Press, 1992), 92.

76 Locke, *Essay* (2.33.5), 395.

77 Ibid., 232.

78 'People, n.6', *Oxford English Dictionary*.

79 'People, n.1–2', *Oxford English Dictionary*.

80 Allen Michie, 'Gulliver the Houyahoo: Swift, Locke, and the Ethics of Excessive Individualism', in *Humans and Other Animals in Eighteenth-Century British Culture: Representation, Hybridity, Ethics*, edited by Frank Palmeri (Burlington VT: Ashgate: 2006), 71.

81 Todd, *Imagining Monsters*, 240.

82 Swift, *Gulliver's Travels*, 228.

83 Nicholas Hudson, 'Gulliver's Travels and Locke's Radical Nominalism', *1650–1850: Ideas, Aesthetics, and Inquiries in the Early Modern Era* 1 (1994), 262; Wertz and Wertz, 'Some Correlations', 267.

84 Locke, *Essay* (3.6.26), 453.

85 de Man, 'Epistemology of Metaphor', 40.

86 Maynard Mack, 'Gulliver's Travels', in *Swift: A Collection of Critical Essays*, edited by Ernest Tuveson (Englewood Cliffs NJ: Prentice-Hall, 1964), 112.

87 Thomas Hobbes, *Leviathan* [1651] (Corvallis: Oregon State University), accessed 27 April, 2012, http://oregonstate.edu/instruct/phl302/texts/hobbes/leviathan-contents.html.

88 Richard Crider, 'Yahoo (Yahu), Notes on the Name of Swift's Yahoos', *Names: A Journal of Onomastics* 41.2 (1993), 103; Zirker, 'Horse Sense'.

89 Crider, 'Yahoo (Yahu)', 104.

90 Swift, *Gulliver's Travels*, 228; Claude Rawson, *God, Gulliver, and Genocide: Barbarism and the European Imagination, 1492–1945* (Oxford and New York: Oxford University Press, 2001), 254, 264.

91 Zirker, 'Horse Sense', 86.

92 W. B. Carnochan, email message to the author, 28 April, 2012.

93 Swift, *Gulliver's Travels*, 246.

94 Jonathan Swift, *Gulliver's Travels* [1726/1735], edited by Albert Rivero (New York: Norton, 2002), 246.

95 Anne Barbeau Gardiner, 'Jonathan Swift and the Idea of the Fundamental Church', in *Fundamentalism and Literature*, edited by Catherine Pesso-Miquel and Klaus Stiertorfer (New York: Palgrave Macmillan, 2007), 38, 36.

96 Goodey, *History of Intelligence*, 1.

97 Ibid., 228–229.

98 J. Paul Hunter, 'Gulliver's Travels and the Later Writings', in *Cambridge*

Companion to Jonathan Swift, edited by Christopher Fox (Cambridge and New York: Cambridge University Press, 2003), 224.

99 David Renaker, 'Swift's Laputians as a Caricature of the Cartesians', *PMLA* 94 (1979), 936–944.

100 Gardiner, 'Jonathan Swift', 36, 39.

101 Swift, *Gulliver's Travels*, Bk 4, chs. 10 and 12.

102 Zirker, 'Horse Sense', 93.

103 Locke, *Essay* (4.4.16), 572.

104 Nokes, *Jonathan Swift*, 328.

105 Real and Vienken, 'Structure of *Gulliver's Travels*', 208.

106 Ernest Tuveson, '*Gulliver's Travels*', in *Swift: A Collection of Critical Essays*, edited by Ernest Tuveson (Englewood Cliffs NJ: Prentice-Hall, 1964), 105.

107 Swift, *Gulliver's Travels*, 245.

108 Laura Brown, *Fables of Modernity: Literature and Culture in the English Eighteenth Century* (Ithaca: Cornell University Press, 2001), 242.

109 Ralph Savarese, *Reasonable People: A Memoir of Autism and Adoption* (New York: Other Press, 2007), 424.

110 Jonathan Swift, 'Battel of the Books', in *Jonathan Swift: The Essential Writings*, edited by Claude Rawson and Ian Higgins (New York: Norton, 2010), 95.

7

SENSATIONALISM AND THE CONSTRUCTION OF INTELLECTUAL DISABILITY

Tim Stainton

It was reasonable to hope, that if ever there appeared a creature similar to those of whom we have spoken [a 'wild child' untainted by society], the sciences in question would bring to bear all the resources of their present knowledge in order to develop him physically and morally, or, at least, if this proved impossible or fruitless, there would be found in this age of observation someone who, carefully collecting the history of so surprising a creature, would determine what he is and would deduce from what he lacks the hitherto uncalculated sum of knowledge and ideas which man owes to his education.

Dare I confess that I have proposed myself both of these two great undertakings?[1]

So wrote Jean-Marc-Gaspard Itard (1774–1838), who, with this goal in mind, began what is often cited as the beginning of educational efforts on behalf of persons with intellectual disability, the education of Victor, the 'Wild Boy of Aveyron'.

The story of Victor, and Itard's efforts towards his education, is at its outset the story of one battle in the struggle to prove the primacy of sensual experience over innate ideas in the development of human understanding. As Itard notes of his observations of Victor, 'If they are collected, methodically classified and correctly evaluated we shall have material proof of the most important truths, truths which Locke and Condillac were able to discover by the power of their genius and the depths of their meditations alone'.[2] With Victor, Itard hoped to deliver the *coup de grace* in this debate by showing that, with the proper sensory stimulation, Victor could be raised from his 'savage state' to join the ranks of the fully human citizen in the new world of revolutionary France.

Locke had anticipated the experiment somewhat in reverse when he argued that if there were innate ideas these '*should appear fairest in and clearest in* those

Persons, ... For *Children, Ideots, Savages,* and *illiterate* People, being of all others least corrupted by Custom, or borrowed Opinion ... one might reasonably imagine, that in their Minds these innate Notions should lie open fairly to everyone's view'.[3] And indeed speculations on the light which children, savages (both the 'wild child' variety and various aboriginal populations), along with animated statues and 'natural man', could shed on these questions abounded in the eighteenth and early nineteenth centuries. 'Ideots', however, were not among the subjects of these real and speculative experiments, except as perhaps in Victor's case, and those other wild children, by accident or mistake. Itard's experiment was squarely in the centre of a number of related debates central to the enlightenment: the source of human understanding; the perfectibility and malleability of man; and, the question of what defined man's true nature and characterized him as a distinct species. As with Locke, though, the 'idiot' was largely an accidental subject in these debates; the 'savage man', however, was a central character and it was to this imputed identity that Itard was drawn. The presence of some form of organic intellectual disability was denied by Itard, despite many who argued to the contrary,[4] and were it not for this belief on Itard's part, Victor would have likely been left, as Itard suggests, to 'die of misery and boredom at Bicêtre'.[5]

In this chapter we will consider the broader context and debates that shaped Itard's work and the theories which underpinned it, notably the work of Locke, Rousseau, and Condillac, whose revision of Locke would create the foundation for the coming medico-psychological hegemony over intellectual disability. We will also consider how these emerging ideas shaped the development of educational and medical efforts related to intellectual disability. Given the amount of work that has been produced on Itard and Victor, we will limit this discussion to the issues most relevant to the broad construction of intellectual disability and the subsequent social response. While the details of Itard's methods will be of interest to those concerned with the history of psychology and education, these are well covered elsewhere[6] and of less interest to our concerns here. To begin, we will turn to Locke, whose theory of sensationalism was the foundation of Rousseau's, Condillac's and, ultimately, Itard's work.

Nihil est in intellectu quod non pirus fuerit in sensu[7]

Sensationalism, the theory that all knowledge was acquired not from innate ideas or principles in the mind, but from the experience and processing of our sensory experience, was certainly not original to Locke, there being both classical and prior contemporary examples of similar theories,[8] but Locke's presentation of the theory was arguably the most influential and, particularly for our purposes, the most commonly noted source influencing the history of intellectual disability.

The *Essay Concerning Human Understanding* begins with Locke's refutation of the 'established Opinions amongst some Men, That there are in Understanding certain *innate Principles*; some primary Notions, ... stamped upon the Mind of Man, which the soul receives in its very first Being; and brings into the World with it'.[9] He initially takes on the argument of Universal Consent – the idea that there are certain principles which are 'universally agreed upon by All Mankind', which therefore must be based on impressions which 'the Souls of men receive in their first Beings'.[10] Locke's refutation begins by arguing that if this were so, then all men would share these principles [Universal Assent], and yet there are those who not only do not assent to them but to whom they are completely unknown. Not surprisingly, it is here that the 'ideot' makes his first appearance in the *Essay*, for, far from there being Universal Assent to certain principles, 'all *Children*, and Ideots, have not the least Apprehension or Thought of them'.[11]

He returns to this in his summation of the argument, adding a slightly different twist. He notes that if these notions were indeed innate, they

> *should appear fairest in and clearest* in [children, ideots, etc], ... For *Children, Ideots, Savages*, and *illiterate* People, being of all others least corrupted by Custom, or borrowed Opinion ... one might reasonably imagine, that in their Minds these innate Notions should lie open fairly to everyone's view .... It might very well be expected, that these Principles should be perfectly known to naturals; which being stamped immediately on the Soul (as these men suppose) can have no dependence on the Constitutions, or Organs of the Body, the only confessed difference between them and others. One would think ... that all these native Beams of Light (were there any such) should in those, who have no Reserves, no Art of Concealment, shine out in their full Lustre ... . But alas, amongst *Children, Ideots, Savages*, and the grosly illiterate, what general maxim are to be found? What universal Principles of Knowledge? Their Notions are few and narrow, borrowed only from those Objects, they have had the most to do with, and which have made upon their Senses the frequentest and strongest Impressions.[12]

In this passage we can see the rejection of the traditional ideas of the truthspeaking idiot and the 'true man' intact within a corrupted earthly body, ideas which he more explicitly rejects later in the *Essay*, severing the remnants of the limited protection of grace. This is consistent with Locke's broader project of establishing the role of human reason and the autonomous individual in opposition to a complete reliance on Divine Will to dictate human action and understanding.[13]

Locke conceived of the mind as a *tabula rasa* or blank slate upon which experience and reflection derived from sensation leave their impression, and from which ideas or knowledge are eventually derived:

> Let us suppose the Mind to be, as we say, a white Paper, void of all Characters, without any *ideas*; How comes it to be furnished? ... Whence has it all the materials of Reason and Knowledge? To this I answer, in one word, From *Experience*.[14]

For Locke there were two sources of knowledge based on experience, the first being *Sensation*:

> *Our Senses*, conversant about particular sensible objects, do *convey into the Mind*, several distinct *Perceptions* of things, according to those various ways, wherein those Objects do affect them: And thus we come by those *Ideas*, we have of *Yellow, White, Heat, Cold, Soft, Hard, Bitter, Sweet*, and all those we call sensible qualities.[15]

The second source of knowledge from experience is reflection:

> The *Perception of the Operations of our own Minds* within us, as it is employ'd about the *Ideas* it has got; which Operations, when the Soul comes to reflect on, and consider, do furnish the Understanding with another set of *Ideas*, which could not be had from things without: and such are, *Perception, Thinking, Doubting, Believing, Reasoning, Knowing, Willing*, and all the different actings of our own Minds; which we being conscious of, and observing in ourselves, do from these receive into our Understandings, as distinct *Ideas*, as we do from Bodies affecting our Senses.[16]

It should be noted, however, that while Locke rejected the idea of innate knowledge, he did not reject the idea of innate *faculties* or powers which allow us to sense and reflect. God, according to Locke, 'hath furnished Man with those Faculties, which will serve for the sufficient discovery of all things requisite to the end of such being; ... a Man by the right use of his natural Abilities, may, without any innate Principles, attain the Knowledge of God, and other things that concern him'.[17] These faculties include perception, retention, and discerning, the ability to perceive two ideas as the same or different.[18] In his chapter on discerning he also discusses several 'Operations' of the mind, including comparison, composition, and abstraction – the absence of which demarks brutes from man and places the changeling somewhere in between. It is these 'innate faculties' which would be disputed by Condillac and others, as we shall discuss below.

Locke also discusses our capacity to experience pleasure and pain, which in turn define good and evil, for what we call good is that which is 'apt to cause or increase Pleasure, or diminish Pain in us; or else to procure, or preserve us the possession of any other Good, or absence of any Evil'; similarly, Evil is that which 'is apt to produce or increase pain'.[19] These in turn are the 'hinges on which our passions turn': love, hatred, joy, sorrow, hope, fear, despair, anger, and envy, and so forth.[20] All of these are rooted in our sense experience rather than an *a priori* notion of good or evil. Our reason naturally leads us to the good as directed by our experience, if we make 'the right use of [our] natural Abilities'.[21] The section on pleasure and pain is immediately followed in the *Essay* by a long chapter on power where Locke discusses, among other things, how the faculties and operations of the mind are applied in determining preferences and making choices. It is this process which makes us free agents. Our liberty to act or forebear as we choose according to our preference can be affected by our passions, which may temporarily constrain our liberty.[22] Our choices are determined by our desire for happiness, which for Locke ultimately consists in the right use of reason which, if applied properly and not distracted by a desire for short-term or more immediate pleasures, will lead us to a Knowledge of God and our ultimate Happiness.

In discussing the nature of liberty, he questions whether the necessity of examining our desires before acting to determine if they are consistent with our ultimate happiness is an infringement of our liberty. In answer to this, he asks:

> would anyone be a Changeling, because he is less determined, by wise Considerations, than a wise Man? Is it worth the Name of *Freedom*, to be at liberty to play the Fool, and draw Shame and Misery upon a Man's self? If to break loose from the conduct of Reason, and to want that restraint of Examination and Judgment, which keeps us from chusing or doing the worse, be *Liberty*, true Liberty, mad Men and Fools are the only Freemen: ... The Constant desire of Happiness, and the constraint it puts upon us to act for it, no Body, I think, accounts an abridgement of *Liberty*, or at least an abridgement to be complained of.[23]

In the above we can of course see a strong logical consistency with the *Treatise of Government*, where those who are unable to perform this process cannot be free agents.

The idea of natural abilities, combining with the basic theory of knowledge derived from our sensation and reflection, opens the possibilities both of a developmental psychology and of an education, both practical and, more importantly, moral, as the greater one's reason and ability to perform the operations of the mind necessary for processing sensory information, the closer one comes to the 'true knowledge of God'. While this formulation does

present a more egalitarian possibility, it also implies both a practical and, ultimately, moral inequality based on variation in one's innate abilities, such as a
failure to develop one's capacity through lack of education or application or a
willful following of one's desires without regard to one's 'true happiness'.

In discussing how God has furnished men with the faculties necessary to
formulate ideas and understanding, Locke notes that God is under no obligations to provide them with innate knowledge:

> God having endued Man with those Faculties of knowing which he hath, was
> no more obliged by his Goodness, to implant those innate Notions in his Mind,
> than that having given him Reason, Hands, and Materials, he should build him
> Bridges, or Houses; which some People in the World, however of good parts, do
> either totally want, or are but ill provided of, as well as others are wholly without
> *Ideas of God*, and Principles of Morality; or at least have but very ill ones. The
> reason in both cases being, That they never employ'd their Parts, Faculties, and
> Powers, industriously that way, but contented themselves with the Opinions,
> Fashions, and Things of their Country, as they found them, without looking any
> farther.[24]

Locke makes a similar point in his later unfinished work *On the Conduct
of Understanding* but, as Goodey notes, he seems more pessimistic in the
potential for those who 'never elevate their thoughts above the spade and
plow ... you will find him no more capable of reasoning than the almost a
perfect natural'.[25] The perfect natural, on the other hand, has no possibility of
improvement whatsoever as he lacks the necessary parts.

As the previous section implies, education is a means of both practical and moral development. Indeed one may even say that education is a
moral duty, since it is only the right use of reason that leads us to knowledge
of God. It is not surprising, then, that Locke developed his own system
of education and addressed it in several works including the *Essay*, the
Conduct of Understanding, and *Thoughts Concerning the Reading and Study
for a Gentleman*. His most significant work on education was, however, *Some
Thoughts Concerning Education*, written while in exile in Holland while he was
also working on the *Essay*.[26] *Some Thoughts* were originally written as a series
of letters to his friend Edward Clarke who sought Locke's advice on educating his children. Eventually they were published on the urging of William
Molyneux, but they retain a very practical if somewhat loosely organized and
repetitive manner.[27]

Locke's educational writings are very much linked to his philosophical and
political writings[28] and are grounded in his sensationalist theory.[29] The focus
on the whole person is evident from the first lines of *Some Thoughts*, where
Locke, following Juvenal, begins with:

A sound mind in a sound body, is a short but full description of a happy state in this world: he that has these two, has little more to wish for; and he that wants either of them, will be but little the better for anything else ... He whose mind direct not wisely, will never take the right way; and he whose body is crazy and feeble, will never be able to advance in it ... .of all the men we meet with, nine parts of ten are what they are, good or evil, useful or not, by their education.[30]

The emphasis on the individual's responsibility for his own development follows from what we have discussed above regarding the possession of faculties and powers which we then must develop. Similarly, he makes it clear that for those who lack such capacities, education is pointless. The importance of developing one's natural endowments is critical to both the development of moral man and of the autonomous agent fit for membership in the civic community envisaged in *Two Treatises*.[31] Not surprisingly, then, Locke has nothing to say about the education of those thought to lack the basic means of joining the ranks of either.

The importance of the environment and the overall sensory experience runs throughout the text. 'I imagine the Minds of Children as easily turned this way or that, as Water, and that little, and almost insensible Impressions on our tender infancies have a very important and lasting Consequences'.[32] He begins with a long discussion of the 'health of the body', which includes the proper clothing (not too tight), diet, exercise and outdoor activities. He also discusses early in the text the need not to let the child have whatever it wishes, in order for the child to develop 'mastery over its desires'. This is to be done at a very early age so that it becomes habit as the child grows. On the other hand, too strict a discipline and too many rules will stifle the child. Locke argues against the use of corporeal punishment as it leads the child to balance one form of corporeal experience, such as the pleasure of misbehaving, with another, the pain of the rod,[33] rather than developing the ability to determine what are the right actions through use of the mind. Learning, for Locke, should be fun and the environment should contain a variety of playthings to stimulate the child.[34] The use of examples is, for Locke, the 'plainest, easiest, and most efficacious' method rather than 'discourse which can be made to them'.[35] This again is consistent with his sensationalism.

Repetition and practice of lessons is preferred over the memorization of rules in order to 'establish habits ... which once being established, operate of themselves easily and naturally, without the assistance of memory'.[36] Imitation is also a critical aspect of education, and hence controlling the environment and those who are around the child is critical to a proper education.[37] For Locke, education is not so much about learning specifics as it is about developing an ability to observe and reflect on experience and making choices which conform to reason. The aims of education are virtue, wisdom, breeding, and lastly, learning. Learning alone, without the prior three, can lead to ill as easily to good, hence the first three are necessary to provide the appropriate context for learning.[38]

Locke emphasizes that education must be appropriate to the child's particular personality and ability:

> in many cases, all that we can do, or should aim at, is to make the best of what nature has given … . Every one's natural genius should be carried as far as it could; but to attempt the putting another upon him, will be but labour in vain.[39]

This follows from Locke's views, discussed above, regarding the variation in natural faculties. He did not believe in unlimited potential, unlike some of the eighteenth-century environmentalists who believed man might learn almost anything,[40] but rather was concerned that a child's natural abilities were developed to their fullest potential. Teaching methods too were to be suited to a child's level of reasoning and adapted to that child's capacities.[41] He also believed that learning should be suited to these ends rather than, for instance, forcing the study of Latin on someone who would have no use of it.[42] Needless to say, the idea of any sort of education for 'idiots' would not have entered into Locke's scheme, despite the suggestion of his former tutor Willis (discussed below) that all people would benefit from some form of education.[43]

Locke's method and theories would not sit too awry with modern approaches to education – a focus on the individual, adaptation of methods and curriculum to the child's ability and interest, and learning through example and repetition rather than rote memorization and lecture. Indeed Locke's educational writings would have a significant impact in England[44] and even more so in France,[45] where, coupled with his sensationalism, they would, albeit somewhat accidentally, have a profound influence on the beginning of attempts to teach the intellectually disabled.

Perfectibility and the natural man

As Goldstein notes, 'under the aegis of sensationalism, the eighteenth century saw – at least in England, its American colonies, and France – something of a pedagogical mania'.[46] The sensationalist view opened the possibility of a developmental psychology and of human malleability and, ultimately, perfection. Indeed, for Rousseau it is this quality of improvement, along with free will, which distinguishes man from beast; 'a faculty', writes Rousseau, 'which as circumstances offer, successively unfolds all the other faculties, and reside among us not only in the Species, but in the individuals that compose it'.[47]

Interestingly he uses people's tendency to lose their mental faculties as they age in furthering his argument, asking 'Why is man alone subject to Dotage?'[48] Is it not because he thus returns to his primitive Condition? And because the Beast, which has acquired nothing and has likewise nothing to lose, continues always in Possession of his Instinct?'[49] He thus asserts man's singular ability through his reason and free will to change and develop both collectively and individually (although for Rousseau this was not necessarily a positive quality).[50]

A proper sensory education was the key to this development and Rousseau, who was profoundly influenced by Locke, sought to illustrate just what constitutes such an education in his great work on education, *Émile*, published in 1762.

> We are born weak, we need strength; we are born totally unprovoked, we need aid; we are born stupid, we need judgment. Everything we do not have at our birth and which we need when we are grown is given us by education.[51]

Rousseau follows Locke quite closely in his view on the role of sensations[52] in developing human understanding but famously departs from Locke, and most of his contemporaries, including Itard, in his view of the role of society. For Rousseau, society is a corrupting influence, as expressed by his famous dictum from *The Social Contract*, 'Man is born free; and is everywhere in chains'.[53] In his *Discourse on Inequality* Rousseau elaborates how man, 'born, equal, self sufficient, unprejudiced and whole' is gradually 'defined by relations of inequality, dependent, full of false opinions or superstitions'.[54] Man in a state of nature is naturally good and happy, but the development of his faculties and mind has led him to civilization, misery, and immorality. 'Good social institutions are those which best know how to denature man, to take his absolute existence [that of the state of nature] in order to give him a relative one and transport the I into the common unity, with the result that each individual believes himself no longer one but part of the common unity'.[55]

In *Émile*, Rousseau seeks to demonstrate a course of education which will build on and protect this natural man, preparing him to resist the corrupting influence of society and develop his natural instincts.

> We are born with the use of our senses, and from our birth we are affected in various ways by the objects surrounding us. As soon as we have, so to speak, consciousness of our sensations, we are disposed to seek or avoid the objects which produce them, at first according to whether they are pleasant or unpleasant to us ... and finally according to the judgments we make about them on the basis of the idea of happiness or of perfection given us by reason. These dispositions are extended and strengthened as we become more capable of using our senses and

more enlightened; but constrained by our habits, they are more or less corrupted
by our opinions. Before this corruption they are what I call in us *nature*.
It is, then, to these original dispositions that everything must be related.[56]

Rousseau's project then is not to educate Émile with specific knowledge, but
to explore how to live an authentic life in tune with his natural inclinations
rather than the dictates of civil society: 'education consists less in precept than
in practice. We begin to instruct ourselves when we begin to live. Our education begins with us ... . to live is not to breathe; it is to act; it is to make use of
our senses, our faculties, of all the parts of ourselves which give us the senti-
ment of our existence'.[57] By following closely the dictates of our senses and
faculties, we are led by our true self, our natural self, which, for Rousseau will
lead to good and happiness.

In Rousseau's view, then, a sensory education is essential for human
equality, freedom, and happiness, just as for Locke our faculties, when used
appropriately, will lead us naturally to God. Rousseau's subject is, of course,
not a 'savage man' but a child, who is educated as natural man, untainted by
civil society until he is secure in himself and the dictates of his own sensations
and faculties. This extends for Rousseau to denying any books but one to his
pupil: *Robinson Crusoe*, Daniel Defoe's tale of 'solitary man in a state of nature,
outside civil society and unaffected by the deeds and opinions of men'.[58] While
Rousseau admits that Crusoe's isolated state will not be Émile's, he notes
that 'it is on this basis that he ought to appraise all others. The surest means
of raising oneself above prejudices and ordering one's judgements about the
true relations of things is to put oneself in the place of an isolated man and to
judge everything as this man himself ought to judge of it with respect to his
own utility'.[59]

Rousseau accepts the sensationalist theory without reservation, including,
it would seem, Locke's notion of innate faculties, though he makes no specific
comment on this. Rousseau's project, however, was not so much to prove the
sensationalist claim, but to demonstrate a course of education using the sensationalist view of human knowledge, with the ultimate goal of ensuring that
man's true nature is revealed as a free, equal citizen uncorrupted by the civil
society, the source of inequality and misery. We can see, however, the core
ideas which would inform Itard's work: malleability, sensationalist education,
and the 'uncorrupted mind'. For Itard, these were found in an 'isolated man'
rather than a child, but both are equally *tabula rasas* ready to be written upon.

Before we leave Rousseau it is worth a comment on what this means for
those whose sensory tools, as it were, may be compromised by disability or
illness.

I would not take on a sickly and ill-constituted child, were he to live until eighty. I want no pupil always useless to himself and others involved uniquely with preserving himself, whose body does damage to the education of his soul ... Let another in my stead take charge of this invalid. I consent to it and approve his charity. But that is not my talent. I am not able to teach living to one who thinks of nothing but how to keep himself from dying.[60]

For Rousseau, this is consistent with the sensationalist doctrine that, 'The body must be vigorous in order to obey the soul'.[61] He makes no direct comment about the mind being strong enough to direct the body, but this would seem to be a reasonable assumption about Rousseau's belief.[62]

While Rousseau's subject was a hypothetical child, others had their isolated man: Voltaire had Candide and a Huron Indian, Buffon had his new Adam, and, as Lane points out, 'La Mettrie and Diderot thought something could be learned from the partial isolation of the deaf-mute'.[63] The most influential immediate intellectual predecessor for Itard, however, and the person most closely associated with a significant shift in the sensationalist doctrine, was Etienne Bonnot De Condillac (1714–80), with his animated statue.[64]

A single source of ideas

Harlan Lane, in discussing Itard's education of Victor, suggests that both directly and through the influence of Pinel, the towering figure of French psychiatry, and de l'Épée, the famed teacher of deaf-mutes, 'Condillac can be called the patron saint of the whole enterprise, from beginning to end'.[65] His sensationalist/empiricist philosophy and methods would both inform and guide Itard's works. Though Itard credits both Locke and Condillac as inspiration, it was Condillac who would be his most direct source.

Condillac was strongly influenced by Locke's *Essay*; indeed he subtitled his early work on sensationalism *Essai sur l'origine des Connaissance Humaines (1746)* (translated as *An Essay on the Origin of Human Knowledge*) as *being a supplement to Mr. Locke's Essay on the Human Understanding.*[66] As Weyant notes, Condillac's *Essay* was the first in a series of works which sought to defend Locke's sensationalist epistemology,[67] the most relevant of which is his later work the *Traite de Sensations* (1754), which developed and clarified his arguments in the *Essay* through the use of a thought experiment where he gradually awakens the understanding of an animated statue by the gradual introduction of various sensory stimulations.

Condillac is critical of prior attempts, such as Buffon's, to prove the sensationalist claim because they invest man with habits which they 'should have made him acquire', and he goes on to claim that his *Treatise* 'is the only work which strips man of all his habits. By observing the birth of sensation, we show how we acquire the use of our faculties'.[68] His use of the statue allows him to begin with not just an isolated man, but a 'proto man' devoid of all human habit and understanding which neither 'savage man' nor children could claim. By the gradual introduction of different sensations – smell, hearing, taste, sight, and touch – he seeks to show how these, working in concert, lead to ideas and memory. Condillac notes, à la Locke, that ideas are both of a simple and complex variety, but Condillac also divides them into sensory ideas, those which 'are currently acting on our senses',[69] and intellectual ideas, which

> represent those that have already disappeared after having made their impressions: these ideas differ from each other only as memory differs from sensation … .
>
> The more memory one has, the more one is consequently capable of acquiring intellectual ideas. These ideas are the stock of our knowledge, just as sensory ideas are its origin.[70]

While it is beyond the scope of this chapter to fully articulate Condillac's theory of how the senses provide the source of all our knowledge, it should be clear at this point that he did not depart significantly from Locke in this regard. While this is generally true, there is one critical aspect in which he disagrees with Locke:

> Locke distinguishes two sources of our ideas, the senses and reflection. It would be more precise to recognize only a single one, either because reflection is underlying only reflection itself, or because it is less the source of our ideas than the channel by which they are derived from the senses …
>
> Thus the philosopher is content to recognize that the mind perceives, thinks, doubts, believes, reasons, knows, wills, reflects; that we are convinced of the existence of these operations because we find them in ourselves, and that they contribute to the progress of our knowledge; but he did not suspect that they could only be acquired habits, he seems to regard them as something innate, and he says only that they are perfected through use.
>
> Judgment, reflection, passion, all the operations of the mind, in short, are only sensation itself variously transformed.[71]

Locke, as discussed above, argued that God 'hath furnished Man with those Faculties, which will serve for the sufficient discovery of all things requisite to the end of such being; …a Man by the right use of his natural Abilities, may, without any innate Principles, attain the Knowledge of God, and other things that concern him'.[72] These faculties include perception, retention, and discerning, the ability to perceive two ideas as the same or different.[73] For Condillac, these all proceed from sensation rather than being innate.

Ernst Cassirer notes the struggle to 'get rid of the last remnants of dualism which had remained in Locke's psychological principles ... to do away with the distinction between internal and external experience and reduce all human knowledge to a single source'.[74] While the English went in the direction of reflection, the French sought to resolve the dualism in reduction to sensation.

This reduction to sensation as a single source of knowledge and faculties essentially reduces the acquisition of knowledge to a physical process, and the subject essentially is a passive recipient of these sensations.[75] Not surprisingly then, Weyant can note the association between Condillac and his fellow *philosophes* and some twentieth-century psychologists such as B. F. Skinner.[76] This connection will be clearer when we discuss Itard's application of Condillac's theory to the education of Victor below. For now, though, we can see how a system which does not presume innate faculties of reason may be conducive to the education of those where such faculties are not readily apparent, such as 'wild men', and by extension or accident, to those with some form of intellectual disability.

Indeed, Weyant notes how Condillac's insistence on sensory processes as the basis of *all* knowledge led later thinkers, such as Helvétius, to argue that all men at birth are in fact equal in capacity and potential, and that all differentiation is simply dependent on the experiences and education a particular person has.[77] This denial of any 'natural' inequality between persons was a complete rejection of any innate differences in ability between persons and also, by implication, of any natural hierarchy of men based on class or breeding, leaving only social causes, on the one hand, and difference in will and ambition on the other, to differentiate between persons. Condillac himself dances around this somewhat. He notes that 'If we examine the difference between one man and another, we will be astonished to see how, in the same period of time, some live so much more than others do'. He goes on to state, 'For we enjoy things not only by sight, hearing taste, smell touch; we enjoy them further through memory, imagination, reflection, the passions, hopes; in short by all our faculties. But these basic sources are not all equally active in all men'.[78] So while Condillac certainly recognized difference amongst men, it is not clear what he means by 'active', which could be taken to be referring to will or, a deficit in experience or in innate capacity. Regardless of Condillac's view on this, it is clear that he takes a step beyond Locke, who recognized innate faculties and their 'natural' differentiation between men (note his views on education suited to station) and the external or sensory basis of developing those faculties essential to reasoning, reflection, imagination and so on.

Douthwaite notes that 'Because of Condillac's insistence on the physical origins of mental processes, the whole economy of the *Traité* is predicated on a passive subject whose actions are essentially reactions'.[79] Victor, and sub-sequently people with intellectual disabilities, would be that passive subject.

Victor and Itard

Let us return now to Victor and Itard. The physical/sensationalist nature of Itard's methods are immediately obvious; for example, in order to enhance Victor's receptivity to sensations, Itard has him given very hot and very cold baths for two to three hours a day. Later in his training, in an attempt to deal with Victor's frequent violent outbursts Itard decides on a rather dramatic approach:

> The occasion soon offered itself in the instance of a most violent fit … Seizing the moment when the functions of the senses were not yet suspended, I violently threw back the window of his room which was on the fourth storey and which opened perpendicularly on to a big stone court. I drew near him with every appearance of anger and seizing him forcibly by the haunches held him out of the window, his head directly turned towards the bottom of the chasm. After some seconds I drew him in again. He was pale, covered with a cold sweat, his eyes were rather tearful.[80]

Dramatic as this is, it is not a far cry from more recent attempts to deal with so called challenging behaviour; indeed, it seems almost humane compared to electric shock and other aversive methods in use today. The roots of such methods are very much in the strict sensationalist tradition of Condillac.

There is much more to be said about Itard and his legacy, but this has been well covered by a number of scholars. For our purpose I hope the connection between sensationalism, its reductionist reformulation by Condillac, and Itard's work is clear. Similarly, the influence of Itard on future educational efforts, notably through Édouard Séguin, often called the father of special education, and other educational innovators such as Maria Montessori is well described in the literature and I won't review it here. But to conclude I would like to return to the second of the two key impacts of sensationalism noted at the beginning of this chapter: that is, how sensationalism, and particularly the radical sensationalism of Condillac, led to the hegemony of medicine and, later, psychology over the intellectually disabled subject.

Medical hegemony

Until the eighteenth century there was little medical interest in 'idiots' or any of the categories roughly associated with our present concept of intellectual disability. The most common early medical sources cited as early medical texts, Paracelsus (1493–1541) and his *De Generatione Stultorum* (The Begetting of Fools), Felix Platter (1536–1614) *Praxeos medicae* (The Golden Practice of Physic) and Thomas Willis (1621–75) *De anima brutorum* (Of the Soul of Brutes) all note the general incurability of idiocy and the limited role of medicine. Paracelsus for example, explicitly rejects any role for medicine, noting 'It is the more difficult that fools are born as there is no disease, they are incurable, have no stones nor herbs whereby they might become intelligent'.[81] He concedes early on that on this question medicine has nothing to say.

Willis is less dismissive; while he generally accepts incurability, he also offers the suggestion that 'though it may not be cured, yet it is often wont to be amended. Wherefore it must be the work both of a Physician and a Teacher, that the wit of such that are so affected, may be somewhat trimmed, and they being at least brought to the use of reason in a little measure, may be accounted out of the number of Brutes'.[82]

Indeed, the general view was that of the incurability and ineducability of idiots, which was certainly the view of Pinel, one of the fathers of psychiatry and moral treatment, and Itard's primary teacher. Itard himself only undertook the attempt at educating Victor because he disagreed with Pinel and most other authorities that Victor was an 'idiot' – believing that he 'was an idiot because he was abandoned in the woods' rather than, as Pinel believed, that 'he was abandoned in the woods because he was an idiot'.[83] It has never been clear whether Victor was abandoned or simply lost; indeed it has never been firmly established that he had anything akin to intellectual disability, though this is the dominant view. Consequently, we can say that Itard's work with Victor as an exercise in the education of the intellectually disabled was wholly accidental.

However, both Itard and his student Séguin (despite the latter being associated primarily with educational interventions) were clear that the work of educating the idiot was primarily the work of medicine. Itard writes that

> in the present state of our knowledge of physiology, the progress of education can and ought to be illuminated by the light of modern medicine which, of all the natural sciences, can help most powerfully towards the perfection of the human species by detecting the organic and intellectual peculiarities of each individual and determining there from what education ought to do for him and what society can expect.[84]

Séguin, despite not completing his medical degree until later in his career, insisted that physicians should control all teaching of idiots.[85] The basis for this was clearly the view that the acquisition of knowledge was, *à la* Condillac, primarily a physical-sensory process and hence, like the parallel of moral treatment for the insane, the work primarily of a physician. The body rather than the mind thus becomes the site of education and as such is appropriately applied by those most familiar with the physical self – the physician. Willis's 'Physician *and* teacher' had become physician *as* teacher. This then sets the stage for medicine to not only engage with 'the idiot', previously thought to be of little interest or worth, but also for the medical oversight of the soon-to-evolve institutions specifically for 'idiots' where the medical gaze would begin to classify and discipline the bodies of the intellectually disabled.

This would also set the stage for the emergence of psychology, most directly behaviourism, which remains the dominant stream concerned with intellectual disability. The similarity of the strict sensationalism of Condillac and the central tenets of twentieth-century behaviourism are self-evident. The rejection of any significant role for mental process goes with an exclusive focus on controlling the stimuli – or sensations – to effect behavioural change. The intellectually disabled subject is essentially the malleable clay to be crafted into moral man (if possible) through control of his sensory experience by external agents.

As noted, sensationalism does open the possibility of a developmental psychology and the belief that humans can grow and change when given the proper environmental and educational stimulation. One cannot help but speculate, though, that these trends have contributed greatly to the historical construction of the intellectually disabled subject as 'less than' human, or only partially human, requiring the expert attention of the medico-psychological régime on their bodies to mold the unformed subject. The hegemony of the medico-psychological regime and its legacies of control is writ most clearly on our physical institutions, but more subtly in our practice of leaving the intellectually disabled subject outside the moral realm, as savage proto-humans whose autonomy and personhood are suspended until a cure for their otherness can be found and applied to their bodies.

Notes

1 Jean-Marc-Gaspard Itard, *The Wild Boy of Aveyron* [1801/1806], translated by George and Muriel Humphrey (New York: Appleton Century Crofts, 1962), xxiii–xiv. This translation contains Itard's *Foreword, The First Developments of the Young Savage of Aveyron* [1801], and *A Report to his Excellency The Minister of the Interior* [1806], and is based on the 1894 reprinted edition of *Rapport et Mémoires sur le Sauvage de L'Aveyron*, Paris. Subsequent references are to the specific report contained in this volume with continuous pagination.

2 Ibid., 49; this passage is from *The First Developments of the Young Savage of Aveyron* [1801].
3 John Locke, *An Essay Concerning Human Understanding* [1689], edited by P. Nidditch (Oxford: Clarendon, 1975), 63–64; Bk. I, Ch. II, S. 27. Emphasis in original (this applies to quotes throughout this chapter).
4 In his report on the subject to the Society of Observers of Man, Pinel concluded that 'the boy was not an idiot because he was abandoned in the woods; he was abandoned in the woods because he was an idiot'. Quoted in Harlan Lane, *The Wild Boy of Aveyron* (London: George Allen & Unwin, 1977), 56. Lane reproduces extensive excerpts of Pinel's report.
5 Itard, *The Wild Boy of Aveyron*, 73.
6 The most comprehensive review of Itard's work with Victor is Lane's *The Wild Boy of Aveyron* (see note 4 above).
7 Nothing is in the understanding that was not earlier in the senses.
8 The Epicureans, Thomas Hobbes, and Pierre Gassendi, who was a key source for Locke, had all put forward similar theories.
9 Locke, *Essay*, 48; Bk. I, Ch. II, S. 1. While Locke does not specify whom he is refuting, it is generally accepted that his main targets were the Scholastics and Descartes; see 'John Locke', *Stanford Encyclopedia of Philosophy*, Revised entry 5 May, 2007. Availabele at http://plato.stanford.edu/entries/locke/.
10 Locke, *Essay*, 48; Bk. I, Ch. II, S. 2.
11 Ibid., 49; Bk. I, Ch. II, S. 5.
12 Ibid., 63–64; Bk. I, Ch. II, S. 27.
13 See Nicholas G. Petryszak, 'Tabula Rasa – Its Origins and Implications', *Journal of the History of the Behavioral Sciences* 17 (1981), 15–27.
14 Locke, *Essay*, 104–105; Bk. II, Ch. I, S. 2.
15 Ibid., 105; Bk. II, Ch. I, S. 3.
16 Ibid., 105; Bk. II, Ch. I, S. 4.
17 Ibid., 91; Bk. I, Ch. IV, S. 12.
18 Ibid., 143–163; Bk. II, Ch. IX–XI. See Petryszak, 'Tabula Rasa', for discussion.
19 Ibid., 228; Bk. II, Ch. XX, S. 2.
20 Ibid., 228–231; Bk. II, Ch. XX, S. 3–13.
21 Ibid., 91; Bk. I, Ch. IV, S. 12.
22 Ibid., 239–240; Bk. II, Ch. XXI, S. 12.
23 Ibid., 265; Bk. II, Ch. XXI, S. 50.
24 Ibid., 91–92; Bk. I, Ch. IV, S. 12.
25 C. F. Goodey, *History of Intelligence and 'Intellectual Disability': The Shaping of Psychology in Early Modern Europe* (Farnham and Burlington VT: Ashgate, 2011), 341.
26 For a review of all Locke's educational writings, see S. J. Curtis and M. E. A. Boultwood, *A Short History of Educational Ideas*, 5th edn (Slough: University Tutorial Press, 1977), Ch. 10.
27 Lawrence A. Cremin, 'Preface', in *John Locke on Education*, edited by Peter Gay

(New York: Teacher College Press, 1964), vii–viii. This contains a complete version of the last version of Locke's text edited by Gay.

28 Peter Gay, 'Introduction', in *John Locke on Education*, edited by Peter Gay, 5–7, 12–14; John W. Yolton, 'Locke: Education for Virtue', in *Philosophers on Education*, edited by Amelie Oksenberg Rorty (London: Routledge, 1998), 173–189.

29 Jan Goldstein, 'Bringing the Psyche into Scientific Focus', in *The Cambridge History of Science, Volume 7, The Modern Social Sciences*, edited by Theodore M. Porter and Dorothy Ross (Cambridge: Cambridge University Press, 2003), 131–153.

30 Locke, 'Some Thoughts Concerning Education' [1693], in *John Locke on Education*, edited by Peter Gay, 19–20; S. 1.

31 Yolton, *Locke*, 174–176.

32 Locke, 'Some Thoughts', 20; S. 1–2.

33 Ibid., 33; S. 48.

34 Ibid., 109–113; S. 148–155.

35 Ibid., 66; S. 82.

36 Ibid., 42; S. 66.

37 Gay, 'Introduction', 7.

38 Locke, 'Some Thoughts', 108; S. 147.

39 Ibid., 42; S. 66.

40 Gay, 'Introduction', 8.

41 Locke, 'Some Thoughts', 65; S. 81.

42 Ibid., 119–121; S. 163–165.

43 Locke attended Willis's lectures at Oxford. See below for Willis's view on the educability of 'brutes'.

44 Curtis and Boultwood, *A Short History of Educational Ideas*, 254.

45 Goldstein, 'Bringing the Psyche into Scientific Focus', 134.

46 Ibid.

47 Jean-Jacques Rousseau, 'A Discourse upon the origin and foundation of the inequality among mankind', in *The Social Contract and Discourse on the Origins of Inequality*, edited by Lester G. Crocker (New York: Pocket Books, 1967), 187. The French original was published in 1755.

48 Rousseau's original French uses the term 'imbécile'.

49 Rousseau, 'A Discourse upon the origin and foundation of the inequality among mankind', 37.

50 Douthwaite suggests that Rousseau sees intelligence as man's frailty, but the context of the quote does not support this contention. Rather it is evidence of man's perfectibility in that he cannot lose what he has not acquired; society, not reason, was for Rousseau the source of Man's downfall. See Julia V. Douthwaite, *The Wild Girl, Natural Man and the Monster: Dangerous Experiments in the Age of the Enlightenment* (Chicago: University of Chicago Press, 2002), 20.

51 Jean-Jacques Rousseau, *Émile, or On Education*, translated and edited by Allan Bloom (London: Penguin, 1991), 38.

52 See, for example, Rousseau, *Émile*, 39.

53 Jean-Jacques Rousseau, *The Social Contract* [1762], in *The Essential Rousseau*, translated by Lowell Blair (New York: New American Library, 1974), 8.

54 Allan Bloom, 'Introduction', in *Émile, or On Education*, translated and edited by Allan Bloom, 3.

55 Rousseau, *Émile*, 40.

56 Ibid., 39.

57 Ibid., 42.

58 Bloom, 'Introduction', 7.

59 Rousseau, *Émile*, 185.

60 Ibid., 53.

61 Ibid., 54.

62 Rousseau was a friend of Jacob Pereire whose work in teaching deaf-mutes he noted. Whether the charity of others refers to this is not clear. See Lane, *The Wild Boy of Aveyron*, 152; Leo Kanner, *A History of the Care and Study of the Mentally Retarded* (Springfield IL: Thomas, 1967), 9–12; Richard Scheerenberger, *A History of Mental Retardation* (Baltimore: Brookes, 1983), 48–50.

63 Lane, *The Wild Boy of Aveyron*, 27.

64 Rousseau, a contemporary of Condillac's, would have been familiar with Condillac's major writings, which were all published prior to *Émile*. At one point in *Emile* he seems to make oblique reference to Condillac: 'Suppose a child born with the size and strength of manhood, entering upon life full grown … such a child-man would be a perfect idiot, an automaton, a statue without motion and almost without feelings'. Rousseau, *Émile*, p. 28.

65 Lane, *The Wild Boy of Aveyron*, 74.

66 Etienne Bonnot de Condillac, *An Essay on the Origin of Human Knowledge: Being a Supplement to Mr. Locke's Essay on the Human Understanding*, translated by Thomas Nugent and introduced by Robert G. Weyant (Gainsville: Scholars' Facsimiles and Reprints, 1971).

67 Robert G. Weyant, 'Introduction', to Condillac, *An Essay on the Origin of Human Knowledge*, vii.

68 Etienne Bonnot De Condillac, 'Treatise on Sensations' [1754], in *Philosophical Writings of Etienne Bonnot, Abbé de Condillac*, translated by Franklin Phillips in collaboration with Harlan Lane (Hillsdale NJ: Lawrence Erlbaum Associates, 1982), 157.

69 Ibid., 168.

70 Ibid.

71 Ibid., 158–159.

72 Locke, *Essay*, 91; Bk. I, Ch. IV, S. 12.

73 Ibid., 143–163; Bk. II, Ch. IX–XI. See Petryszak, 'Tabula Rasa', for discussion.

74 Quoted in Weyant, 'Introduction', viii.

75 Douthwaithe, *Wild Girl*, Chapter 2.

76 Weyant, 'Introduction', xii–xiii.

77 Ibid., xiii–xiv.

78 Condillac, *Treatise*, 338.

79 Douthwaite, *Wild Girl*, Chapter 2.

80 Itard, *The Wild Boy of Aveyron*, 44; this incident is recounted in 'The First Developments of the Young Savage of Aveyron' [1801].

81 Paul F. Cranefield and Walter Federn, 'The Begetting of Fools: An Annotated Translation of Paracelsus', *The Bulletin of the History of Medicine* 41 (1967), 57. This work is a translation of Paracelsus's *De Generatione Stultorum* (1603).

82 Paul F. Cranefield, 'A Seventeenth-Century View of Mental Deficiency and Schizophrenia: Thomas Willis on "Stupidity or Foolishness"', *Bulletin of the History of Medicine*, 35 (1961), 291–316; p. 302. This article includes Samuel Pordage's 1683 translation of Willis's chapter XIII 'Of Stupidity and Foolishness', which is not without considerable problems. For a critique of Pordage, see C. F. Goodey, '"Foolishness" in Early Modern Medicine and the Concept of Intellectual Disability', Medical History 48 (2004), 289–310.

83 Lane, *The Wild Boy of Aveyron*, 56. Lane reproduces extensive excerpts of Pinel's report on the subject to the *Society of Observers of Man*.

84 Douthwaite, *Wild Girl*, 61.

85 James W. Trent, *Inventing the Feeble Mind: A History of Mental Retardation in the United States* (Berkeley: University of California Press, 1995), 40.

8

PETER THE 'WILD BOY': WHAT PETER MEANS TO US

Katie Branch, Clemma Fleat, Nicola Grove, Tim Lumley Smith, and Robin Meader

Openstorytellers is a company of storytellers who have learning disabilities, and is based in Frome, in Somerset, UK. As a group we do performances, workshops, and training, and are interested in stories about people like ourselves from history and legend. One of our projects is about Peter the Wild Boy, a figure from the eighteenth century who attracted much attention in his lifetime, becoming a focus of debate about the relationship between language and the soul, nature and nurture. In this chapter the group talks about how we came to create our performance, and our views and feelings about the story and its importance. The chapter is written by Nicola, with a round table discussion with members of the group, whose contributions are individually acknowledged. All attended special schools, and live variously independently, with family, or in a residential facility. They run the storytelling company, devising shows, giving talks, and organizing workshops. Three of the group also worked on a project to develop personal stories with people with profound and multiple disabilities. They are thus very familiar with legends, folktales, and life stories.

Peter the Wild Boy

In 1725 a boy was discovered living in the forest near Hamelin, in northern Germany; some reports have him being discovered by a hunting party led by George I of England, who was originally from this region of Germany, while others say he was captured by local peasants. The so-called 'wild boy' did not speak and apparently walked on all fours, and he elicited much conjecture on how he had survived in the woods – including whether he had been raised by wolves or bears. At any rate, after his capture he was sent to the nearby town of Zell [Celle] and kept in the local prison for almost a year. Eventually, though,

Peter (as he was named by his captors) was sent to England by order of King George I (who had also had Peter to his court in Herrenhausen, in Germany). In London Peter quickly became an object of curiosity, with people visiting him to see the 'wild boy' for themselves and many writing speculative articles on his history, and discussing how he might be important for understanding what made people 'human'. In time, popular interest in Peter subsided, and he lived with a series of caretakers, notably James Fenn, a farmer in Hertfordshire, and, after James died, with his brother Thomas Fenn; he was living with Thomas in 1751 when he went missing, reappearing a month later in a jail in Norwich, 100 miles away. After Thomas's death, Peter moved into the care of a Mr Brill, who had inherited Fenn's farm; Peter was supported by Brill for the remainder of his years, and performed manual labour on the farm; among his illustrious visitors in these years were the novelist Maria Edgeworth and her father, Richard Lovell Edgeworth, in the 1770s, and the philosopher James Burnett, Lord Monboddo, in 1783. Peter died on 22 February, 1785, having refused food and comfort following the death of his care-giver Brill; he was likely in his early seventies. His gravesite can be seen in Northchurch in the churchyard at St Mary's.

Developing the story

We came across the story of Peter by accident in the autumn of 2010. Nicola's granddaughters had been to an exhibition at Kensington Palace and her daughter noticed some information about Peter and told her. So Nicola looked up the website, since removed, and found that there was an imaginary blog authored by Peter. The website was very creative, but it made her ask a lot of questions. So she looked up some information about Peter. She felt that the persona on the website was very untrue to what his actual experience must have been. She took the issue to Openstorytellers and asked for their views – and although they too thought the website was very interesting, their experience with people who do not communicate in words led them to challenge this representation as well.

Here is some of the text from the website:[1]

> Peter the Wild Boy is a digital character in the Enchanted Palace. He is a gossipy and irreverent commentator on the palace's past and present – offering exclusive online access to the fashion, fairytale and 300 years of palace intrigues.

The blog is said to be 'by Peter the Wild Boy'. One of the featured events is 'the Wild Boy's Ball' with photos of people who attended. There are eighteen blogs, from April 2010 till November 2011. The final blog shows a contemporary etching of William and Mary, with a party hat and party blower superimposed. The text for this blog reads:

> Between 1691 and 1694 William III and Mary II held more than 14 elaborate, all-night winter balls at Kensington Palace, with the lamps of Hyde Park kept alight to illuminate them. The food and drink supplied were lavish – including beer, ale, cider, mead, port and other wines, as well as bread, fruits and confectionary (a 'square piramede of the best confeccons'), meat, poultry and seafood. The expenses for one of these came to £332, equivalent to nearly £30,000 in today's money.

At the time (2010) there were film clips which showed Peter appearing and disappearing as a tricksy playful character who was full of surprises.

Some of our questions were: How could someone who did not talk write these blogs? Was he really a tricksy person? Or would he have been confused and unhappy? Did the website give us any sense of who Peter really was?

We emailed Kensington Palace to tell them what we thought, and this led to a commission to produce an educational resource about Peter which presented the story in a different way. We then developed our performance, which involved doing some research about what people had said at the time – we mostly used Daniel Defoe's pamphlet *Mere Nature Delineated or A Body without a Soul*:

> The world has for some time been entertained … with a strange appearance of a Thing in human shape … .[2] A youth is brought over hither, said to be taken up in the forest. He was found wild, naked, dumb, known to and knowing nobody.[3]
>
> December 11th 1725 The Intendant of a House of correction has brought a boy hither, supposed to be about 15 years of age, who was catched some time ago in a forest or wood near Hamelin, where he walked upon his hands and feet, ran up trees as naturally as a squirrel, and fed upon grass and the moss of trees. By what strange fate he came into the wood is not known, because he cannot speak … .[4] [He is] dumb or mute without the least appearance of cultivation or of having ever had the least glimpse of conversation among the rational part of the world … .[5] [He was] showed to His Majesty and is since brought over to England and every day to be seen.[6]

Robin Meader tells the story (as reflected in our performance) from memory, as follows:

He was a boy who was brought up in the forest with all the animals with the flowers, they were his friends. Suddenly he was captured one night and taken off to London where they started making fun of him and asking him to speak. They dressed him but he kept throwing the clothes off. People were interested because they had never seen a boy like him before. And they were dancing with him and Princess Caroline took pity on him. Then he went to a farm where there was a bloke called Farmer Fenn. He used to work for the farmer and he would do jobs like milking cows and clearing up the hay and feeding the pigs and chickens. And then one day he ran away and into the market town of Norwich.

And then people would see him in the market place. And because people had never seen a person with a learning disability before because he didn't speak they thought he was a Spanish spy or something so they called a policeman, so they put him in some really early handcuffs and marched him into a cell and then they kept him there for a night when suddenly there was a fire, people didn't know what to do and because he kept looking at the fire someone took him out the prison cell. He was in the newspaper, and Princess Caroline and the others said 'Peter come home' and then Farmer Fenn took him and put the collar around him. And then he got older and he died. So people then put flowers on his grave.

In our workshop we stop the action at points to ask questions such as:

- How did Peter manage to live in the forest? He must have had some skills to survive.
- How did it feel for him to be suddenly confronted by the noise and bustle of the court?
- People tried to teach him to speak – and failed. But there are many ways in which people who do not speak can communicate; can you think of any?
- Why did he run away from Farmer Fenn? Was he hoping to get back to the forest?
- People thought he might be a spy because of the strange noises he made. Do we still treat some people as suspicious nowadays? Who are they?
- Someone risked their life to save Peter from the fire – what does that tell us?
- When Peter came home, people were worried that he might put himself in danger again – can you think of any ways that they could have kept him safe without shutting him up?

We finish our performance with the much more positive images of Peter in old age: for example, the writer Maria Edgworth said that 'In old age, he looks like the bust of Socrates'.[7]

Finally we quote Defoe's thoughtful meditation on whether people who are nonverbal have souls – he says of Peter 'I must allow him to have a soul':[8] 'He that without the help of speech can pray / Must talk to Heaven by some superior way'.[9]

Peter and the Pitt Hopkins Society

In 2011 we were interested to read the research by Lucy Worsley,[10] the histo-rian at Kensington Palace, who believes from her conversations with geneticist Phil Beale from the Institue of Child Health, that Peter may have had a specific syndrome: Pitt Hopkins Syndrome. Then the Pitt Hopkins society, based in the Netherlands, contacted us because they were interested in what we were doing. We found out that they are trying to reclaim the image of Peter as a gentle person, not someone who is wild. Sue Routledge, whose son has been diagnosed with the syndrome, had been to visit the churchyard where Peter is buried. She met the vicar who told her that Peter is remembered in the village as 'Gentle Peter', and asked if this was typical of children with the syndrome. She was very moved by this folk memory and by his question. However, she and other geneticists she has corresponded with are sceptical of the post hoc diagnosis, for several reasons: one being that breathing problems are very common in these children and the diagnosis would be more likely if there had been some mention of this, and the other that none of the children she knows about (160 have a diagnosis worldwide) would be able to survive in the wild or to journey from Hertfordshire to Norwich. So rather than trying to identify his condition, it's more important to look at the story for what it tells us about Peter as a person, how he was viewed and what people said about him at the time, and what his experiences mean for us today.

Reflections on the story of Peter

These are our thoughts about the meaning of the story. We started by discuss-ing how Peter comes across through the historical records, and what we guess about his reactions.

TLS. *He was brought to England against his will – we don't know but we think he may have wanted to stay living in the forest (because he ran away and because he ran away later).*
CF. *He couldn't speak.*
RM. *He had learning difficulties.*
TLS. *He didn't know how to communicate.*
KB. *He could hear – he liked the ticking clock and he liked music.*
    He couldn't learn to talk.

Then we talked about how he appeared to others. This led us to reflections on our own experiences and how we deal with difficulties and challenges.

TLS. *When he first arrived he did behave like an animal because he didn't know how to behave any differently.*

RM. *He was like people who run around like a King Kong movie, an out of control chaos society. It makes someone look more like a barbaric warrior not a normal citizen.*

People would lock up doors.

There are ways of managing behaviour – you get people to sit down in a chair and you count to ten to calm down and if they don't you call their parents.

NG. *Robin, you've had experience of that from school, I remember you talking about one of your friends there, in the special school.*

RM. *Yes that's right.*

KB. *One of the boys was jealous and he tried to strangle me.*

CF. *If you've got epilepsy, you stay where you don't touch people who are having fits.*

KB. *If I cannot hear people I tell them to talk to me face to face.*

People now would see specialists and have hearing check and hearing aids, speech therapy, eye checks, medical checks and blood tests.

TLS. *He was probably whacked when he did something wrong. May've been whipped.*

Tim is correct in this assumption: the Daily Mail article (see below) quotes a contemporary source stating that he was sometimes 'beaten on the legs with a broad leather strap to keep him in awe'. This made Tim recall his own caning as a schoolchild:

When I was at school corporal punishment was still in. Kids were caned if they misbehaved. Special school – I was about 8 – I didn't know how to write my name and I didn't, and he [the teacher] *caned me.*

Thinking about punishments raised the issue of the treatment of people with severe disabilities: the group had viewed the BBC Panorama film showing the abuse of people in a residential institution, and had written to support a campaign about it.

RM. *Nowadays you get hate crime for people with disabilities and lots of mickey taking. Some cases of being stabbed and starved.*

TLS. *People treat people with disabilities badly because they think they're benefit cheats. Might be accused of stealing and things.*

RM. *I didn't like being abandoned from my own mother.*

TLS. *I think even today people can be treated like Peter. I used to have a job in a*

riding stable, and I wasn't allowed to have coffee with the girls, I had to sit sepa-
rately as if they didn't want to be associated with me.

We looked at Defoe's first description and at how the image was manipu-
lated. Some of the contemporary images of Peter are quite shocking – and
the one of him posted when he went missing certainly looks very wild and
unkempt. It is a distressing portrait.

RM. *When he ran away it reminds me of a company called Missing – on milk*
cartons and websites.
CF. *He looked like a tramp.*
RM. *The description of him as a thing in human shape says he might be an animal.*
Something creepy like a hunchback or werewolf.
KB. *It isn't very nice. It may mean that they are not treated well.*
RM. *Like press wanting to get a good story so they slant things in order to get the*
story they want, not truth.
TLS. *I think what interested them is that they had never seen a boy as wild as that.*
     He is ending up as a trophy in a cabinet.

The sensationalist depiction of Peter goes on to this day. For example, when
the *Daily Mail* wrote up an account of Lucy Worsley's findings, they employed
highly derogatory language. A comparison of the language used by the two
journalists to describe Peter from *The Mail* (David Leafe) and the *Guardian*
(Maev Kennedy), reporting the same research, is instructive (see Figure 1).[11]
In fact, reading *The Mail*, one may well ask if some journalists have made any
advances at all in the last three hundred years in the sensitivity with which they
report on such stories. Although there is some awareness of the fear that he
must have felt when rescued from the fire, the picture presented is monstrous.
By comparison the *Guardian*'s report is highly restrained and factual. In
response, Sue Routledge from the Pitt Hopkins Research Foundation posted
a comment, which she forwarded to us, and which we discussed in the group.

> Happy, content and loving are better words used to describe children with Pitt
> Hopkins Syndrome in the 21st Century. I realise that these are not the words
> used in the 18th century even by the learned Rousseau, Defoe and Blumenbach,
> but I'd have hoped the *Mail* would have used less emotive words than 'Half
> human, scampered, gorilla, pet, wild, strange'. I have a son with Pitt Hopkins
> Syndrome and though raising awareness of PTHS is something I and families
> and doctors I know are keen to do, there are more appropriate words to be asso-
> ciated with our children. I prefer to use 'Gentle Peter' in messages to the online
> support group that I co-manage, as he was also described. I'm pleased he was

well cared for and happy on the farm where he spent most of his life. I doubt he had PTHS but he obviously did have severe learning difficulties. We will never know for sure, but in our era let's remember him as a gentle man in his long life, cared about enough to have a gravestone and floral tribute.

TLS. *I think that's very good, a great deal of compassion for Peter.*
RM. *I think that's a lot nicer than the newspaper.*
TLS. *The newspapers seem to do that they turn things to get a good story.*
KB. *We write down what we want and we expect them to write them down* [to respect what we say]. *I wouldn't call anyone those names, I would call him Gentle. I agree with what she wrote about her son, not with what they wrote in the newspaper. It's like you don't judge a book by its cover, you find out what they are like.*

Then we discussed the other side of the story:

CF. *Peter is a boy who is brought up in a wild nature environment, so this explains why he's doing things like eating off the floor, climbing trees.*
KB. *He is a boy with learning disabilities.*
CF. *Do not take the mickey out of him just because he can't speak and behaves differently to you – doesn't mean he is different.*
TLS. *He is misunderstood.*
CF. *He has a problem with picking things up.*
RM. *He can't speak because the messages don't get through from his brain to his mouth. His brain won't think.*
KB. *If I couldn't speak I would sign.*
RM. *He is a seventeenth-century citizen, not a prehistoric man wolf.*

Reflecting on his treatment:

CF. *Not Ok because he may have an impairment problem. He's not like that, he may be just like a family and want friends – and if you look inside Peter's heart you might see that he is caring about people.*
NG: *What do you think is important about other people – that they can think and speak, or that they care about you?*

In response, everyone said caring for others is the most important thing. (Again, this insight is born out by the history. Peter is reported to have died soon after the death of Farmer Brill with whom he lived, pining and refusing food.)

The Mail

Title: 'The Child Savage Kept as a Pet by King George'

From the opening paragraph:
an astonishing sight ...
a strange half-human figure silhouetted against the burning building ...
Its excessively hairy appearance and animal-like grunting immediately
gave rise to speculation that it was some kind of gorilla or orangutan. As
the creature scampered towards them on that October night in 1751, the
locals backed away in terror. Yet a closer look at its face revealed that
this was no animal but a fully-grown man, more frightened of them than
they of him ...
Before long, he was coaxed by the locals to come timidly towards them,
and they were able to take care of him. As they puzzled over his identity
in the days to come, they found that he could speak — but he could say
only two things: strangled versions of the names Peter and King George.

Attributes and descriptions later in the article:
an unfortunate ... kept as a much-celebrated 'pet' ... the creature ... The
monarch watched with appalled fascination as Peter, napkin at his neck,
gorged himself on vegetables, fruit and raw meat, eating noisily from his
hands ... Frustrated by Peter's wild ways ... The grinning, bushy-haired
boy entranced courtiers with his refreshing lack of ceremony, scuttling
about like a chimp and scampering up to the King ...
Although short, he was remarkably strong and, with gleaming white
teeth and 'a roving look' in his green eyes, often giggled during solemn
proceedings.

Guardian

Title: 'Peter the Wild Boy's Condition Revealed 200 Years After his
Death'; 'Feral German child who was kept as a pet'

From the opening paragraph:
Peter's charming smile, seen in his portrait painted in the 1720s by
William Kent on the king's grand staircase at Kensington Palace, was
the vital clue.

Attributes and descriptions later in the article:
Peter's strange life ... description of his physical characteristics and odd
habits ... curvy Cupid's bow lips, short stature, coarse hair – the portrait
shows him with a thick, curly mop – drooping eyelids and thick lips ...
His mental development would also have been affected

*enough to explain why he was **abandoned by his family,** and once captured
in the forest **like a wild animal, treated like a performing dog** rather than **a
damaged little boy.***

1 Comparison of language used to describe Peter in two newspaper accounts,
March 2011

RM. *Peter's got human rights – there's the declaration of independence.*

We discussed the website again later and expressed two views. Robin said he felt the representation was wrong, and Katie and Clemma agreed with him:

RM: *No, because Peter the Wild Boy wasn't there at the time of the write up. You cannot underestimate people who weren't present at the time* [i.e. of writing].
CF and KB: *It wasn't the truth – Peter wasn't there then.*
  He couldn't write.

But Tim saw it as just an interpretation:

TLS: *I think it was Ok because they didn't really know the truth – they didn't know the true story, it's an interpretation, and in that sense it's fine.*

Labels: then and now

We had a brief discussion about the labels people carry. How does it feel to be identified as someone with a 'learning disability'? Here the group reflects on how it may help, but how ultimately we need to learn about each other as individuals – and that applies just as much to the interactions of people without disabilities as it does as to those with people who are disabled.

TLS. *It's helpful because it makes people understand why we've got learning disabilities. I don't think back then people know about disabled people. It's interesting to learn – they think he's a wild animal but he isn't. Maybe if members of the public may not know you're disabled they don't know how to handle us, know how to approach us.*

KB. *In my generation I say to people I've got a disability, which is a bit like Peter the Wild Boy. Because I've got deletion of chromosome 12 – when they tested my body they found there was a deletion. That's the sort of disability I've got. It's to do with the balancing.*

NG. *Do you find it's useful to know about the chromosome deletion, or not?*

KB. *Yes it is. We need people to give us support and help us with all the things we find difficult. My mum helps me but I've got to figure it out for myself. When I tell people I can't hear things, or carry things, I tell people in confidence and I trust them. I don't tell everyone I've got a chromosome deletion, but if I put my back out, I am putting myself at risk, it helps to explain. I don't go round in public saying I've got a disability because people might laugh at you the way they did at Peter.*

Robin reflected that discrimination does not just happen to people with disabilities:

RM. *It's hard to tell what's underneath the able-bodied person. A person with learning disabilities might look straight at everything, but you always got to judge who to speak to and who not to speak to. People with LD get discriminated against but so do able-bodied people who are drunk. They don't judge below the surface whether they're intelligent or not. If you're working with people who are hyperactive like me or people with Down Syndrome or people with cerebral palsy, it's hard to tell who's energetic, who's Ok. People have to be aware that those people need important medication or care and advice.*
KB. *The lesson is you cannot judge people by their appearance. We should treat people the same even if they do behave like an animal or like a human. We all get treated individually.*

History and legend: why stories are important

Finally the group discussed the importance of historical figures who may be thought of as having learning disabilities – and how we see the significance of history.   Nicola started by asking how the group saw the difference between history and legend. All agreed with Tim that:

History is something that really happened, legend is something that's made up, could be true we don't know.

Then Nicola asked if historical stories were important, and if so, why?

RM. *Because it will show you like what your ancestors were like a long time ago. 'Cos my disability could go back to prehistoric times. A type of cave man who is not able-bodied.*
NG. *How do you feel about the story of Peter?*
TLS. *Makes me feel good, it's interesting, even back when Peter was born. Good because it makes people aware – of people who achieved things.*
KB. *History is a good thing because it makes you follow like people's footsteps. Like people's parents, they follow their footsteps, because if you don't you won't have a bigger picture.*

Katie went on to make a connection between the bigger picture and contemporary events:

'Cos my cousin belongs to Afghanistan, they're fighting and some people might come back with no legs and arms.

She then linked this to her own struggle for recognition and empowerment.

That's what I'm doing – I'm not fighting, I'm using my voice, to talk to staff and say what's not good. 'Cos like in Openstorytellers we've got a jigsaw puzzle, everyone's got their own little role and we help each other to fix the jigsaw puzzle together and that's what [the service] should do. If people were like Openstorytellers and helped each other out you wouldn't have this problem. I think people without disabilities should listen to disabled people and not put them down.

The group revisited their mission statement and considered how it is furthered by telling the story of Peter:

• Making a safe place for people to grow through stories; strengthening minds.

KB. *For me there's two sides of the story. It tells you you've got to be strong and get on with your life. It gives me a sad feeling when I tell the story.*

NG. *Yes, you find it a big challenge to tell because it used to upset you quite a bit, didn't it?*

KB. *It helps me to deal with the sad feeling. There are some bits that are happy, like the ticking of the clock and the dancing. Helps me because it does have a good end. And when Peter doesn't want his clothes, it's like [a family member], when she sometimes doesn't want to get dressed in the morning and I'm trying to help her – it helps me understand her.*

• Improving the identity of vulnerable people.

NG. *By vulnerable you mean ...?*

TLS. *People with learning disabilities who can't speak for themselves and people with challenging behaviour. The story helps people to understand them.*

• Helping people feel at ease in the community.

RM. *It gives them a lift, it makes people aware of people like him. It challenges people without disabilities and helps them understand people like us. I think of that time when Peter went to prison I can't think he's committed a crime. The story helps*

people to understand that people can be treated badly for no reason or discrimi-
nated against.

• Enrich, enhance, enchant.
We concluded that the questions raised by Peter's story are the same today as
they were then. We need to celebrate difference.
KB. *If we were all the same we'd be totally boring.*

Epilogue

Sue Routledge contributes her own thoughts on the story and the research as
a parent:

> I first heard about Peter when information popped into my inbox as a Google
> alert one Sunday afternoon in March 2011. 'Wild Peter diagnosed with PTHS
> 200 years after his death!' I was absolutely flabbergasted as two years ago there
> were only about 160 members of our group as PTHS is so rare. I read all I could
> get on Peter, talked to the group, and wrote to two renowned geneticists asking
> their opinion. Our group decided to call him 'Gentle Peter', as he was not wild
> in character but a wild boy believed to be brought up by animals in the woods.
> I was worried that 'wild boy' might be the first thing that people found on new
> diagnoses of PTHS but this doesn't seem to be an issue. I watched the BBC pro-
> gramme, then visited Kensington Palace, spoke to people there, and was shown
> the original papers! We visited Peter's grave and church, with its Plaque. It was
> moving that villagers still remember him. The Rector asked us if children with
> PTHS were gentle! That was pretty poignant! It's comforting to know that Peter
> was looked after and happy until old age, as it is a worry to parents how their
> child will be cared for when they are no longer around. I find 'Gentle Peter' abso-
> lutely fascinating and would love to know if he really had PTHS or not! Cannot
> imagine my son Christoper doing what Peter could do (e.g. getting to Norwich,
> etc.) but do know of other children with PTHS who could I think.

Sue also shared with us the correspondence with a parent of an autistic child
who responded to her online posting, taking her to task for 'political correctness' and suggesting she 'chill out a bit and don't try to find offence when none
is intended'. She continues:

> I was a bit offended by her PC stuff as she was missing the point, as the author
> *didn't have to use those words,* as new parents were going to see them if they did
> a Google search. I know the author wasn't intending to offend but he should
> stop and think of who might be reading the words eventually, so I replied: 'I
> was using this as a forum to express views which some parents of children with

PTHS and a geneticist share. Autism is a very broad diagnosis and heard of, if not understood, by most of the general public but Pitt Hopkins Syndrome is a very rare syndrome with only 150 documented cases world wide with very little public awareness. When I first saw the article in the *Guardian* online on Sunday afternoon I had mixed feelings, incredulous that PTHS had come up for a diagnosis but concerned about the "wild" connection upsetting new parents. Our children are not wild! Peter's life is actually extremely well documented in literature of the time. It's actually fascinating to read what is there about him. Quotes were put in quote marks but the words I picked out were the author's choosing. Political correctness has its place but I still think it would be fitting for Peter to be remembered not for the misled thought that he was a feral child but for the endearing person he seems to have been'.

Notes

1 Unfortunately, this site and the accompanying blog are no longer available online.

2 Daniel Defoe, *Mere Nature Delineated, or A Body without a Soul* (London: T. Warner, 1726), 1.

3 Ibid., 2.

4 Ibid., 10.

5 Ibid., 3.

6 Ibid., 16.

7 Maria Edgeworth and Richard Lovell Edgeworth, *Practical Education*, Vol. 1 [1823] (New York and London: Garland, 1974), 63. See also See Lucy Worsley, 'Peter the Wild Boy', *The Public Domain Review*, 7 November, 2011. Accessed 15 March, 2017, https://publicdomainreview.org/2011/11/07/peter-the-wild-boy/.

8 Defoe, *Mere Nature*, 20.

9 Ibid., 53.

10 See Lucy Worsley, *Courtiers: The Secret History of the Georgian Court* (London: Faber, 2011).

11 David Leafe, 'The Child Savage Kept as a Pet by King George', *Daily Mail*, 24 March, 2011. Accessed 15 March, 2017, www.dailymail.co.uk/news/article-1369387/The-child-savage-kept-pet-King-George.html. Maev Kennedy, 'Peter the Wild Boy's Condition Revealed 200 Years After his Death', *Guardian*, 20 March, 2011. Accessed 15 March, 2017, https://www.theguardian.com/artanddesign/2011/mar/20/peter-wild-boy-condition-revealed.

9

'BELIEF', 'OPINION', AND 'KNOWLEDGE': THE IDIOT IN LAW IN THE LONG EIGHTEENTH CENTURY

Simon Jarrett

The Tudor formation of the powerful Court of Wards from 1540 had brought a more sharply formalized focus to what constituted incapacity, and what constituted idiocy, in English law, after the loose and sporadically used guidance of the medieval Prerogativa Regis.[1] This court, through to its demise in the 1640s, consolidated and shaped the conventions and practices of the legal treatment of those deemed incapacitated into a form that persisted through the eighteenth and nineteenth centuries. Despite its abolition after the Restoration in 1661, the functions of the court simply passed over to the Court of Chancery.[2] As the law on capacity strengthened and formalized, however, it faced growing challenges from families to eliminate the use of 'idiocy grants' – confiscation of the lands and assets of people deemed idiots in law – which were seen as unfair and punitive. This pressure rose as the early Stuarts, James I and Charles I, milked the court for everything they could gain from it. Gradually, in response to this pressure, terms and conditions for idiots moved into line with those for lunatics, meaning that estates were not permanently confiscated, there was proper accounting for profits, and maintenance of both idiots and their families had to be in line with their degree and estate in life.[3]

The jurist Lord Coke had broadened the conceptual framework of idiocy in 1628. As the first of his four categories of *non compos mentis*, those of unsound mind, he named the idiot: 'Idiota ... from his nativitie, by a perpetuall infirmitie'. However, to his categories he then added a catch-all complication: 'all other persons, who from *natural imbecility*, disease, old age or any such causes, are incapable of managing their own affairs'.[4] These 'natural imbeciles' were a new legal concept. They were not idiots, but with an impaired mind from birth, and a question mark over their capacity: on which side of the capacity border did they lie? Along with Coke, lawyers and the public interested themselves in the conundrum of what constituted idiocy, and the shifting idea of imbecility, which was passing from a generic concept of mental and physical weakness to a more specific notion of a person born mentally feeble, but not quite idiotic.

Thus the idiot arrived at the beginning of the eighteenth century, characterized in law and through the processes of the Court of Wards and then Chancery as a 'solitaire': a person unable to understand money, numbers or social relationships and lacking self-awareness and memory. Many around them, in the burgeoning mercantile economy, learned, traded, and left the idiot class of the labouring poor behind. The static, residual unchanging idiots were joined by the scanty outline of a new imbecile class, the simpleton group challenged by the dynamism of this commercializing, learning, progressing world. Through 'mere weakness of understanding',[5] their right to social status was being questioned. The idiot in law was coming into sharper social focus, becoming a complex and important matter, with the exclusionist legal discourse shaped by the Court of Wards contested by a countervailing familial narrative of informal protection and opposition to ruthless expropriation.

At this juncture in 1700 the lawyer John Brydall produced a summary of idiocy law laying out, for the first time, the legal canon as it related to idiocy and *non compos mentis* generally.[6] The system for 'begging an idiot' (referred to as 'our old English proverb'[7]) remained intact under the Court of Chancery, as did the monarchical right to identify idiots and take possession of lands.[8] Idiots could be discerned by appearance,[9] and could not make a promise or a contract, marry, make a will or give voluntary consent.[10] They were distinguished from lunatics and others of unsound mind in that they were 'wholly destitute of reason ... by a perpetual infirmity, as... *Fools Natural*'.[11]

Brydall then introduced a paradox and an area of ambivalence. The paradox was that idiots could sometimes appear perfectly reasonable and 'it may appear, then such a one is no idiot naturally'.[12] They were capable of glimmers of light when they appeared *compos mentis*. If so, and they used their reason when making any contract, then 'the same might then be allowed as lawful'.[13] Yet if 'they are an idiot indeed', then this could not be.[14] Brydell solved the paradox by asserting that such moments were a divine act, 'because Almighty God doth sometimes so illuminate the Minds of the foolish they are not much inferior to the wise'.[15] There was the appearance of reason, but not its substance. How could the law distinguish between the two? He looked to the ability to understand abstractions; ideas and meanings rather than simple facts. An apparently reasonable testament made by an idiot was not good because 'a Testament is an Act to be performed with Discretion and Justice. But a natural fool, by the general presumption of law, doth not understand what he speaketh, tho' he seem to speak reasonably'.[16] Despite the occasional illuminations granted by God, 'the Law doth not presume the same by occasion of Words only'.[17] The words of idiots, like those of a parrot, lacked meaning because they lacked understanding or intention and meant no more than 'a Parrot speaking to the Passengers [passers-by]'.[18] Brydall, however, still left room for conjecture. If further proof could be provided and 'indeed if it may appear by sufficient conjectures, that they had the use of Reason or Understanding', then an idiot's testimony could stand.[19] He destabilized the conceptualisation of idiocy by speculating as to whether idiots could indeed reason, judge, and speak a truth, rather than parrot it. Strictly in law they could not, but Brydall hedged his bets and left a trace of doubt.

He also introduced a further twist to Coke's concept of natural imbecility. There was, he argued, a human type 'that only is of mean capacity or understanding, or one who is, as it were betwixt a man of Ordinary Capacity and a Fool', who it appeared could make a testament.[20] However this should only be with the proviso 'that he understands the nature of a Testament – if not, [he] is not fit to make a Will'.[21] The mental shortcomings of the person of 'dull capacity ... lacking virtue moral and theological, or to be of a quick understanding'[22] did not in themselves justify depriving them of their legal rights. Yet nor did it mean they were automatically entitled to them. The lifelong imbecile class took further shape under the gaze of the law, and provided a challenge to it. The law must in future consider how to respond to their complexity.

How was legal knowledge about idiocy being formed and transmitted? The idiot not only had a legal identity by the beginning of the eighteenth century, but also occupied a space in the minds of people, defined in lay terms and talked about in jokes, slang, and everyday conversation. As well as using case law and earlier legal theory, Brydall drew on this popular cultural wisdom, this 'common sense' and cultural understanding about what constituted idiocy. He acknowledged the interplay between the demotic and formal, legalistic definitions:

> Idiot signifies commonly an unlearned or illiterate person, but among the English Jurists is a term of law, and taken for one that is wholly deprived of his Reason and Understanding from his birth and ... in our common speech is called a *fool natural*.[23]

To explain the idea of the 'glimmer of reason' that could occur with idiots he described at great length a 'merry accident' that occurred in Paris when an idiot was asked to judge a dispute between a diner and a cook.[24] This apparent real-life account had in fact appeared, much more concisely, in a jest book thirty years earlier:

> A fellow in a Cook's shop in France filled his belly only with standing by whilst the meal was dished up, and the Cook would be paid for a meal. So it was left to

the decision of the next Passenger, which happened to be an Idiot, who said that the man's money should be put between two dishes, ringing it for a time, and the Cook should be content with the jingling of the money as the man was satisfied with the smelling of the meat.[25]

The joke was that the idiot had wisely, yet also naively, judged that if the customer was only smelling the food, the cook should only hear the money. The same jest, presented as an illustrative case, had also appeared in Swinburne's *Wills and Testaments* in 1590.[26] As Brydall acknowledged, the 'case' had been recounted by 'divers credible writers', as had further anecdotes he recounted concerning the apparent wisdom of fools.[27] Knowledge passed both ways between popular lay discourse and legal theorisation. The idea of the idiot having a lucky, random, lucid thought would take hold; 'Well Mr Random, a lucky thought may come into a fool's head sometimes', Smollet's hero was told half a century later.[28] That idiocy could be discerned in appearance was a common shared belief, and ordinary Londoners captured Brydall's ideas of 'dull capacity', 'dunce', and 'dull pate' with a rich vernacular terminology as they confidently described the idiotic when giving testimony in criminal cases: 'he was a soft-pated fellow', 'He was of such a slow and dull apprehension'.[29] It surfaced in everyday street language where the 'dullard', 'dull swift', 'dulpickle', 'addle-pate', 'leaden pate', and all the other 'windy fellows' (those without sense or reason) were identified, targeted, and teased by Londoners of all classes.[30] The concepts of idiocy and capacity lived in the minds of people as well as in legal theory, and the ideas passed upwards from the streets into lawyerly discourse as well as down from the legal caste. Notably, no flow of knowledge came from medical men – idiocy was a matter for the lawyers, and the public, to determine.

Brydell's synthesis of legal theory and popular wisdom presented the early eighteenth-century idiot as irrational, vulnerable, imposable, lacking understanding of everyday social commerce, and, in theory at least, owned by the monarch. As the Strasbourgeois visitor Archenholz later succinctly put it, the king 'is the guardian of all the fools in the kingdome, and he inherits the estates of all those who die without heirs'.[31] Yet this same idiot could have glimmers of reason and, however apart in mind, was very much physically amongst England's families and communities. Next to the idiot stood a perplexing group: dull, slow, soft and weak, imbecile from birth, somewhere between the sound and the unsound.

Idiocy in the eighteenth-century courtroom

How did Brydall's characterisation manifest itself in the discourses of the eighteenth-century courtroom? Suspected idiots and imbeciles appeared before ecclesiastical or civil courts to prove whether or not they had capacity, to determine the legitimacy of marriages, or to do the same for wills. This meant that they were of course from families that had property and other assets, and therefore almost entirely from amongst those Defoe called 'the great who live profusely, the rich who live very plentifully and the middle sort who live well',[32] rather than 'the poor that fare hard ... the miserable that really pinch and feel want'.[33] However, because important issues of inheritance and bloodline were at stake, civil cases, despite their narrow class composition, offer revealing insights into legal and public thinking about idiocy.

It was in this context that the strange life and last testament of Sir John Leigh, wealthy property owner in Surrey, came under the legal gaze in the ecclesiastical courts from 1739. He was alleged by his solicitor never to have had sufficient judgement, capacity, or understanding, and to be no more capable than a child of seven years.[34] He had married and had a son but, once widowed, his son 'aware of the weakness of his father's capacity and understanding', managed his estate for him.[35] Sir John spoke strangely and monosyllabically, saying 'yes yes yes by Christ no no no by Christ' and was seated separately from the family when dining.[36] On hearing in 1731 that his only son had died young, Sir John showed no reaction,[37] yet this was to be a turning point; as a fifty-eight-year-old weak-minded man with 'very unsound and imperfect judgement',[38] without a known heir and with a considerable estate, he was an obvious target for predators. A group of family friends attempted to protect and oversee him but this stable grouping of support was quickly displaced by a band of local gentlemen who moved in to take over the house and estate. They called themselves, without legal sanction, Sir John's commissioners and spent their time in 'rioting, drinking and other excesses'.[39]

William Vade, an apothecary who moved in when Sir John developed pain in his foot in 1732, appeared to exert growing power and control over him. Sensing his credulity, after his toe was amputated Vade assured Sir John that it would grow again. In fact his whole foot was then amputated but Sir John vented his fury on others. Vade dominated him, allowing no visitors without his permission, including two previously unknown cousins, now next of kin, tracked down by Sir John's solicitor, whom Vade persistently obstructed and barred from admission.[40] In 1733, despite Sir John having recently exclaimed 'Chris[t] God! I to be married? I know nothing of going to be married!'[41] Vade took him to London by stagecoach for just that purpose. A marriage ceremony was performed between sixty-year-old Sir John, made drunk to the point where he fell over, and his new sixteen-year-old bride. The new Lady Elizabeth was none other than Elizabeth Vade, William's daughter.[42] On hearing of this marriage Sir John's cousins took out a commission to prove incapacity and enable annulment of the marriage. However, because he could answer some questions 'tolerably' and now had a wife to help manage his affairs, he was found of sound mind.[43] From this point William Vade took total control of Sir John's life. In 1736, Lady Elizabeth, aged just eighteen, died suddenly.[44] Vade's hold on Sir John's estate for himself and his family was again threatened. Three days later he called Sir John to a part of the house where he had grouped an attorney and several witnesses; servants heard shouting, and by the end of the day there was a new will, leaving all to William Vade. When John Leigh died the next year, Vade inherited.[45]

At the final appeal of the lengthy case against the will brought by Sir John's cousins, Lord Hardwicke pronounced it 'the greatest instance of weakness he had ever met with'. He accepted the finding of the 1733 Commission that Sir John was not idiotic, but stated that the boundary was so narrow between a person *non compos mentis*, and one as weak as Sir John, that he upheld the complaint.[46] This was a dramatic expansion of the territory of incapacity and imbecility, because it drew even those just beyond Coke's boundaries of unsoundness of mind into the orbit of those whom the law must protect, encompassing Brydall's people 'neither of the wisest sort, nor of the foolish'st but … betwixt a wise man and a fool'.[47] To Brydall's challenge of whether such a group should be deprived of or entitled to their legal rights Hardwicke's answer was on the side of deprivation. The case drew the weak-minded imbecile further into the realm of incapacity.

The instinctive inclination towards Sir John, despite his clear vulnerability, had been to value individual liberty over statutory interference. His gentleman acquaintances had sought to create an informal network of protection, and the commission jury opted for non-intervention. The locus of care for those who could not support themselves was still perceived to rest in the informal realm of family and acquaintances, not with the state or institution. However, in his case these informal networks failed or became, in the case of his bride, an instrument of the exploitative forces ranged against him. Seeing this, Hardwicke's verdict effectively asserted the right of the state legal apparatus to intervene in an expanding territory of imbecility. The state's right to protect assets and bloodlines was asserted over the claims of neighbourhood and familial protectors. As Arthur Onslow, speaker of the House of Commons, who knew Sir John's family, told him, his duty was 'to ensure that what had descended *to* him descended correctly *from* him'.[48] It was his inability to preserve bloodline and familial entitlement that led to Hardwicke's judgement.

The complex association of the idiot with value in relation to heritable assets dominated civil legal proceedings. Idiots could represent value in that they could be commodified, associated with inherited wealth. They also represented a threat to value in that they were thought not to understand or appreciate their assets, and thus through profligacy, simplicity or vulnerability could squander estates and end bloodlines unless the law intervened. Finally they also represented valuelessness, in the sense that the common human comforts, luxuries, and opportunities that money could bring were perceived not to have any meaning for them. Their inability to understand, or value, money was key in this perception. For a group of people not to value what was valued by common human assumption was unnerving, and raised questions about human status.

These themes loomed large in the case of Henry Roberts who, according to an anonymous polemical broadside published after his death, 'by unparalleled cruelty was deprived of his estate under the pretence of idiocy'.[49] Roberts inherited a very large fortune, including Barbados slave estates. After the death of his sister and heir in 1742, a commission was brought on the grounds of his 'weak mind'.[50] The anonymous author described farcical proceedings as Roberts was bullied and heckled in the Exeter courtroom, then taken forcibly by a mob to a tavern where he was manhandled to the balcony and displayed to a baying crowd, his wig removed.[51] At an equally colourful appeal, witnesses testified that Roberts lacked 'common humanity' and that any correct answers he gave resulted from a system of nods and winks from his supporters.[52] Childlike behaviour was the main evidence given of his idiocy: shooting with a bow and arrow, blowing feathers, tossing up his hat and catching it, kicking pebbles and needing help to sign his name.[53] Roberts complained bitterly that he had been confused by the jurors: 'They came round me and asked their Questions together, without giving me Time to answer. They asked me what a *Lamb*, and what a *Calf* was called at one, two and three years old. They gave me a Sum of Money to tell, which I miscounted, and then I heard them say, he is not capable of managing his affairs, we will return him incapable'.[54] This combination of childlike behaviour, simplicity and eccentricity was sufficient for an 'unsound' finding.

In 1743 Roberts, worth £400 a year, passed into the hands of his appointed guardian, Dr John Lynch, Dean of Canterbury,[55] a 'notoriously acquisitive accumulator of preferments'.[56] Lynch swiftly moved to add the estate of Roberts's sister and the Barbados plantations.[57] The certificate confirming that Roberts was of unsound mind was signed by his Archbishop.[58] Roberts, now an imbecile caught in a classic web of eighteenth-century corruption, was lodged at the top (the poorest part) of an 'ordinary house' in Canterbury, with one servant. Falling ill in 1746, he deteriorated rapidly and died aged twenty-eight. His estate, which with the Barbados plantations was now worth £3,000 a year, descended to Dr Lynch.[59]

Roberts's journey from a life of wealth and ease when his family was alive to legalized imbecility, poverty, and a lonely death, was not unique. In an acquisitive and corrupt economic culture where many sought preferment and easy wealth, a vulnerable, unprotected idiot with a large, or even modest, estate was an obvious target. The wealth, status and well-being of newly parentless idiots could be drained, despite a system ostensibly designed to protect them; the idiot was a commodity to be plundered. In mid-century, Andrew Birkbeck, an idiot, lived with his stepmother for a year after the death of his wealthy father. The stepmother then put him out to lodgings with a 'keeper' where he would receive 'meat, drink, washing and lodging and ... necessary care' for five shillings a week. Soon he was moved elsewhere at 3s 6d per week, and within a year to yet another keeper at 2s 6d per week. By this time it was necessary for 'the Parish over and above [to] find him cloaths' through Poor Law funds.[60] The value, both physical and moral, of the idiot declined as assets were stripped and the right to physical comfort and luxury denied. Despite ostensible personal wealth, it was seen as natural that the Poor Law, designed to give minimum ease to the most destitute, should release funds to sustain the delegitimized idiot inheritor.

Exploitative designs came in many forms, both from within and outside the family. There was always a counterbalancing group, seeking to protect idiots and maintain their human and fiscal status. In the case of Sir John Leigh and Henry Roberts this involved informal friendship groupings battling predatory outsiders. In the extraordinary case of Fanny Fust it was her family who led the battle, in a complex case highlighting the disputed demarcation lines between choice and protection, freedom and vulnerability.[61] In 1786 Fanny, aged twenty-two, was heiress to several substantial family fortunes.[62] Living near Bath, with servants, carriages, and a well-connected family, she was also, according to her mother, an idiot, 'in a state of total ... imbecility of mind and is in every respect of as weak a state of mind as she was when only three years of age'.[63] Evidence of her idiocy was her inability 'of counting twenty, of knowing her right hand from her left, one kind of animal or vegetable food from another, the Sun from the Moon, the value and difference of the most common English coins, of knowing the days of the week and the difference of times and seasons'. Once when out walking in a storm and seeing lightning 'she called out in a very childish manner "do it again" meaning that the people with her should make the lightening happen again'.[64] As well as lacking basic knowledge and understanding, essential foundations of human participation, she exhibited dangerously transgressive behaviour that threatened both class and sexual propriety; she had 'in the presence of men servants pulled up her petticoats with an intention of making water'.[65] She needed constant attendance to help with dressing, eating, and protection from danger, such as falling into the garden pond. After seven years schooling she could do no more than write her name, with help.[66]

Henry Bowerman, an army lieutenant[67] who scarcely knew Fanny, was accused of hatching an elaborate plot with co-conspirators to kidnap and marry her, to obtain her fortune. The plot involved enticing her to tea at the house of a former school companion. Five conspirators waiting there took her, on the pretence of going to eat strawberries and cream, to a nearby village. There, a post-chaise with two horses was waiting. Fanny was separated from the trustworthy companion her mother had insisted should accompany her and taken to the Bath-London road where Bowerman was waiting with three further conspirators and a coach and horses. The entire group, with Fanny, then drove through the night to Dover and sailed to France, where Bowerman made frantic attempts in Calais, Lille, and Tournay to find a priest to perform a marriage.[68] None agreed to do so, Fanny's idiocy apparently evident to them through her appearance and behaviour. Bowerman eventually found a troubled Church of England priest in Lille who at first refused to conduct a ceremony but was plied with alcohol and persuaded to perform it, having been carried home intoxicated and then fetched from his bed at dawn to conduct the nuptials.[69]

Meanwhile Fanny's well-resourced mother discovered she was in France and dispatched four investigators, one armed with a request from the Secretary of State for Foreign Affairs to Louis XVI in Paris to make an order for Fanny's return. The order was granted, Fanny tracked down to a private house in Lille rented by Bowerman and, accompanied by three French Cavaliers and the investigators, returned to Calais, and thence to her mother in Bath.[70] Fanny, when asked why she had come to France, replied that 'she came to eat strawberries and cream'.[71] A long hearing in the Ecclesiastical Court of Delegates eventually resulted in the annulment of the marriage. Bowerman appealed, claiming Fanny had consented and only appeared idiotic because her mother gave her strong alcoholic drinks.[72] In 1787 Fanny's mother reluctantly took out a commission of lunacy for guardianship. Having avoided this previously because it would be too distressing for her 'on account of her maternal affection and extreme tenderness for her daughter', she was now 'by experience convinced how ready and desirious the wicked part of mankind were to take advantage of such the imbecility of her daughter'.[73] The Commission declared Fanny of unsound mind as she answered affirmatively when any man in the jury or public gallery was pointed out to her and she was asked if she wished to marry him. When 'shewn four of five guineas and asked if she would hand over her large property for that amount, she said yes'.[74] Deemed unable to understand money or marriage, her marriage was annulled and Fanny Bowerman became Fanny Fust again, now officially an adult idiot in the custody of her mother. The case formally ended in 1790.[75]

The Fust case gives an important insight into the late eighteenth-century conceptualisation of idiocy. In over a thousand pages of testimony no reference is made to medical evidence of her imbecility. Instead appeals are made throughout to 'common sense', to the circular notion that Miss Fust must be an idiot because she appears to be an idiot and behaves like an idiot, lacking what the witness testimony refers to as 'common capacity'.[76] She was observed by all, claimed the deposition, to be 'short, fat, deformed, squinting and weak in her understanding'.[77] The judges in France determined the case on 'the appearance of Fanny Fust' as well as her strange behaviour and irrational answers'.[78] The public could easily determine her idiocy. The crew on the channel steamer were 'convinced by Fanny's gestures, manners and appearance that she was insane or an ideot'.[79] French passers-by spontaneously exclaimed what a fool she was, 'not merely from the bodily infirmities … but from the mental defects which very visibly appeared in her manner and deportment'.[80]

There was common sense about idiocy: the legal profession simply confirmed what the public already discerned. If a woman would sell her property for four guineas, urinate in front of men servants and did not understand the science of lightning, she could not understand the abstractions of money, property, propriety, and scientific understanding underpinning polite and commercial society. However, this visible idiocy was discernible not only to those who sought to support and protect Fanny, but also those who wished to exploit her, 'the wicked part of mankind'. Those operating informal social or familial networks of support came under siege from rapacious predators hunting assets. Fanny's mother had to resort to law to fight the pervasive, sophisticated corruption ensnaring the asset that was her daughter. The informal system, widely accepted as the proper means of idiot support, was threatened, and institutional legalism was the best resort for families able to afford it. A new acceptance of institutional process to manage idiocy was evident. Courts had been reluctant to provide protection to Sir John Leigh and Henry Roberts either through a reluctance to interfere in individual liberty (Leigh) or through a corrupt bias in favour of those mining an idiot's wealth (Roberts).

In the case of Fanny Fust, the family fought back and bent the legal process to their own will.

At the end of the eighteenth century, therefore, the original early modern legal idea of idiocy was still intact but its stability and borders threatened by exploitative corruption and crumbling informal networks. The trends discernible in trials were reflected in legal treatises on idiocy by Highmore in 1807[81] and Collinson in 1812.[82] There had been greater focus as the century developed on the levels of knowledge and understanding necessary to constitute full human understanding and permission to participate in the 'offices of life'. These had moved far from the ability to count to twenty and recognize one's mother and father. Legal theorists began to take greater interest in idiocy and, more broadly, imbecility with a growing canon of case law and law reports on which to build. The borderlands of idiocy became more fluid as the contested new class of lifelong imbecile was consistently reinvented. Collinson was clear that things had moved on since Hardwicke's pronouncement on Sir John Leigh's case, which situated him just the other side of the border of unsound-mindedness. Now 'non compos mentis comprehends, not only idiots and lunatics, but all other persons who from *natural imbecility* ... are incapable of managing their own affairs'.[83] The courts were extending to 'persons incapable of managing their own affairs through mere weakness of understanding ... the same relief as to lunatics'. Lord Chancellor Eldon had pronounced that he was not prepared to correct any judgement that had classified the naturally weak of mind, but non-idiotic, as *non compos mentis*, giving legal status to the lifelong imbecile.[84]

Alongside this extension of the boundaries, however, state intervention in idiocy became less revenue-driven and arose more from family concerns about exploitation or inheritance. Collinson noted that 'the king's interest in the property of idiots has long been considered a hardship' but added that in fact 'few instances can be given of the oppressive exertion of it'.[85] Juries were increasingly likely to return a finding of 'unsound mind' rather than idiocy to avoid the sequestration consequences of legally defined idiotism. Even when idiotism was found, it was increasingly rare for the crown to claim its confiscation entitlement.[86] There was a wider political reluctance to interfere with individual and private decision-making, thereby undermining individual liberty of conscience and action. Collinson urged 'to take care not to extend the prerogative of the crown so as to restrain the liberty of the subject, and his power over his person and property, further than the law allowed'.[87] He argued that 'there cannot be an act of greater oppression than to interfere with the economy of domestic life'.[88] Informal family and friendship networks were, however, coming under siege from perceived acquisitive exploiters: families, as in the Fanny Fust case, began to see legal intervention and state protection as a new, more formal and effective option.

However significant these changes, Highmore and Collinson's concept of the idiot remained broadly recognisable: instantly discernible by the layman, evident in appearance as much as action or thought (or lack of it),[89] easily imposed upon, cut off by their mental incapacity from the norms and assumptions of daily society, of questionable value as a person. The idea of idiocy was constructed as much by popular perception as legal theorisation. Collinson even recycled the now very ancient joke about the idiot in the Paris cookshop to illustrate that the idiotic could sound reasonable but 'to do a sensible act, is no certain proof of a sound mind'.[90] Institutionalisation was never mentioned, expert medical opinion never sought. There was no intimation that idiots as a class were dangerous. As Highmore put it, 'Ideots are afflicted with no turbulent passions; they are innocent and harmless, and often excite pity, but never occasion fear'.[91] They could, though, be a danger to themselves, and face danger from others. The purpose of the law, in the eyes of the legal theorist, was to 'secur[e] them against injury from their own hands and from the self-interest of others'.[92] Families provided for them and friends rushed to defend them. The law saw one of its primary aims as ensuring that the 'interests of their families are preserved'.[93] Idiots remained at the heart of their community: challenged, vulnerable, perceived as different, and lacking capacity, but with sufficient personal capital in the eyes of others to be worth defending.

A new medico-legal discourse in the early nineteenth century

While a non-medicalized legal discourse on idiocy subtly interwove public notions of dim-wittedness into English jurisprudential theory, something very different was happening in France, where idiocy had attracted greater medical interest. Large institutionalisation programmes at the Salpêtrière and Bicêtre in Paris had brought idiots, as well as the mentally ill, prostitutes, and other urban 'detritus', under the medical gaze.[94] Medical jurisprudence was already established in France, an area of law where, as the legal writer and physician Fodéré happily pointed out, the French were ahead of the English.[95] In 1800 Pinel, the 'founder of psychiatry' in France,[96] and Salpêtrière chief physician, called for the application of medical jurisprudence to idiocy and lunacy, lamenting that 'in the present state of our knowledge it is the jurisprudence in relation to the different lapses of reason that seems least advanced to me'.[97] It would, he claimed, illuminate doubtful cases, disputes over soundness of mind where medical men could 'enlighten jurisprudence'.[98]

Fodéré had in fact already produced a legal medicine treatise during the turmoil of the revolutionary 1790s and then published a much expanded edition in 1813.[99] Claiming he was embarrassed by the quality of medical reports he had seen in previous cases, he promised to codify medical jurisprudence.[100] Medicine would bring jurisprudence scientific exactness, a new medicalized light shining from the reason of the Enlightenment.[101] He dismissed traditional legal approaches as speculative and unscientific[102] and denounced lay knowledge as gossip and folklore. Ridiculing the idea that neighbours could identify causation, curability, or incurability, he asked:

> what authority can be competent, other than that of doctors? ... What comparisons can there be between the assertions of a large number of, if you like, ignorant people, only judging according to their own manner of being, little interested in the thing itself, and easily persuaded; and the motivated decisions, given with knowledge of cause by truthful, upright, enlightened doctors, with a deep knowledge of the strength and weakness of the human condition, and having as a guarantee their reputation and the dignity of their position.[103]

To show what this medical authority could bring to the determination of idiocy, Fodéré offered a nosology, hierarchically ranked, bringing apparent scientific precision to vaguely defined legal ideas of unsoundness of mind. He defined three areas of mental disorder – mania (*manie*), dementia (*démence*), and imbecility (*imbécillité*) – each depriving a person of the ability to judge and compare, making them incompetent to manage their affairs and naturally excluded from the social order.[104] Imbeciles, from birth, were 'absolute strangers ... like monsters amongst the human race',[105] and could be further sub-divided into three categories. The first of these lacked the simplest association of ideas, parroting words meaninglessly and, by chance, sometimes mouthing something of 'wondrous divinity', only to jump immediately to an unconnected triviality.[106] This group was harmless. The second group could manage some simple ideas and tasks, comparable to a seven-year-old. The third group, with some rudimentary education, could form slightly better ideas. There was, however, no connection between their sometimes impressive words and their actions. Lacking judgement, they had no sense of morality; they could appear to talk about abstract moral concepts like injustice, but it was like listening to an automaton.[107] Amongst these could be found a misbehaving group of 'pre-pubescent charlatans and rascals'.[108]

The importance of Fodéré's classification was its claim to a new legal taxonomic modernity, cutting through the Gordian knot of vague legal musings evolved over centuries of case law, brushing aside the dull stupidity of lay 'common sense', and producing a finely tuned hierarchy of dullness to measure levels of personal responsibility and capacity. It directly challenged the loose

subjectivity and assumed certainties of the existing legal process, this collaboration between the law and the people using speculation to define incapacity.
Here was neatly defined, evidence-based fact, driven by the Enlightenment
quest for reason, bringing precision and certainty to the administration of
justice. Nevertheless, however hard Fodéré tried to excise the past and introduce a new clinical, scientific rationality to legal decision-making, old tropes
and folk wisdom surfaced in his work. He quoted the old adage that we are
all mad: 'Le monde est plein de fous / et qui n'en veut pas voir,/ doit se tenir
tout seul /et briser son miroir'.[109] This had in fact appeared in a 1731 English
graffiti collection, attributed to a mirror scratching in Paris's Rue Boucherie,
and translated as 'The world is full of fools and asses / to see them not ... retire
and break your glasses'.[110] It echoed a question asked by the jurist Thomas
Powell in 1623 about those who 'beg' fools: 'which is the Gardian, or which
the foole?'[111] When Fodéré wrote about the idiot's characteristic elision from
banal trivia to 'wondrous divinity', he was incorporating into medical sympto-
mology the long-running joke about the Parisan cook house idiot. His description of a 'new' class of lifelong imbecile, with some abilities but still lacking
capacity, added little to Collinson and Highmore, his categories offering no
causative theory or, indeed, treatment. His claim was simply that medical men,
with their fine observational skills, professional probity and sensibility, would
see the idiot more clearly than any layman, including the lawyer.[112] He did,
however, introduce one new concept, the idea of the dangerous idiot, linked
to natural moral depravity. His first and second classes, the most intellectually
absent of the family of idiots, were specifically not dangerous, because they
lacked the necessary thought. The dangerousness of the third class was their
ability to deceive by parroting moral language while not understanding it. It
was this class that contained his 'charlatans and rascals'.[113] Medicine had now
laid claim to the new criminal class of the moral imbecile.

Fodéré's notion of the moral imbecile as a legal category was now developed by Etienne Georget, Salpêtrière alienist and former pupil of Pinel, in his
1820 De la folie[114] and his 1826 Discussion médico-legale sur la folie ou alienation
mentale.[115] Firstly Georget added a new layer of complexity and sophistication
to Fodéré's three-level taxonomy of idiocy by inserting a fourth. Those of the
first degree had no mental existence at all and would die if not cared for. The
second degree had some feelings (sensations) but could not meet their own
needs, acting unreflectively and without purpose. These first two degrees were
a splitting of Fodéré's first grouping of harmless but mindless idiots. He then
described a third degree, equivalent to a child of seven who could recognize
some people and objects, could make their needs known through gestures,
and had a sense of who might help them. Like parrots, this grouping had the

ability to assimilate and then perform the words of songs. Finally there was the fourth degree, imbeciles with some feelings and memory, who could judge and perform simple acts but, lacking discernment, could only express themselves in basic language to meet ordinary needs.[116] To Fodéré's criminalisation of the imbecile class, Georget added disgust and revulsion for the idiot class. Urinating and leaving faecal matter wherever they were to be found and highly prone to masturbation, they were also short-lived and riddled with disease.[117] The implication of both characterisations, the imbecile as deterministically criminal and amoral, the idiot as helpless, ill, and not in control of their bodies, was that both needed some form of long-term custodial medical care. Georget explicitly claimed the superiority of medical truth over popular wisdom and lawyerly discourse, accusing lawyers who, in his opinion, talked 'most assuredly' about mental alienation of making the biggest mistakes and of being strangers to medicine.[118] He argued that punishing imbeciles for their crimes would have no effect because they and their peers had no moral understanding and once released they would return to crime, the natural impulse of their condition. Only by their lifelong institutionalisation could public security be protected.

Analysing a recent arson case, Georget neatly triangulated the three currents of thought – lay, legal, and medical – in legal decision-making on idiocy and imbecility, and explained the superiority of the medical discourse. Pierre Joseph Deléphine, standing trial in Paris in 1825, was a sixteen-year-old gardener accused of eight counts of arson. Once he had attached lighted tapers dipped in inflammable liquid to a bird's tail and launched it into a neighbour's garden.[119] Neighbours signed a statement referring to his disordered thoughts, lapses of concentration and habit of running naked around his father's garden. They all agreed that he was not imbecile but rather, claimed one, wicked (*méchant*) or, in the words of another, evil (*beaucoup de malice*).[120] The tribunal agreed with the laity's assessment and Deléphine was sentenced to death. Georget dismissed the neighbourly evidence which he said had simply presented Deléphine through an account of his bizarre ideas and strange actions and words, with no analytical appraisal. For Georget these citizens could describe surface behaviours but nothing more. Their inability to interpret, signify or pathologize led them to irrational and superstitious notions of evil and wickedness.[121]

Deléphine's lawyer agreed that the neighbours' demonic claim was absurd. For him this was a matter of mental incapacity caused by monomania, Deléphine's pyromaniac *idée fixe*, revealed by his unhealthy pallor and sad eyes.[122] He denounced the stupidity of the neighbours' unrefined views, the propensity of the 'vulgar' to dismiss the whole idea of mental alienation as a fiction, a ruse to escape conviction.[123] He issued a rhetorical challenge:

'open the medical annals, consult the tribunal case records, go into the insane hospitals', and there they would learn that nature visits the mind with just as many misfortunes as the body.[124] He argued successfully for commutation of the death sentence on the grounds of lunatic irrationality. But for Georget the lawyer's argument was no better, as he was not interpreting evidence; he was simply reporting and labelling behaviours. Georget, in fact, had the necessary evidence in his hands, as he wrote, proving Deléphine a miserable and villain-ous imbecile. His evidence was the copy of the act of accusation Deléphine had held in front of him throughout the trial. It was covered in his scrawl: endless signatures, meaningless letters, doodles, and ink stains. If he had really under-stood the enormity of his crime, asked Georget, and knew that he was facing a capital charge, would he really give himself over to such infantile pursuits?[125] This indisputable evidence denoted not only the insensibility of the criminal but also the mind of a child under eight years, which meant stupidity (*bêtise*) or silliness (*niaiserie*).[126] This insight was fruitless, Georget added causti-cally, as at no time during the trial were medical professionals asked to assess Deléphine's mental state.[127] Even French justice was not fully ready to accept medicine's ownership claim over imbecility.

The importance of this episode lay not in the outcomes of Deléphine's trial but in the reasoning of Georget's analysis. A framework of medical truth and scientific analysis was placed around abject public superstition and unin-formed legal speculation to provide a mirror onto what could have been. The justice system was corrupt, a synthesis of crude popular 'common sense' and ossified, arcane, unscientific legal processes. Georget offered a new, enlight-ened way forward: the medical man would take the imbecile villains and mischief makers who clogged up the courts and fed the guillotines into the lifelong care of the institutions, where many of their peers already lived. The judicial system was wasted on this hidden criminal class with no knowledge or understanding of law and morality.[128] Rather than a courtroom, there needed to be a statutory process of identification and dispatch to the institution, where the imbecile would be kept out of mischief, the repulsive idiot cared for, and the threat to society diminished. Thus was the medical case on idiocy in 1826. A sceptical legal profession, and a sceptical public, were yet to be convinced, but the drumbeat of medical demand for greater powers to confine the idiot and the imbecile was becoming more insistent.[129]

Influence of medical jurisprudence on English legal thought

Fodéré had been keen to point out the tardiness of English law in adopting medical jurisprudence and his challenge was taken up by the physician and apothecary John Haslam's 1817 treatise, *Medical jurisprudence as it relates to insanity according to the laws of England*.[130] Promising not to encroach on lawyers' territory, Haslam did just that as he set out a design to enable the advocate 'to adapt the facts of nature to the scale of justice' in cases of unsoundness of mind, assuring lawyers that they 'will be instructed to institute appropriate enquiries for the discovery of truth'.[131] Haslam certainly had time, and motive, in 1817 to write his book and establish a new potentially lucrative field of medical authority. Formerly the physician at Bethlem hospital, he had been called before a select committee in 1814, with the superintendent Monro, to answer allegations of cruelty and ill-treatment, culminating in his dismissal by the governors in 1816.[132] The under-employed Haslam embarked on writing his treatise in an attempt to rebuild his career and open up new opportunities as an expert medical witness.

Haslam acknowledged that 'when idiocy is plain to see the physician has an easy duty to perform'.[133] Some idiots might be able to 'whistle tunes correctly, and repeat passages from books which they have been taught by ear', but they would not fool the medical man, who would know that 'they are incapable of comprehending what they repeat'.[134] However it was at the interstice, that enduring strip of uncertainty between the idiot mind and the perfect mind, where medical men could apply their professional skills and scientific certainty. He identified two conflicting degrees of intellect, one of which, 'although mean when compared with superior minds ... will enable a human being to take charge of himself and transact his affairs'. There was also, though, 'an inferior degree, which incapacitates him from the performance of these affairs'.[135] Through 'patient examinations and repeated interviews' (implying that the potential imbecile would be under medical supervision for some time), the specialist physician would determine on which side of this divide their patient lay, 'for the mind of any man may be gauged both as to its acquirements and its capacity'.[136] How exactly, and with what evidence, it would be gauged, Haslam did not reveal, as he produced a circular definition of imbecility:

> a state or degree of mental incapacity equivalent to idiotcy, a degree which renders him incompetent to the management of himself and his affairs; and which degree, by observation and enquiry may always be ascertained. The degree, satisfactorily measured, does, in my opinion amount to unsoundness of mind.[137]

In short, imbeciles were imbeciles because a medical expert pronounced them to be so.

Anticipating Georget, Haslam assessed and compared the three sources of knowledge that competed in the courtroom. He dismissed the lay knowledge of the jury, who 'have in common with the mass of mankind formed their opinions [and] … always adopted the popular and floating opinion' through ignorance.[138] He was yet more dismissive of the 'blandishments of eloquence and the subtil underminings of lawyers', basing their arguments on past legal authorities who had never produced any definition or direction how to discover unsoundness of mind.[139] The medical profession would bring, in contrast, 'sagacity, experience, and truth' to the task of 'explaining and characterising the person's intellect'.[140] Lawyers only wanted to know if a person could conduct their own affairs; they were not interested in physiological defects, which led to absurdities where parrot-like counting qualified as capacity. The medical man could tell the court whether the person understood the abstract concept of number, or had the capacity to acquire this understanding, something never taken into consideration by the lawyer.[141] After breaking his promise not to invade lawyers' territory Haslam acknowledged the civilizing value of the law, 'established for the protection and happiness of the community', but asserted that 'knowledge of the human intellect, in its sane and disordered state, may be expected from medical opinion'.[142]

The discredited Haslam, a professional outcast who eventually died poor in 1844,[143] did manage to construct some sort of career as a rather belligerent and testy expert medical witness, but the impact of his treatise was not as he had hoped. It was not until the 1830s that other medical men, and lawyers, began to examine the English medical claim to explain and define idiocy in court, and it was done with markedly less enthusiasm than Haslam had evinced. Andrew Amos, England's first professor of medical jurisprudence,[144] drew on case law and the jurists Coke, Hardwicke, and Eldon to grapple with the definitional problem of imbecility and its link to incapacity.[145] He acknowledged that he was 'rather ashamed to say' that these were the principle sources of legal authority,[146] and agreed with Haslam that medical witnesses were needed in court to detect witnesses making false imbecility claims,[147] but advanced no greater claim.

The reclusive barrister and legal writer Leonard Shelford[148] specifically re-stated the lawyerly claim over idiocy and was distinctly muted in his assessment of what medical jurisprudence might offer.[149] Shelford asked, on the question of identifying unsoundness of mind and its degree, 'can no one else do this but a medical man?' He acknowledged that 'popular bias' on these matters infiltrated the courts and influenced juries, who although 'of the intelligent class' were prone to inconsistent decision-making through their 'popular and ill-defined notions', which a professionally conversant medical man should avoid.[150] However, he warned, 'of all evidence in courts of justice, that of medical men ought to be given with greatest care, and received with utmost caution'.[151] Against Haslam's notion of the silver-tongued lawyer bamboozling juries with beguiling eloquence, Shelford set the opinionated, jargon-strewn evidence of the medical man. Medical evidence about the mind was only acceptable if 'comprehensible to laymen and explicit in facts, tender, slow and circumspect in opinion'.[152] Legal power still rested very much with the lay person. The job of medical men was to convince juries that there was such a 'radical perversion of intellect ... that a person was bereft of ... reason'.

Shelford restated the claim of individual liberty, as advanced by Collinson and others, against medicalized statist encroachment, and regretted that vague definitions around imbecility in particular would 'invade the liberty of the subject and the rights of the people'.[153] Where imbecility existed, it needed to be determined with great accuracy, because there was no reason why an imbecile person who could remain 'orderly and mannerly' should not retain some self-dominion.[154] Here Shelford gave a new discursive emphasis to the old trope of the idiot as child. Important indicators of both idiocy and imbecility were childlike behaviours such as preoccupation with frivolous pursuits, fondness for trifles, shyness, easy submission to control, and acquiescence under influence.[155] He argued against the total deprivation of rights for the person deemed to lack capacity through idiocy or imbecility, for even such a person might 'spend his own little income in providing for his wants, as a boy spends his pocket money', despite being vulnerable to imposition.[156] The idiot could be permitted to sit astride his own legal kingdom, a tiny world in which only trifles mattered and nothing of real import required decision.

The early nineteenth-century battle between law and medicine

A flurry of texts on idiocy and imbecility now emerged on both sides of the Atlantic. British writers remained highly sceptical towards the claims of Georget, Fodéré, and Haslam to medical authority in this field. In 1834 the barrister Chitty mocked the pretentions of the new practitioners of medical jurisprudence to superiority over lawyers in the area of the mind, seeing medical jurisprudence as better employed in clearly scientific fields such as toxicology and post-mortem. 'Medical professors', he wrote, 'who naturally have investigated every subject relative to the distressing defects in the human understanding more laboriously than lawyers or jurymen can do ... have long sub-divided and assigned particular appropriate names for every deviation from mental perfection'.[157] Rejecting these claims to scientific precision, Chitty warned 'it is very clearly established that the question whether idiot or not, must be decided by a jury, after hearing all the evidence'.[158] His reference to 'all the evidence' was pointed; medical testimony alone was not sufficient. Noting how the four definitions of incapacity had now evolved into 'idiotcy', lunacy, insanity, and then 'any such degree of imbecility as to incapacitate a party to take care of his own property',[159] Chitty argued that juries no longer had to worry about medical technicalities so long as *they thought* that the person's mental faculties were 'so enfeebled as to render him incompetent to act for himself'.[160] He acknowledged that medical evidence was 'unquestionably admissible'[161] (advocates of medical authority would have been puzzled that this should have to be acknowledged at all), but ranked medical authority on idiocy only on a par with other competing claims, including the common sense judgement of the jury member. He praised the law's generally accurate view of the progressive and ascending scale in the development of the mind'.[162] Chitty did, however, contribute to the rising alarm being sounded by medical men about potential threats from idiots as a class, and highlighted a new cause for anxiety: 'idiots are in in general inoffensive but particularly as regards the female sex, sometimes there are dangerous exceptions'.[163] This introduced the dangerously unrestrained, promiscuous and amoral female imbecile to the legal picture.

The medicalization of legal discourse on idiocy was advocated more assertively in the US, where Georget and Fodéré's work was influential. Theodric Beck, Professor of medicine at the College of Physicians and Surgeons of Western New York, drew heavily on Georget in his 1836 work.[164] He evidenced the necessity of medical judgement in cases of idiocy and imbecility with numerous case histories, some from Georget, identifying common disorders in criminal trial defendants and asylum residents. Beck drew attention to the new 'disputed form of disease' of moral imbecility, where a person's intellectual functions are quite sound but their feelings and affections are 'perverted and depraved', which in turn destroys or severely impairs their power of self-government.[165] Highlighting this group's ingenuity and ability to hide their disorder, Beck noted that only trained medical professionals who knew what to look for could identify it, and proposed that they needed the authority to do so urgently.

In 1839, Isaac Ray's treatise laid down the medical claim even more emphatically.[166] Ray was an American psychiatrist and was to become medical director of the State Hospital for the Insane in Augusta. He wished 'to challenge those practices passed down on the authority of our ancestors',[167] scorning the law's preference for ancient wisdom over new modes of medical knowledge when these were 'facts, established by men of undoubted experience and good faith'.[168] He attacked the law's 'crude and unsound notions' about the human mind[169] and its 'blind obstinacy' when (medical) truth disproved its established maxims and decisions.[170] He ridiculed juries, which, far from Shelford's 'intelligent class',[171] were simply 'a number of men, who may have had very little education of any kind ... [sitting] in judgement on the manner of a man's understanding'.[172] How could the dull, he implied, judge the dull? The law was 'still loose, vacillating, and greatly behind the present state of knowledge' of idiocy and other conditions of mind.[173]

Ray called for the introduction of expert medical witnesses, as employed in France, who would be in a permanent state of readiness to be called by the courts.[174] Such men could settle the complexities of capacity and understanding amongst the imbecile class who possessed 'some intellectual capacity, though infinitely less than is possessed by the great mass of mankind'.[175] He added a further complication: the stupid person. Ordinary imbeciles were aware of their intellectual deficit but the stupid person 'imagines himself equal, if not superior to other men in his intelligence'. The stupid person was consequently far more dangerous, as they were prepared to act 'precipitately and without reflection' while shy, unconfident imbeciles could never make up their mind to do anything for fear of consequences.[176] The stupid person, appearing suspiciously like the moral imbecile, thus joined the increasingly crowded space occupied by persons of dubious capacity between the perfect mind and the perfect idiot. Ray echoed Georget on the futility of penal sanctions against imbecile offenders, for whom deterrence was meaningless. Perpetual confinement in a medical institution was the only sensible course, to protect society and their own welfare.[177] It was futile to expect courts and juries to act correctly in these puzzling cases.[178]

Towards the mid-nineteenth century, therefore, there were strong currents of thought in France and America, each only recently emerging from wider social revolutions, advocating a revolutionary medicalized modernisation of judicial process, where expert witnesses would set scientific fact against the fanciful opinions of juries and the past-worshipping manipulations of the lawyer. In France this was driven by a new faith in scientific evidence and medical testimony in the recent Napoleonic code.[179] In England, there was predictably reactionary suspicion, as Ray saw it, against this new knowledge. English medical jurisprudence focused more pragmatically on forensic science, with its poisons, knife wounds and fake life assurance claims, than on the speculative art of fathoming people's minds.[180] There was greater concern also about the personal liberty implications of state intervention in the name of protection. The population of idiots seemed to be growing exponentially as old, loose categories of unsoundness of mind hardened into notions of the lifelong imbecile, sometimes a harmless, timid person with a small but insufficient intellect, but sometimes moral imbeciles, with their ability to pass as non-idiotic, masking degenerate morals and criminality and threatening the fabric of society from below. The 'perfect' idiot was mostly helpless and pitiable, sometimes disgusting and repulsive. Both idiots and imbeciles could be very childlike, but simultaneously degraded and threatening. From some parts of the medical world arose an insistent call for a judicial process by-passing mainstream courts and creating a direct route into lifelong medical supervision, offering care for idiots and protection both for and from imbeciles. In both cases, the separation between the idiot and the imbecile and their original community would be complete and final.

In the battle for courtroom authority over the idiot in England throughout the nineteenth century, the medical men would not have it all their own way. Despite the strong currents of enthusiasm from the US and France, and a small group of practitioners in England, who claimed the medical right to identify, treat, and manage those deemed idiotic, such claims would be resisted under English law. Resistance came in the form of a persistent libertarian rear-guard, lawyers (and some doctors) who valued the freedom of the individual to live a life unimpeded by state interference over any exploitation risks caused by weak mental faculty. Sometimes doctors would be called to give their opinion in legal cases, but as late as the 1860s their testimony was given only as much credence as lay testimony, and frequently treated with disdain or suspicion by lawyers, judges, and even fellow medical men.[181] In the English courtroom at least, the inevitability of the great incarceration was far from assured.

Notes

1 H. E. Bell, *An Introduction to the History and Records of the Court of Wards and Liveries* (Cambridge: Cambridge Univeristy Press, 1953), 1, 85–86.

2 Ibid., 163.

3 Richard Neugebauer, 'Treatment of the Mentally Ill in Medieval and Early Modern England: A Reappraisal', *Journal of the History of the Behavioural Sciences* 14 (1978), 164–166.

4 Sir Edward Coke, *Institutes of the laws of England*, 1628, cited in George Dale Collinson, *A treatise on the law concerning idiots, lunatics, and other persons non compotes mentis* (London, 1812), 57–58. Emphasis added.

5 Collinson, *A treatise on the law concerning idiots, lunatics, and other persons non compotes mentis*, 59.

6 John Brydall, *Non compos mentis: or the law relating to natural fools, mad folks and lunatic persons inquisited and explained for the common benefit* (London, 1700).

7 Ibid., preface A4.

8 Ibid., 13–15 and 17–18.

9   Ibid., 16.
10 Ibid., 8, 10, 12.
11 Ibid., preface A2.
12 Ibid., 8.
13 Ibid., 38.
14 Ibid., 10.
15 Ibid., 35.
16 Ibid., 38.
17 Ibid.
18 Ibid.
19 Ibid.
20 Ibid., 8–9.
21 Ibid., 9.
22 Ibid., 3, 6.
23 Ibid., 6. Emphasis in original.
24 Ibid., 35–36.
25 William Hicks, 'Selections from *Oxford Jests*' [1671], in *A nest of ninnies and other English jestbooks of the seventeenth century*', edited by P. M. Zall (Lincoln: University of Nebraska Press, 1970), 240.
26 Henry Swinburne, *A treatise of testaments and last wills* [1590], 8th edn (London, 1743), 80–81.
27 Brydall, *Non compos mentis*, 36–38.
28 Tobias Smollett, *The adventures of Roderick Random* [1748] (London: Everyman, 1975), 253.
29 Old Bailey Proceedings (*OBP*), July 1723, 'Trial of Thomas Allen' (t17230710–39) & *OBP*, July 1775, 'Trial of Joseph Muggleton, William Jackling, James Lewis' (t17750712–49)
30 In B. E. (Gent), *A new dictionary of the terms ancient and modern of the canting crew in its several tribes, of gypsies, beggars, thieves, cheats & c.* (London, 1699), and Francis Grose, *A dictionary of the vulgar tongue* (London, 1788).
31 Johann Wilhelm von Archenholz, *A picture of England: containing a description of the laws, customs, and manners of England*, Vol. 1 (London, 1789), 31.
32 Daniel Defoe, *Review*, 25 June, 1709, cited in Dorothy George, *London Life in the Eighteenth Century* (London: Penguin, 1992), 363–364, note 48.
33 Ibid.
34 *Bennet v Vade*, 1742, TNA PROB 18/54/18.
35 *Bennet v Vade*, 1739, TNA PROB 18/51/5.
36 Ibid.
37 Ibid.
38 Ibid.
39 Ibid.
40 Ibid.
41 Ibid.

42 *Bennet v Vade*, Deposition, 1740, TNA PROB 18/52/11.
43 *Bennet v Vade*, 1739 TNA PROB 18/51/5.
44 Ibid.
45 Ibid.
46 Collinson, *A treatise on the law concerning idiots*, 60–61.
47 Brydall, *Non compos mentis*, 6.
48 *Bennet v Vade*, 1739 TNA PROB 18/51/5. Emphasis in original.
49 Anon., *The case of Henry Roberts, Esq, a gentleman who by unparalleled cruelty was deprived of his estate under the pretence of idiocy* (London, 1767).
50 Anon., *The case of Henry Roberts*, 4.
51 Ibid., 6.
52 Ibid., 8.
53 Ibid., 9.
54 Ibid., 11–12. Emphasis in original.
55 Ibid., 12.
56 Richard Sharp, 'Lynch, John (1697–1760)', *Oxford Dictionary of National Biography* (Oxford: Oxford University Press, 2004), www.oxforddnb.com/. Accessed May 2009.
57 Anon., *The case of Henry* Roberts, 12.
58 TNA C211/22/R34.
59 Anon., *The case of Henry Roberts*, 13–14.
60 *Birkbeck v Birkbeck*, 1750/51, TNA E 134/24/Geo2/Mich 9.
61 *Bowerman v Fust*, 1789, TNA DEL 1/644.
62 Ibid., 132–135.
63 Ibid., 136.
64 Ibid., 136–137.
65 Ibid., 141.
66 Ibid., 138–139.
67 Ibid., 369.
68 Ibid., 147–181.
69 Ibid., 259–269.
70 Ibid., 195–214, 295–329.
71 Ibid., 311.
72 Ibid., 365.
73 Ibid., 333–335.
74 Ibid., 348–349.
75 'Westminster Hall', *Times* (London, England), 22 April, 1790: 3; The Times Digital Archive, accessed 18 June, 2014.
76 *Bowerman v Fust*, 1789, TNA DEL 1/644, 164.
77 Ibid., 203.
78 Ibid., 212.
79 Ibid., 67.
80 Ibid., 312.

81 A. Highmore, *A treatise on the law of idiocy and lunacy* (London, 1807).
82 Collinson, *A treatise on the law concerning idiots*.
83 Ibid., 58. Emphasis added.
84 Ibid., 65.
85 Ibid., 100.
86 Ibid.
87 Ibid., 63.
88 Ibid., 65.
89 This was in contrast to lunacy, which could be hidden. 'Idiocy … may be discerned, but lunacy cannot'. Highmore, *A treatise on the law of idiocy*, 36.
90 Collinson, *A treatise on the law concerning idiots*, 43–46.
91 Highmore, *A treatise on the law of idiocy*, vi.
92 Ibid., xii.
93 Ibid., xii.
94 Michel Foucault, *Madness and Civilization*, translated by Richard Howard (London: Routledge, 1989), 229–264.
95 F. E. Fodéré, '*Traité de médecine légale et d'hygiène publique ou de police de santé: tome premier*' [1792] (Paris, 1813), xii.
96 Deborah B. Weiner, 'Foreword', in Philipe Pinel, *Medico-philosophical treatise on mental alienation*, [1800], [1809], translated by Gordon Hickish, David Henly, and Louis C Charland (Chichester: Wiley-Blackwell, 2008).
97 Pinel, *Medico-philosophical treatise*, 72.
98 Ibid., 72.
99 F. E. Fodéré, *Traité de médecine légale et d'hygiène publique ou de police de santé: tome premier*' [1792], 2nd edn (Paris, 1813).
100 Fodéré, *Traité de médecine légale*, v, ix.
101 Ibid., xxxiv.
102 Ibid.
103 'Quelle comparaison peut-il y avoir entre les assertions d'un grand nombre, si l'on veut, de personnes ignorantes, ne jugeant que d'après leur manière d' être, peu intéressés â la chose, et se laissant facilement séduire; et les décisions motivées, rendues avec connaissances de cause, par des médecins vrais, probes, éclairés, connaissant â fond le fort et le faible de la nature humaine, ayant pour garantie leur reputation et la dignité de leur état.' Fodéré, *Traité de médecine légale*, 192–193 (author's translation).
104 Ibid., 186.
105 'absolument étrangers … comme des monstres parmi la race humaine.' Fodéré, *Traité de médecine légale*, 186 [Author's translation].
106 'Divinité fabuleuse.' Fodéré, *Traité de médecine légale*, 202 (author's translation).
107 Ibid., 203.
108 'Les charlatans et les fripons.' Fodéré, *Traité de médecine légale*, 203 (author's translation).
109 Ibid., 184.

110 Hurlo Thrombo, *The merry thought: or the glass-window and bog-house miscellany* (London, 1731), 43–44.

111 Thomas Powell, *The attourney's academy, or the manner and forme of proceeding practically upon any suite, plaint or action whatsoever, within this kingdome: especially in the great courts at Westminster* (London, 1623), 216–217.

112 Ibid., 285.

113 Ibid., 203.

114 Etienne-Jean Georget, *De la folie: considerations sur cette maladie* (Paris, 1820).

115 Etienne-Jean Georget, *Discussion médico-legale sur la folie ou alienation mentale* (Paris, 1826).

116 Georget, *De la folie*, 103–104.

117 Ibid., 104–105.

118 Georget, *Discussion médico-legale*, 1.

119 Ibid., 132.

120 Ibid., 134.

121 Ibid., 132, 139.

122 Ibid., 135–136.

123 Ibid., 136.

124 'Ouvrez les annales de la medicine, consultez les registres des tribunaux, entrez les hospices d'alienés': Georget, *Discussion médico*-legale, 136–137 (author's translation).

125 Ibid., 138.

126 Ibid.

127 Ibid., 141.

128 Ibid., 140.

129 Ibid., 175–176.

130 John Haslam, *Medical jurisprudence as it relates to insanity according to the law of England* (London, 1817).

131 Ibid., ii–iii.

132 Andrew Scull, Charlotte Mackenzie, and Nicholas Harvey, *Masters of Bedlam: The Transformation of the Mad-Doctoring Trade* (Princeton: Princeton University Press, 1996), 31–37.

133 Haslam, *Medical jurisprudence as it relates to insanity*, 3.

134 Ibid., 97–98.

135 Ibid., 98.

136 Ibid.

137 Ibid.

138 Ibid., 8–9.

139 Ibid., 4, 8.

140 Ibid., 3.

141 Ibid., 94–96.

142 Ibid., 103.

143 Ibid., 10, 42.

144 Thomas S. Legg, 'Amos, Andrew (1791–1860)', *Oxford Dictionary of National*

Biography (Oxford: Oxford University Press, 2004); online edn accessed 26 June, 2014.

145 Professor Amos, 'Lectures in medical jurisprudence delivered in the University of London: on insanity', *London Medical Gazette* 8 (July, 1831), 418–419.

146 Professor Amos, 'Lectures in medical jurisprudence', 418.

147 Ibid., 420.

148 E. I. Carlyle, 'Shelford, Leonard (1795–1864)', rev. Jonathan Harris, *Oxford Dictionary of National Biography* (Oxford: Oxford University Press, 2004); online edn accessed 26 June, 2014.

149 Leonard Shelford, *A practical treatise on the law concerning lunatics, idiots and persons of unsound mind* (London, 1833).

150 Shelford, *A practical treatise on the law concerning lunatics*, 45.

151 Ibid., 46.

152 Ibid.

153 Shelford, *A practical treatise on the law concerning lunatics*, 4.

154 Ibid., 5.

155 Ibid.

156 Ibid.

157 J Chitty, *A practical treatise on medical jurisprudence*, London 1834, 344.

158 Chitty, *Practical treatise*, 345.

159 Ibid., 343.

160 Ibid., 344.

161 Ibid., 353.

162 Ibid., 341–342.

163 Ibid.

164 Theodric Beck, *Elements of medical jurisprudence* (London, 1836).

165 Ibid., 402.

166 Isaac Ray, *A treatise on the medical jurisprudence of insanity* (London, 1839).

167 D Spillan, 'Introduction', in Ray, *A treatise on the medical jurisprudence of insanity*, x.

168 Ibid., xxviii.

169 Ray, *A treatise on the medical jurisprudence of insanity*, 3.

170 Ibid., 4.

171 Shelford, *A practical treatise on the law concerning lunatics*, 45.

172 Ray, *A treatise on the medical jurisprudence of insanity*, 24.

173 Ibid., 49.

174 Ibid., 54–55.

175 Ibid., 71.

176 Ibid., 75.

177 Ibid., 115.

178 Ibid., 117.

179 John Peter Eigen, *Witnessing Insanity: Madness and Mad Doctors in the English Court* (New Haven: Yale University Press, 1995), 112.

180 See, for example, William Guy, *Principles of forensic medicine*, 2nd edn (London: 1861).

181 See, for example, the cases of *Ingram v Wyatt* (1828), TNA, DEL 1/725, *Bagster v Newton*, 'Commission of Lunacy, Bagster v Newton', *London Medical Gazette* 10 (21 July, 1832), and *Windham v Windham* 1861. See also 'The case of Mr W. F. Windham', *Times* (London, England, 17 December, 1861), 3, TDA and various *Times* articles 1861–62.

10

IDIOCY AND THE CONCEPTUAL ECONOMY OF MADNESS

Murray K. Simpson

Intellectual disability has long had, and indeed continues to have, an uneasy and inconsistent position in the nosology of mental illness. This situation has coupled with a generally under-problematized historical linkage between 'intellectual disability' and 'idiocy', resulting in a severely weakened understanding of the historical descent of the latter and the overstatement of its connection to the former. Hitherto, very little attention has been given to the significance of the conceptual location of idiocy within medical psychology and madness. Even by the end of the eighteenth century the position and constitution of idiocy in relation to other mental diseases was still not consistent, either in location or definition. Whilst Wright contemplates the relatively marginal interest given to the history of idiocy within the historiography of madness and psychiatry,[1] this in itself does not address two key issues: firstly, whether any such separation is historically legitimate, and, secondly, whether this impoverishment of historiography actually invalidates a good deal of what we believe about the history of psychiatry. Leaving out what might be perceived as uninteresting aspects of insanity undermines our capacity to understand what gave it any coherence in the first place. This chapter attempts to redress this marginalization and to relocate an understanding of idiocy within the economy of madness and alienism.

As will be demonstrated through an admittedly rather selective study of the conceptual 'locations of idiocy' within medicine and, more specifically, psychiatry, its relational position has been highly varied and complex. Furthermore, the very capacity of psychiatry logically and consistently to sustain intellectual disability as an object of study and therapeutic target is questionable.

In 1792, William Pargeter's 'Observations on maniacal disorders' drew strong connections between madness and modern lifestyles – excess, poor diet, 'unnatural' sleep patterns and so forth. Idiotism figured, for Pargeter, as one of the potential symptoms and sequelæ of this.

> When we behold the most shining characters – our relations – our dearest friends and companions, whose reason lies either 'buried in the body's grave', or who linger out an hapless existence in a rueful state of idiotism or fatuity, we cannot but be affected with the most lively sensations of pity and regret. Under the influence of passions and reflections, which occurrences of this nature are apt to excite, we are sometimes undutifully inclined to withdraw from Providence that veneration and respect which it claims from all; as if it were possible for Heaven to be deficient in integrity of design – wisdom of appointment, or uniformity of conduct. But why should we charge God foolishly, with what is generally occasioned by an unreasonable indulgence of our sensual appetites, or a too servile compliance with the prevailing manners.[2]

Insofar as idiotism is concerned, Pargeter was typical of his day, which is, perhaps, to say lacking in any clear conceptual typicality at all. Aside from not approaching his subject from a perspective of classifying idiotism as a species of insanity, Pargeter does not regard its appearance exclusively, or even primarily, as congenital. However, less than a century later, it would become an anachronism and an absurdity to regard idiocy as anything other than developmental.[3] The 'developmental' approach to idiocy differed significantly to simple 'congenital' models. First, it expanded the concept of idiocy beyond conditions arising before, during, or shortly after birth, to the whole *developmental period*. Second, it became an impairment *of* development, not merely during it.

Only in the nineteenth century did anything resembling current conceptual models and systems of classification begin to crystalize. The position of idiocy is both symptomatic and illustrative of this fact. Thomas Arnold's nosography, for instance, was based on a primary division between 'ideal' and 'notional' insanity; the former having four types and the latter nine, none of which correspond to idiocy. Although classification was the primary, and most successful, response of medicine to the heterogeneity of insanity, it was not the only one. William Battie proceeded by adopting a restrictive definition of madness and excluding any conditions that did not fit it. Battie distinguished madness from foolishness (a conflation which he attributed to the French), and, other than to distinguish 'original' from 'consequential' madness, his treatise contained no system of differentiation to speak of.[4]

> that man and that man alone is properly mad, who is fully and unalterably persuaded of the Existence or of the appearance of any thing, which either does not exist or does not actually appear to him, and who behaves according to such erroneous persuasion.[5]

In certain other schemes a binary division exists, but idiocy and insanity remain linked by some other common rubric. Thus, with 'lunacy' providing the over-arching term, Francis Willis was to suggest:

> Lunacy [...] resolves itself into a question of *compos* or *non compos mentis:* the
> conduct of the individual is the evidence of his competency or incompetency
> [...] whether the latter has existed *ex navitate* [idiocy], or been created by
> disease [insanity].[6]

However, by the time that alienism begins to take shape at the very end
of the eighteenth century, positions such as Battie's begin to disappear.
Nonetheless, as this chapter will demonstrate, a variety of distinct forms of
arrangement existed, linking idiocy with other forms of mental illness. None
of these dominated to exclusion and none of them can be said to have been
swept aside by improved scientific knowledge of respective conditions. The
aim of this chapter is not to try and trace the history, much less the *progress,* of
idiocy within the disciplinary history of medicine. Neither is it to answer the
question as to whether intellectual disability should or should not be regarded
as a psychiatric condition. Rather, its central goal is much more restricted;
it is to describe the relations between psychiatry and idiocy at various historical points and to consider some of the numerous factors that might have
impinged on their development. As will be seen, this relationship is one of
the most revealing aspects of psychiatry's epistemological trajectory over the
period. It also says a good deal about the practical and conceptual directions in
which the fledgling discourse on idiocy was able to move.

   This chapter will also explore some of the various positions that idiocy
occupied in various nosological frameworks of psychiatry and medicine generally from the late eighteenth century to the end of the nineteenth. This exploration will demonstrate the lack of any consistency in its position or in its general
direction. Instead, the positioning ranges from random, through consequent,
to opportunist. The choice and coverage of these conceptual frameworks and
classificatory schemes is not exhaustive, and neither is it intended to cover all
of the major periods of either psychiatry or idiocy. Instead, their selection is
designed to demonstrate the contention that there is no underlying consistency, logic, or essential basis to them, only the exercise and relations of power.

Cullen and fragmented dispersal

The nosological impulse in medicine that arose in the eighteenth century was
largely an extension of taxonomic thinking in biology. It had begun in earnest
in 1731 with the work of Boissier de Sauvages, and continued its development
largely along those same taxonomic lines established in botany.[7]

   Between 1777 and 1784, William Cullen published his seminal four volume
First Lines in the Practice of Physic, which set out one of the most systematic
and influential nosologies of its time. The outline version, *Synopsis Nosologiæ*

```
┌─────────────────────────────┬───────────────────────────────────────────┐
 Pyrexiae                                    Cachexies          Local diseases


                        Neuroses


┌──────────────┬──────────────────┬────────────────────┐
 Comata         Adynamiæ           Spasmodic            Vesaniæ


   ┌ Apoplexy     ┌ Syncope          ┌ Tetanus            ┌ Mania
   └ Palsy        ├ Dyspepsia        ├ Epilepsy           ├ Melancholy
                  └ Hypochondriasis  ├ Chorea             ├ Amentia
                                     └ Etc.               └ Oneirodynia
```

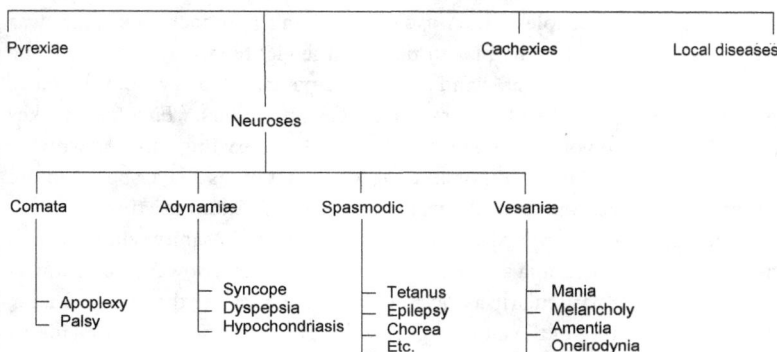

2 Idiocy in Cullen's nosography

Methodicæ, first appeared in 1769, and does not entirely correspond in every aspect in the original schema.[8] In it, 'amentia' appears as one of four species of 'vesaniæ'. The vesaniæ, in turn, were a branch of the neuroses – one of the four disease classes (see Figure 2). This grouping of the fairly familiar types of insanity would seem to suggest a strong link to the later nosographies of insanity produced by Pinel and Esquirol. In Pinel's case, the *Nosographie philosophique ou méthode de l'analyse appliquée à la médecine*, published in 1798, takes an essentially 'flat' approach to insanity (see Figure 3, below).[9] Pinel was a strong admirer of Cullen, translating his *First Lines* into French. However, 'fatuity' plays multiple functions in Cullen's work, of which constituting a variety of disease is only one – the others being as symptoms and sequelæ of a variety of other diseases.

However, it is the incorporation by Cullen of idiocy into the vesaniæ and neurotic illnesses that is of greatest significance in the positioning of idiocy within the conceptual framework of psychological medicine from its earliest stages. *Neuroses*, then, comprise:

> all those preternatural affections of sense or motion, which are without pyrexia as part of the primary disease; and all those which do not depend upon a topical affection of the organs, but upon a more general affection of the nervous system, and of those powers of the system upon which sense and motion more especially depend.[10]

The *vesaniæ* encompassed diseases involving 'the lesions of our judging faculty'. Such lesions are divided broadly into *delirium*, 'erroneous judgment', and *fatuity*, or 'weakness or imperfection of judgment'.[11] Such a division seems redolent of Locke's division of the insane and idiot; however, it does not occupy a central role in the nosology. Cullen's approach to insanity was part of a wider shift that had taken place in the eighteenth century, with the incorporation of both organic and psychic elements, and away from the more purely psychical definitions of Locke, Sauvages, and others.[12] *First Lines* makes a further separation of delirium into those conditions existing with and without pyrexia (fever), making it impossible for it to function as a layer between the general class of vesaniæ and its specific diseases – delirium existing as both a common symptom of pyrexiæ, and as constitutive of 'insanity', under which heading are located mania and melancholia.[13] Even here, however, delirium is a symptom most particularly associated with mania, rather than melancholia, whilst consideration of the latter begins with a general review of 'partial insanity', which would later be more clearly categorized as 'monomania' by Esquirol and others.[14] In addition, 'phrensy', 'hypochondriasis', 'hysteria', and 'canine madness' sit outside the whole framework of the vesaniæ ('inflamations', 'adynamiæ', and 'spasmodic affections' respectively). Clearly, then, it was not only idiocy that remained fluid and ambiguous in the constellation of the nascent medico-psychological complex.

As to idiocy, Cullen clusters 'Imbecility of the judgment' into three types:

> Amentia *congenital*, continuing from birth.
> Amentia *senilis*, from decay of perception and memory, in old age.
> Amentia *acquisita*, induced by evident external causes in men of sound judgment.[15]

Perhaps one of the most important things that Cullen's nosography reproduces and reinforces is the general ambiguity of the position of idiocy. On the one hand, it is located within a general medical conceptual economy, and specifically of insanity; on the other, it is bracketed as unworthy of attention. Hence, *First Lines* concludes consideration of the vesaniæ stating:

> Having now delivered my doctrine with respect to the chief forms of insanity, I should in the next place proceed to consider the other genera of Amentia and Oneirodynia, which in the Nosology I have arranged under the order of Vesaniae: But as I cannot pretend to throw much light upon these subjects, and as they are seldom the objects of practice, I think it allowable for me to pass them over at present; and the particular circumstances of this work in some measure requires that I should do so.[16]

Similarly, Alexander Crichton, in his influential treatise of 1798, included 'fatuitas' as one of the six categories of 'amentia' – itself one of three subcategories of derangement – in his nosography.[17] However, it occupies almost none of the rest of the book.

For Cullen, the other functions played by fatuity were as symptoms and sequelæ of other diseases. In the case of palsy, for instance, 'some degree of fatuity' is posited as 'symptomatic'. As sequelæ, repeated epileptic fits are identified as proximate causes of fatuity, whilst in some cases of rachitis 'stupidity or fatuity prevails'.[18] Similar views can be found elsewhere. William Perfect does not identify amentia as a species of insanity, but outlines the case of a man with 'a depravity in the habitual constitution of the mind [and who eventually] [...] dwindled into a total decay as he approached the verge of idiotism, in which dark abyss I must leave him',[19] thus contributing to the radical exclusion of the idiotic from the very idea of humanity.

Idiocy and alienism

As noted, the influential nosologies of madness of Pinel and Esquirol were essentially flat, with species of insanity set out horizontally and with no vertical hierarchical sub-divisions (see figure 3 for Pinel's nosology).[20] Even by its third and final edition in 1807, Pinel's categories of 'neuroses of brain function' had merely expanded – apoplexy, epilepsy, hypochondria, melancholia, mania, dementia, idiocy, somnambulism, and hydrophobia – whilst remaining flat.[21]

Among the last of those taking such a flat approach was John Conolly with his influential 1856 scheme for asylum construction and governance. Conolly did not present a nosology, strictly speaking, as the main body of his work considers only acute mania, chronic mania, melancholia, general paralysis, and mental disorder combined with epilepsy, with no apparent place for idiocy. Whilst there is an appended report on the 'Instruction of the insane at the Bicêtre in Paris, and of the idiot and imbecile at Earlswood, near Reigate, and Essex Hall, Colchester', the focus is not on 'treatment without restraints' – the subject of the book – but merely education and training, and even that is not constituted in the terms of medico-pedagogy, established by Séguin. Similarly, whilst Pinel and Esquirol had incorporated idiocy within their schemata, the emphasis on moral treatment, and the action on the will, left it largely neglected in practice. By the time of Conolly's work, pedagogical optimism had altered this picture somewhat, though it still was not included within his framework of moral treatment.[22]

However, within a few decades, more complex systems of classification emerged. Henry Maudsley published several variants of his nosology in the

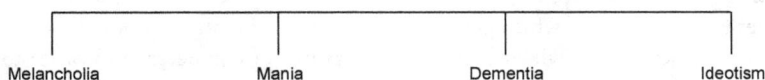

Melancholia	Mania	Dementia	Ideotism

3 Pinel's nosographic framework

1870s, but all shared the common element of having more than one level of division (see Figure 4). In addition to locating idiocy and imbecility within the general taxonomy, Maudsley describes in some detail different species, causes, pathological anatomies, and consequences of amentia. In so doing, he draws heavily on degeneration theory; hereditary taint resulted in 'the insane temperament'.[23] Degeneration theory provided the basis for the connection between idiocy and the other species of insanity.

> Insanity, of what form soever, whether mania, melancholia, moral insanity, or dementia, may be looked upon then philosophically as a stage in the descent towards sterile idiocy.[24]

Idiocy, then, sat alongside a range of conditions, even beyond insanity – immorality, alcoholism, consanguine marriage, hypochondria, and so forth – as the hereditary outcome of progressive inter-generational degeneration. Of course, Maudsley comes neither first nor last in relation to degeneration theory and insanity.[25]

Another example of organic approaches to insanity, though without degeneration theory, was E. C. Spitzka's 1883 *Manual on Insanity*. A neurologist, Spitzka outlined a theory and nosology of insanity based on organic pathology, rather than psychology. For this reason, as with the degenerationists, he reversed the view that idiocy was, at best, a marginal area in the treatment of insanity. Arguing against the view that idiocy, imbecility, and cretinism were not even to be considered as species of insanity at all, he asserted:

> the typical psychoses of the neuro-degenerative series may arise on the basis of the same or similar developmental defects as those which are so characteristic of the states of arrested and perverted development.[26]

Krafft-Ebing's binary division of 'arrested development' from all other forms of insanity was also summarily dismissed by Spitzka for failing to take account of pathological connections between idiocy and other forms of insanity. Spitzka cited various commonalities between idiocy and other species, particularly with monomania, for instance. Unsurprisingly, perhaps, Krafft-Ebing proceeded to ignore arrested development in the volume on clinical practice.[27]

Spitzka incorporated three grades of arrested development – idiocy, imbecility, and feeble-mindedness – though his nosography of insanity included only the first two (see Figure 5). His approach evidences superficial similarities to other systems which graded degrees from, for example, idiot, imbecile, and simpleton,[28] or which used crude measures of competence in order to classify, such as Ireland's three-level division of idiots and five-fold division of imbecility.[29] In these cases, the descriptors for each grade serve as proxy

Affective insanity
or
insanity without delusion

    a. instinctive
    b. moral

Ideational insanity

Melancholia ⎡ acute
⎣ chronic

Mania ⎡ acute
⎣ chronic

Monomania ⎡ acute
Dementia ⎣ chronic

Amentia

Imbecility ⎡ moral and
Idiocy ⎣ intellectual

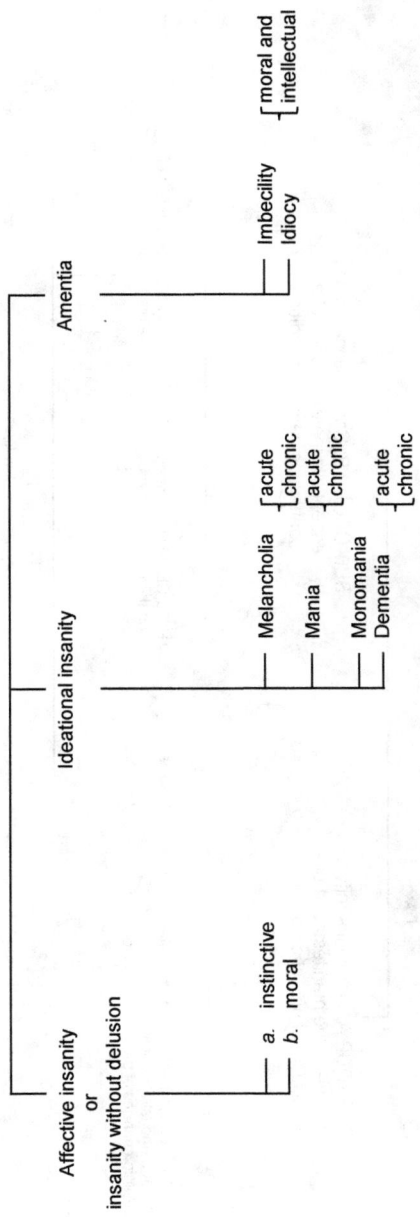

4 Maudsley's nosology of insanity

Insanity

GROUP FIRST: PURE INSANITIES

GROUP TWO: COMPLICATING INSANITIES

SUB-GROUP A: Simple insanity, not essentially the manifestation of a constitutional neurotic condition.

SUB-GROUP B: Constitutional insanity, essentially the expression of a continuous neurotic condition

FIRST CLASS: Not associated with demonstrable active organic changes of the brain

SECOND CLASS: Associated with demonstrable active organic changes of the brain

THIRD CLASS: Dependent on the great neuroses

FOURTH CLASS: Independent of the great neuroses

Genus 19: Periodical insanity

Order: arrested development
Genus 20: Idiocy and imbecility
Genus 21: Cretinism

Genus 22: Paranoia (monomania)

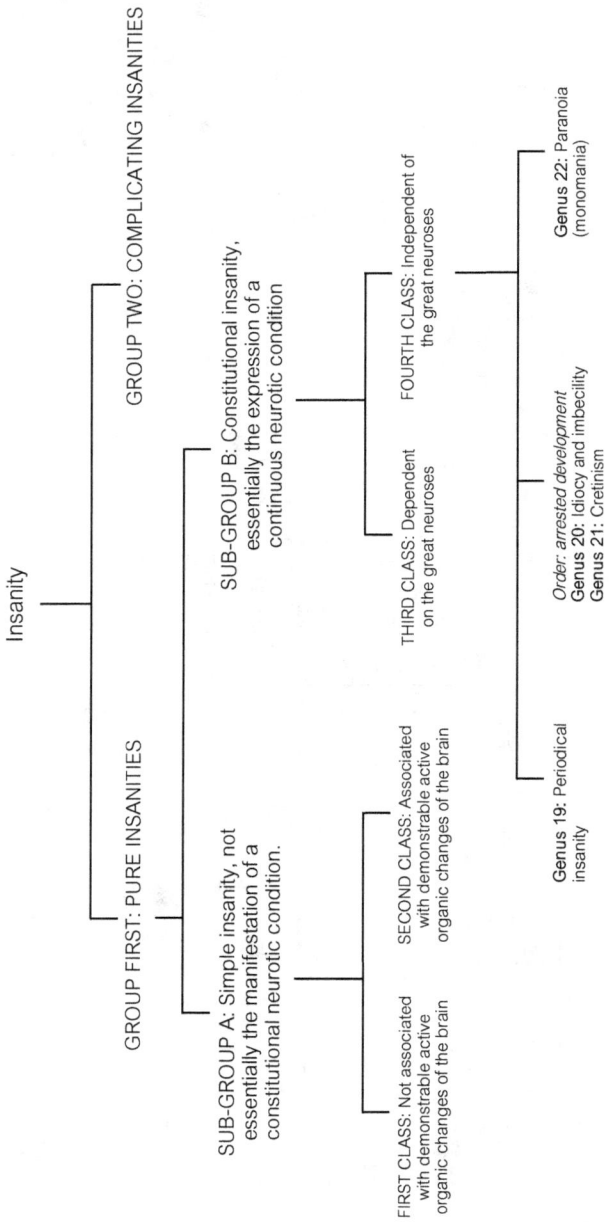

5 Spitzka's nosology of insanity

indicators for 'psychic' states.[30] For Spitzka, by contrast, the continuum from idiot to feeble-minded was entirely organic, anatomical, and physiological.

> There is a complete series of transitions, beginning at the lower end with the non-viable anencephalous monster and passing up through the brain-monstrosity, the microcephalous, the idiot, the imbecile, and the feeble-minded, to the normal person. This transition is at once structural and physiological.[31]

However, the flatter, simpler schemata did not die out. In 1890 Mercier contended that 'it is fruitless to endeavour to draw up an elaborate scheme of classes, orders, and genera, into which cases of insanity are to be grouped. No such divisions exist in nature'.[32] His five 'forms' divide into: idiocy and imbecility; sleep, old age, and drunkenness; melancholia; exaltation; and dementia. Mercier's central justification for his position is that symptoms deemed definitive of one species are invariably present to lesser degrees or as sequelæ of other species; all cases of insanity exhibit *similitudo dissimilis*.[33]

In the cases of 'congenital' idiocy and imbecility, Mercier distinguishes them from mental defect arising after someone has reached an 'average degree of intelligence', which he refers to as 'insanity proper'.[34]

> Thus it will be seen that in idiocy and weakness of mind, the process of development has not been carried *far enough*; while in insanity, the process has been carried far enough, but has diverged into the *wrong direction*.[35]

Clearly, Mercier has difficulty inserting idiocy unambiguously into his classification of insanity, and yet it is identified as a form nonetheless. Even in later work, Mercier continues to include idiocy as a form of insanity. The states of sleep, old age, and intoxication share a similarly ambiguous position as 'approximations to insanity', whilst still being identified as forms.[36] However, although Mercier dismisses aetiology as a basis for the classification of insanity, there is no mention at all of any specific pathological types of idiocy. On this point, the broader direction of psychiatric classification developed with little reference to an expanding nexus of institutional practices and knowledge-centred exclusively on idiocy. It is to this that we now turn.

A discourse on idiocy

From around the 1840s, a largely autonomous discourse and institutional archipelago for idiots and imbeciles had arisen. Centred initially on pedagogical concerns and new techniques, by the mid-century, this had become reintegrated within medicine as medico-pedagogy.[37] As it developed further, institutionally, professionally, and conceptually, the essential link with education – as treatment or as target – was weakened or broken. The emphasis began to shift, with the emergence of systems of classification and the study of pathology. Even before this, Séguin, through an extensive series of case studies, identified idiocy with 'microcephaly', 'hydrocephalus', 'cretinism', 'epilepsy', and so forth, without producing a classification.[38]

The emergence of these more sophisticated nosologies of idiocy depended entirely on the prior establishment of institutional populations comprising exclusively idiots and imbeciles. Having accomplished that, typing became almost inevitable. Séguin argued that scientific study was one of the central purposes of the institution: 'our love for them and their fellows must follow them with scalpel and microscope beyond life, to mark the peculiarities of their organs as we have done those of their functions'.[39]

One of the most notable of the new nosologies was that of William Ireland, who, unlike Down, for example, based his classification on pathological anatomy, rather than racial atavism.[40] In this respect, it leaned more towards modern medicine than degeneration theory. Whilst accepting the principle of hereditary degeneration, he was sceptical of the levels of determinism often cited. That said, he did identify idiocy as the mental disease most susceptible to hereditary transmission. Signalling a shift away from the restriction of medical intervention to physiological treatment, which did not differentiate by pathology, Ireland tried to establish a nosology that had the potential to lead to differential treatment:

> all kinds of idiocy have not the same future, nor ought to be treated in the same way. To group them all together is as absurd as to go on measuring the heads of the microcephalic and hydrocephalic idiots, and to generalise the results into one useless average.[41]

Ireland identified ten types of idiocy: genetous;[42] microcephalic; eclampsic; epileptic; hydrocephalic; paralytic; cretinism; traumatic; inflammatory; idiocy by deprivation. In the absence of being situated in a more general medical or psychiatric nosology, the system is, again, entirely flat.

However, although this network re-integrated idiocy into medicine, the alignment with alienism was somewhat tenuous. None of the medico-pedagogues – Brockett, Guggenbühl, Howe, Saegert, Séguin[43] – situated either idiocy, or their own work, within the framework of insanity and its treatment. Even Séguin, drawing explicitly upon moral treatment, did not reposition idiocy as a target of alienism *per se*.[44] Nor did the later writers, such as those mentioned above, position their pathological species of idiocy within the nosologies of alienism. Ireland, in particular, saw no real pathological similarity between idiocy and insanity, suggesting:

The most grievous hardship which idiots suffered from ... [the Lunacy Laws] was their imprisonment in lunatic asylums. Naturally gentle and timid, they were shut up in the same wards with the insane, people subject to furious fits of passion and dangerous delusions, and whose conversation and example are often suggestive of evil. From their imitative tendencies they soon learned all the shameless indecencies brought before their eyes.[45]

By the time of Alfred Tredgold in the early twentieth century, the picture has started to reform once more, with some explicit, if muted, acknowledgement of the place of idiocy within the wider economy of insanity. Hence:

In the literal sense of the word 'insanity,' all aments may be looked upon, and are often described, as 'congenitally insane.' But nowadays there is a tendency to restrict the term to those cases in which there is a perversion of the *ego*, and it is in that sense that it is used here.[46]

In this instance, it was not the shifting terrain of idiocy that put it at a distance from the mainstream of psychiatry, but the advent and impact of psychoanalysis on psychological medicine. Whilst Tredgold discusses insanity among aments, a psychoanalytic nosology has no place for diseases that are not ego-related. Thus, though psychoanalysis was presented as the medical treatment of nervous patients, and the *General Introduction to Psychoanalysis* outlines a 'General theory of the neuroses', because it decisively excluded somatic approaches, there was no place for idiocy or dementia. 'Neurosis', for psychoanalysis, had little to do with organic lesion in the nervous system; rather, it concerned itself with the 'forms' and 'burdens' of *symptoms*.[47] That said, psychodynamic theories and practices have themselves had a shifting and ambiguous relationship to the mainstream of psychiatry. What the semi-autonomous field of idiocy did do was largely to eliminate *idiotic insanity* and reproduce it as *idiocy*.

In addition to the impact of conceptual changes, the place of idiocy within medical psychology was also affected by more practical matters within the profession of psychiatry. Thomson notes that retirement and war left Britain with just 661 members of the professional body of psychiatry, the Medico-Psychological Association, in 1919, making recruitment into the already unattractive area of mental deficiency even more difficult. Ultimately, the primary role of the mental deficiency colony for psychiatry was to push mental deficiency to the margins of its therapeutic and conceptual ambit in order to focus on the real business of mental illness.[48] Consequently, as a result of an internal pull from those working within the field of idiocy, then the external pressure to remove them from the business of general psychiatry, mental deficiency was already well-established as a largely autonomous field by the inter-war period.

Idiocy and the historiography of madness

For over fifty years, the critical historiography of psychiatry has forced a reorientation of the field and the opening of new lines of investigation. Such developments have forced even the more supportive histories to become less Whiggish in their approach.[49] However, the striking feature of these accounts – and the more critical in orientation they are the more this appears to be true – is the general lack of attention to intellectual disability.[50] In his study of psychiatric nosology, Kendler's historical examples only include 'schizophrenia, major depression, dysthymia, generalized anxiety disorder, intermittent explosive disorder or narcissistic personality disorder'.[51] Munsche and Whittaker examine four prominent nosological frameworks from the eighteenth century (including that of Cullen). They identify eight mental diseases common to all four, including amentia. However, of them all, only amentia is not discussed in relation to DSM–IV and, in fact, their discussions go little beyond repeating the definitions and terms provided by the four taxonomists. Similarly, Shorter presents a historical discussion of psychiatric nosology up to DSM–V, leading to a proposal for a 'history-based nosology', whilst omitting idiocy entirely from discussion. Castel, in his turn, goes as far as to suggest that the alienists prevented any species of insanity from being split off into separate institutions, and yet this is precisely what happened with idiocy, though he completely misses this fact. It is a mistake to read straightforwardly into the past modern notions of a fundamental distinction between intellectual disability and mental illness, even where superficial resemblance exists. However, this brief review highlights that this error continues to exist in historical, sociological, and nosological investigations.[52]

This retrospective exclusion is at its most radical where the very institution of psychiatry is under attack. This is particularly clear in Thomas Szasz's sustained assault on psychiatry:[53] 'deception and coercion are intrinsic to the practices of mental health professions. The core concept of psychiatry [...] rest[s] on the medicalization of malingering'.[54]

Needless to say, those 'few' conditions with definite organic change are excluded from the critique of psychiatry. In so doing, Szasz offers no clear means of understanding how psychiatry was constituted overall, i.e. including those elements that do not fit his critique. Rather than an understanding of psychiatry, we are instead confronted with strategic manoeuvres of professional power.

There was an increasing challenge of non-medical psychology throughout the twentieth century for control of a variety of areas: phobias, eating disorders, addictions, and other non-organic conditions.[55] Even Scull's study of the emergence of professional rivalries between medical and non-medical psychologies makes no mention of mental retardation, even though this was one of the principal points on which non-medical psychology challenged psychiatry.[56] Scull repeats the familiar presentist mistake of projecting an assumed separation of psychiatry from intellectual disability onto the historical economy of concepts they are ostensibly studying.

In another example of the shifting of some conceptual elements, Rafalovich contends that 'moral imbecility', which arose from the discourse on idiocy and imbecility, became separated off from it, and fed into the conceptual foundations of *encephalitis lethargica*, which was the first formulation of the symptomatic grouping that we now call ADHD.

> The discussion of *encephalitis lethargica* provided a specific diagnosis of the symptoms for which imbecility had limited utility. Imbecility became quickly antiquated in medical discourse partially because organic causes of the condition could not be found.[57]

However, imbecility most certainly did not disappear and, in fact, it expanded with the moron/feebleminded – of which Rafalovich makes no mention, even though it appears in several of his consulted primary sources.[58] In addition, the organic classification of idiocy and imbecility was not done on a psychic basis, even with the advent of intelligence testing. Pathological types, such as Mongolism, cretinism, and microcephaly, included individuals who were both mentally imbecile and idiot. The distinction between the two, for which he cites Ireland, is entirely on degree of mental capacity, which is not significantly different to Esquirol.[59] Rafalovich misses altogether the fact that the pathological classifications of idiocy and imbecility, which were being developed within medicine at that time, operated 'horizontally', so to speak, rather than merely on a 'vertical' scale of mental capacity or intelligence, however loosely defined.

Needless to say, the failure to adequately connect idiocy and psychiatry is also a prominent feature of the historiography and sociology of intellectual disability. Key texts in the field fail singularly to situate idiocy within psychiatry and medicine other than at an institutional level, that is to say, there is little exploration or understanding of how it comes to be that psychiatry assumed this control, firstly, at a conceptual level. Noll's seminal text on institutional provision for the feeble-minded in the American South contains no discussion of the conceptual framework of mental illness, psychiatry, or medicine. O'Brien's recent work on feeble-mindedness and eugenics makes little mention of mental illness and none of psychiatry. Thomson discusses the importance of the development of professional psychiatry in Britain and makes a significant contribution to understanding mental deficiency in relation to the social adjustment to democracy, though even here there is no real discussion of conceptual issues. Conversely, Jackson takes Thomson to task for giving insufficient consideration to the construction of medical categories and concepts of mental deficiency. Paradoxically, however, Jackson himself fails to situate the medical assemblage of 'mental deficiency' within the wider theoretical fields of either psychiatry or medicine. As a consequence, he gives greater prominence to the strand of thought that emphasized mental deficiency as racial atavism, and relatively little to more orthodoxly *medical* approaches, such as that of William Ireland, whose pathological classification receives almost no attention. So, for instance, whilst for Down the Kalmuc/ Mongolian type was definitive of the whole theory, because Ireland could not identify its aetiology, it remained part of the undefined 'genetous' class.[60]

Conclusion

The diverse, incompatible, and highly contingent conceptual economy of psychiatry demonstrates that the presence, exclusion, function, and positioning of idiocy have varied primarily on the basis of how its overall concepts, targets, and methods of intervention are conceived and constructed. For Cullen, amentia linked to other diseases of the nervous system and preceded developmental approaches. Pinel and Esquirol notionally held onto idiocy, but held little therapeutic optimism, and it was left marginalized in the framework of moral treatment. Degenerationist and neurological approaches in the latter half of the nineteenth century linked idiocy and insanity organically. The methods and aims of the medico-pedagogues and later physicians of idiocy were, again, quite different. It was advantageous to attain autonomy and to redefine and reposition idiocy outside of psychiatry. Psychoanalysis, Garrabé suggests, obliterated the systems of Cullen and Pinel altogether.[61] The fact that it was not possible for idiocy to be constituted as a target of intervention for psychoanalysis led again to its exclusion. Then, by the time eugenics began to hold sway, and specifically target the moron/feebleminded, psychiatry once more competed with psychology for professional control.[62] Mercier, for example, had focused in 1890 on idiocy mainly in relation to the danger that idiots and, to a lesser extent, imbeciles posed to themselves through their lack of social competence; but by 1911, his focus was on feeblemindedness as the species of insanity most heavily linked with crime, second only to drunkenness: 'deficient in self-control; restrained by no definite sense of morality; such persons take easily to crime'.[63]

This general pattern of contingency continued through the twentieth century, into the twenty first. The existentialist orientation and general focus

on schizophrenia of the anti-psychiatrists also resulted in the marginalization of intellectual disability, which, again, did not fit the target of its critique.
Studies of schizophrenia in families by Laing, Esterson, and Cooper specifically excluded anyone of obviously subnormal intelligence. More recently,
phenomenological approaches to psychiatry, including the 'neo-Jasperians',
predicate theory and practice heavily on consciousness, both in the definition
and treatment of mental disorder.[64]

> Abnormal mental phenomena, ie, disorders of experience and expression, are
> 'the object' of psychiatry [...] A psychological description involves converting
> the patient's experiences (lived in the first-person perspective), or translating
> certain aspects of his/her expression and behavior, into specific categories of
> symptoms and signs that defined in third-person terms, thus providing 'objec-
> tive', sharable information for diagnosis, treatment, and research.[65]

Other neo-Jasperians, such as Marková and Berrios, argue that for psychiatry
to understand its own epistemological configuration, it must recognize the
contextuality of its objects: temporally and socially, as well as biologically
and psychologically.[66] They propose that psychiatry deals with two objects:
'mental disorders' and 'mental symptoms'. The emphases on subjectivity and
dialogue in relation to symptomatology immediately pose problems, particularly for those with more profound intellectual disabilities. However, intellectual disability is not a condition that anyone who was assessed or diagnosed as
having could experience as intrinsically pathological in any case. And, though
Marková and Berrios identify the conceptual objects of psychiatry as rooted
in the nineteenth century, it seems implicit that intellectual disability does not
figure in their frame of reference.[67] For this reason, then, intellectual disability
must be radically excluded from phenomenological and 'hybrid' models of
psychiatry. Whilst there remain a range of definitions and concepts about what
intellectual disability might or might not be, including social constructionist
ones, none are predicated on the interpretation and mediation of subjective
experience by the psychiatrist.

In a more recent development, Kendler, whilst recognizing that 'The creation and revisions of the DSM are firmly entrenched in a particular historical
context',[68] still believes that 'accuracy' can be achieved in psychiatric nosology
through a process of 'epistemic iteration', which is

> getting us from our historical starting point toward progressively more accurate
> approximations of the reality of psychiatric illness. However, for this process
> to achieve its aim, it will require a relatively stable consensus about the goals of
> psychiatric diagnosis.[69]

However, Kendler over-estimates the level of agreement, or perhaps consistency, in the objects that psychiatry is trying to define and arrange to begin with.

Ultimately, as Garrabé notes, 'The purpose of classification is power'.[70] Whilst studying the relations of power specifically has not been the central purpose of this chapter, it has been impossible for them not to have spilled out in the very act of examining the place of idiocy in the conceptual economy of madness. Garrabé's observation holds as true today as for historical study. Where, how, and by whom intellectual disability becomes constituted is a matter of power: the power to produce, control, and regulate objects of knowledge; to identify targets for intervention and modes of governance; to create lines of separation and points of connection; what it means to be sane, insane, intellectually disabled, and, ultimately, what it means to be human.

Notes

1 David Wright, 'Mongols in Our Midst: John Langdon Down and Ethnic Classification of Idiocy, 1858–1924', in *Mental Retardation in America: A Historical Reader*, edited by Steven Noll and James W. Trent, Jr. (New York: New York University Press, 2004), 92–93.

2 William Pargeter, 'Observations on maniacal disorders' [1792], in *Patterns of Madness in the Eighteenth Century: A Reader*, edited by Allan Ingram (Liverpool: Liverpool University Press, 1998), 180.

3 Murray K. Simpson, 'The Developmental Concept of Idiocy', *Intellectual and Developmental Disabilities* 45 (2007).

4 Thomas Arnold, *Observations on the Nature, Kinds, Causes, and Prevention of Insanity, Lunacy, or Madness*, 2 vols. (Leicester: Robinson & Cadell, 1782–86); William Battie, *A Treatise on Madness* (London: J. Whiston and B. White, 1758), 4.

5 Battie, *A Treatise on Madness*, 6.

6 Francis Willis, *A Treatise on Mental Derangement* (London: Longman, Hurst, Rees, Orme, and Brown, 1823), 229–230.

7 See K. S. Kendler, 'An Historical Framework for Psychiatric Nosology', *Psychological Medicine* 39 (2009), 1937; Roy Porter, *The Greatest Benefit to Mankind: A Medical History of Humanity from Antiquity to the Present* (London: HarperCollins, 1997), 261; Volker Hess and J. Andrew Mendelsohn, 'Sauvages' Paperwork: How Disease Classification Arose From Scholarly Note-Taking', *Early Science and Medicine* 19 (2014).

8 We will be working from William Cullen, *First Lines of the Practice of Physic* (Edinburgh: C. Elliot, 1789) and *Nosology: Or, A Systematic Arrangement of Diseases by Classes, Orders, Genera, and Species* (Edinburgh: C. Stewart and Co., 1800).

9 Phillipe Pinel, *A Treatise on Insanity* [1806], translated by D. D. Davis (New York:

Hafner, 1962); Jean-Étienne Dominique Esquirol, *Mental Maladies: A Treatise on Insanity* [1854] (New York: Hafner, 1965). Esquirol's classification is essentially the same as Pinel's except that it separates dementia from idiotism.

10 Cullen, *First Lines*, Vol. II: 122 [MXCI].

11 *Ibid.*, Vol. IV, 114–115 [MDXXIX].

12 John Locke, *An Essay Concerning Human Understanding* [1689], edited by Peter Nidditch (Oxford: Clarendon, 1975), 160–161; Bk. II, Ch. 11, S. 12–13; François Boissier de Sauvages de la Croix, *Nosologia methodica*, Vol. 2 (Amsterdam: Fratrum de Tournes, 1768), 248–249; Porter, *The Greatest Benefit*: 271.

13 Cullen, *First Lines*, Vol. IV, 119 [MDXXIX].

14 Ibid., Vol. II, 115 [MXCI]; Esquirol, *Mental Maladies*.

15 Cullen, *Nosology*, 130.

16 Cullen, *First Lines*, Vol. IV: 188 [MDXCVIII].

17 'Imbecility of all the faculties of the human mind, particularly those concerned in associating and comparing ideas; accompanied with want of language, a stupid look, and general bodily weakness'. Alexander Crichton, *An Inquiry into the Nature and Origin of Mental Derangement*, Vol. II (London: T. Cadell, Junior, and W. Davies, 1798), 344.

18 Cullen, *First Lines*, Vol. IV, 341 [MDCCXXIV]. Rachitis, or rickets, is not even a neurotic illness, lying as it does under the cachexies.

19 William Perfect, *Select Cases in the Different Species of Insanity, Lunacy, or Madness, with the Modes of Practice as Adopted in the Treatment of Each* (Rochester: Gillman, 1787), 67, 71. See also, Battie, *A Treatise on Madness*; John Smith, 'Distress of mind in old age' [extract from *King Solomons Portraiture of Old Age* (1666)], in *Three Hundred Years of Psychiatry, 1535–1860*, edited by Richard Hunter and Ida Macalpine. (London: Oxford University Press, 1963), 182–183; Cullen, *First Lines*, Vol. III, 175 [MCXLV]; Ibid., Vol. IV, 341 [MDCCXXIV].

20 Esquirol's was similar in approach, though the species differed slightly: lypemania (melancholy), monomania, mania, dementia, and idiocy and imbecility.

21 Jean Garrabé, 'Nosographie et classifications des maladies mentales dans l'histoire de la psychiatrie', *L'Évolution psychiatrique* 79 (2014), 10.

22 John Conolly, *The Treatment of the Insane Without Mechanical Restraints* (London: Smith, Elder & Co., 1856), x; Édouard Séguin, *Idiocy and its Treatment by the Physiological Method* (New York: William Wood & Co., 1866).

23 Henry Maudsley, *The Pathology of Mind*, 3rd edn. (London: Macmillan & Co., 1879), 186.

24 Ibid., 114.

25 F. Carbonel, 'L'idéologie aliéniste du Dr. B. A. Morel: Christianisme social et médecine sociale, milieu et dégénérescence, psychiatrie et régénération. Partie I', *Annales Médico-Psychologiques* 168 (2010); Volker Roelcke, 'Biologizing Social Facts: An Early Twentieth-Century Debate on Kraepelin's Concepts of Culture, Neurasthenia, and Degeneration', *Culture, Medicine and Psychiatry* 21 (1997).

26 Edward Charles Spitzka, *Insanity, its Classification, Diagnosis and Treatment: A*

Manual for Students and Practitioners of Medicine (New York: Bermingham and Co., 1883), 275.

27   Richard von Krafft-Ebing, *Lehrbuch der Psychiatrie auf Klinischer Grundlage für Practische Ärtze und Studirende* Vols. 2–3 (Stuttgart: Verlag von Ferdinand Enke, 1880).

28   Samuel Gridley Howe, *On the Causes of Idiocy* [1848] (New York: Arno Press and The New York Times, 1972), 7.

29   William Wotherspoon Ireland, *On Idiocy and Imbecility* (London: J. & A. Churchill, 1877), 263; Charles Mercier, *Crime and Insanity* (London: Williams and Northgate, 1911), 286–287.

30   Ireland, *On Idiocy and Imbecility*, 38.

31   Spitzka, *Insanity, its Classification, Diagnosis and Treatment*, 275.

32   Charles Mercier, *Sanity and Insanity* (London: Walter Scott, 1890).

33   Ibid., 285.

34   However, the description Mercier gives is developmental, rather than strictly congenital.

35   Ibid., 287, emphasis in original.

36   Ibid., 329.

37   Murray K. Simpson, *Modernity and the Appearance of Idiocy: Intellectual Disability as a Regime of Truth* (Lampeter: Edwin Mellen Press, 2014).

38   Désiré-Magloire Bourneville, *Recherches cliniques et thérapeutiques sur l'épilepsie, l'hystérie et l'idiotie*, 26 vols. (Paris: Bureaux de Progrés Médical and Felix Alcan, 1872–1907) *passim*; John Langdon Down, 'Observations on an ethnic classification of idiots', *Clinical Lecture Reports of the London Hospital* 3 (1866); Ireland; Séguin.

39   Séguin, *Idiocy and its Treatment by the Physiological Method*, 1866, 75. See also Ireland, *On Idiocy and Imbecility*.

40   Ireland, *On Idiocy and Imbecility*; John Langdon Down, 'Observations on an ethnic classification of idiots', *Clinical Lecture Reports of the London Hospital* 3 (1866).

41   Ireland, *On Idiocy and Imbecility*, 39.

42   The genetous class includes all cases for which no pathological explanation can be found, at least not while the individual is alive. They constitute the largest category and include the 'Kalmuc' (Mongolian) type, which would constitute a class of its own had Ireland been able to identify pathological causes.

43   See R. C. Scheerenberger, *A History of Mental Retardation* (Baltimore: Paul H. Brookes, 1983), for further details.

44   See, for example, P. Martin Duncan and William Millard, *A Manual for the Classification, Training, and Education of the Feeble-Minded, Imbecile, and Idiotic* (London: Longmans, Green and Co., 1866); Howe, *On the Causes of Idiocy*; Séguin, *Idiocy and its Treatment by the Physiological Method*.

45   Ireland, *On Idiocy and Imbecility*, 341.

46   Alfred Tredgold, *Mental Deficiency (Amentia)*, 2nd edn (New York: William Wood & Co., 1915), 342. Emphasis in original.

47 Sigmund Freud, *General Introduction to Psychoanalysis* [1916–17], translated by G. Staneley Hall (New York: Horace Liverwright, 1920), 221.

48 Mathew Thomson, *The Problem of Mental Deficiency: Eugenics, Democracy, and Social Policy in Britain c.1870–1959* (Oxford: Oxford University Press, 1998), 126, 144.

49 See, for example, Edward Shorter, *A History of Psychiatry: From the Era of the Asylum to the Age of Prozac* (Chichester, NY: John Wiley, 1997).

50 Phylis Chesler, *Women and Madness* (London: Allen Lane, 1972); Michel Foucault, *Madness and Civilization*, translated by Richard Howard (London: Routledge, 1967); Roy Porter, *Madmen: A Social History of Madhouses, Mad-Doctors and Lunatics* (Stroud: Tempus, 2006); Andrew Scull, *The Most Solitary of Afflictions: Madness and Society in Britain 1700–1900* (New Haven: Yale University Press, 1993).

51 K. S. Kendler, 'An Historical Framework for Psychiatric Nosology', *Psychological Medicine* 39 (2009), 1939.

52 Heather Munsche and Harry A. Whittaker, 'Eighteenth-Century Classification of Mental Illness: Linnaeus, de Sauvages, Vogel, and Cullen', *Cognitive and Behavioral Neurology* 25 (2012); Edward Shorter, *What Psychiatry Left out of DSM–V: Historical Mental Disorders Today* (New York: Routledge, 2015); Robert Castel, *The Regulation of Madness: The Origins of Incarceration in France* (Cambridge: Polity Press, 1988), 134.

53 Thomas Szasz, *The Myth of Mental Illness: Foundations of a Theory of Personal Conduct* (New York: Hoeber-Harper, 1961); *The Manufacture of Madness: A Comparative Study of the Inquisition and the Mental Health Movement* (New York: Harper Row, 1970); 'Mental Illness as a Metaphor', *Nature* 242 (1973).

54 Thomas Szasz, *Psychiatry: The Science of Lies* (Syracuse: Syracuse University Press. 2008), 1.

55 Nikolas Rose, *Governing the Soul* (London: Free Association, 1999), 234–238; Mathew Thomson, *Psychological Subjects: Identity, Culture, and Health in Twentieth-Century Britain* (Oxford: Oxford University Press, 2006), 250–288.

56 Andrew Scull, 'Contending Professions: Sciences of the Brain and Mind in the United States, 1850–2013', *Science in Context* 28 (2015); Murray K. Simpson, 'Medicine vs. psychology: The emergence of a professional conflict in development disability', *Journal on Developmental Disabilities/Le journal sur les handicaps du développement* 8 (2001).

57 Adam Rafalovich, 'The Conceptual History of Attention Deficit Hyperactivity Disorder: Idiocy, Imbecility, Encephalitis and the Child Deviant, 1877–1929', *Deviant Behavior* 22 (2001), 99.

58 'Feebleminded' is used here in the UK sense of the term, to mean a class of mental defectives higher than imbeciles; this is broadly equivalent to the 'moron' in North America.

59 Rafalovich, 'The Conceptual History of Attention Deficit Hyperactivity Disorder', 99.

60 Steven Noll, *The Feeble-Minded in our Midst: Institutions for the Mentally Retarded in the South, 1900–1940* (Chapel Hill: University of North Carolina Press); Gerald V. O'Brien, *Framing the Moron: The Social Construction of Feeble-Mindedness in the American Eugenic Era* (Manchester: Manchester University Press, 2013); Thomson, *The Problem of Mental Deficiency*; Mark Jackson, *The Borderland of Imbecility: Medicine, Society, and the Fabrication of the Feeble Mind in late Victorian England* (Manchester: Manchester University Press, 2000), 9.

61 Jean Garrabé, 'Nosographie et classifications des maladies mentales dans l'histoire de la psychiatrie', *L'Évolution psychiatrique* 79 (2014), 13.

62 Steven A. Gelb, 'Social Deviance and the "Discovery" of the Moron', *Disability, Handicap and Society* 2 (1987); James W. Trent Jr., *Inventing The Feeble Mind: A History of Mental Retardation in the United States* (Berkeley: University of California Press, 1994).

63 Mercier, *Crime and Insanity*, 57.

64 R. D. Laing, *The Divided Self* (London: Tavistock, 1960); R. D. Laing, and Aaron Esterson, *Sanity, Madness and the Family* (London: Tavistock, 1964); David Cooper, *Psychiatry and Anti-Psychiatry* (Abingdon: Routledge, 1967); German E. Berrios, 'Jaspers and First Edition of *Allgemeine Psychopathologie* – reflection', *British Journal of Psychiatry* 202 (2013); Jose de Leon, 'One Hundred Years of Limited Impact of Jaspers' *General Psychopathology* on US Psychiatry', *The Journal of Nervous and Mental Disease* 202 (2014).

65 Josef Parnas, Louis A. Sass, and Dan Sahavi, 'Rediscovering Psychopathology: The Epistemology and Phenomenology of the Psychiatric Object', *Schizophrenia Bulletin* 39 (2012), 270.

66 Ivana S. Marková and German E. Berrios, 'Epistemology of Psychiatry', *Psychopathology* 45 (2012).

67 This, of course, is not necessarily a criticism, since, as they observe, other things once considered 'disorders', such as homosexuality, are no longer considered such. Indeed, this reinforces their argument regarding contextuality.

68 Kendler, 'An Historical Framework', 1937.

69 Ibid., 1941.

70 'Le rêve de tout classificateur est de pouvoir' (author's translation): Garrabé, 'Nosographie et classifications', 15.

11

VISITING EARLSWOOD: THE ASYLUM TRAVELOGUE AND THE SHAPING OF 'IDIOCY'

Patrick McDonagh

In his 1860 *A Visit to Earlswood*, the Reverend Edwin Sidney opens with a description of landscape as seen from a rail car:

> The traveller by railway from London to Brighton is carried over a tract of country of great physical and moral interest. The picturesque undulations of the rising grounds on either side, belong to formations where once roamed many of the strange-looking creatures whose restored forms are seen in the garden of the Crystal Palace – itself the most wonderful object seen on the journey. Instead of the wild regions where erst ranged these gigantic brutes of a bygone period, we see now the highest cultivation, the most tasteful mansions, villas, parks, gardens, and cottages, with fields where are pastured the gentler animals destined for the special service of civilized man. But more than this, large and well-built structures meet the eye in succession, and the inquirer learns with pleasure that they are the homes of the fatherless, the outcast, and the imbecile, raised by Christian philanthropy. To the last of these my visit was directed, by the invitation of its managers .... [1]

Sidney's introduction to his 26-page pamphlet marks a passage across borders: across time, from the age of dinosaurs to the present civilized society; from urban London to the rural outskirts of Surrey; and from English society to the enclosed community of the asylum. His readers journey with him across terrain that is not only geographical but also temporal, intellectual, and moral, before arriving at the destination: the Royal Earlswood Asylum, also known as the National Asylum for Idiots.

The late 1850s and the 1860s saw the publication of a number of pamphlets and magazine and newspaper articles describing visits to Earlswood, which had opened in 1854 in the small town of Redhill, Surrey. [2] The intended readership – usually wealthy or at least middle-class, presumably rational and intelligent – lived far beyond the institutions, in terms of identity if not geography. As with Sidney's pamphlet, these reports of visits to Earlswood (and other 'idiot' asylums) often served as public relations exercises that advocated the new forms of care and pedagogy provided by these institutions; usually they also served as tools for soliciting funds or other support.

The writings we will consider here were conceived and presented as travel narratives, or travelogues, describing visits to the Royal Earlswood Asylum. As the first large 'idiots asylum' in England, Earlswood received many visitors and prominent press coverage. While other institutions also received visitors, some of whom wrote travelogue-narratives of their visits, Earlswood was by far the most documented in this manner, especially in its early years, and thus provides the clearest opportunity for comparing visitors' reports; it is also the most thoroughly documented Victorian 'idiot asylum' in current historiography.[3] For these reasons, the main focus of this chapter falls on the Royal Earlswood Asylum and its literary visitors.

Earlswood travelogues share certain observations, rhetoric, and, most notably, a common set of interwoven narrative strands. The Reverend Sidney was a frequent visitor, writing four pamphlets in support of Earlswood (three of which were travelogues reporting on specific visits); others who composed Earlswood travelogues include J. C. Parkinson, a prominent journalist, and Cheyne Brady, a lawyer and asylum advocate, as well as a number of anonymous writers. The most famous English asylum visitor, Charles Dickens, anticipated the others by travelling not to Earlswood but to the National Asylum for Idiots' first site at Park House in 1853. As Murray Simpson has noted, 'prior to the mid-nineteenth century, nothing existed which could meaningfully be said to constitute a cohesive discursive field of idiocy. All that existed were a few isolated fragments in medicine, law and philosophy with no overall coherence or consistency'; given the lack of a cohesive body of commentary on idiocy, these travelogues become important elements in a nascent 'discourse on idiocy'.[4]

Travel writing, notes Barbara Korte, is characterized by 'generic hybridity and flexibility' with one consistent formal feature: the use of narration to describe a journey.[5] Carl Thompson describes the genre broadly, suggesting that if 'all travel involves an encounter between self and other that is brought about by movement through space, all travel writing is at some level a record or product of this encounter'.[6] The Earlswood travelogues certainly meet these definitions. In terms of their literary context, they also draw on the concurrent publications by or about British writers exploring what was soon to become known as 'the dark continent', Africa, and on writings documenting the activities of British missionaries there and in India, North America, and Australia. At the time, most readers received these publications as describing intrepid British adventurers and missionaries, with little ethical concern over the colonizing of indigenous peoples; today, of course, the imperialist ideology informing these writings is explicit.[7] Similarly, Earlswood travelogues consistently reiterate the notions that the task of the asylum leadership is to civilize as much as possible the idiot mind, and to introduce light into its darkness; as such, the 'idiot' residents of the asylum parallel the inhabitants of Africa and other outreaches of the British Empire, and the imagery used to describe Earlswood recalls that used to describe the task of rendering colonized peoples, frequently identified as childlike, as grateful subjects of the British crown.

The travelogue is, as Korte observes, a 'hybrid' genre, and the Earlswood travelogue is interlaced with objective physical description, anthropological analysis, domestic narratives, character sketches, and even the occasional glimpse of utopia. Earlswood visitors share rhetorical strategies in their narratives, often in terms of 'before' and 'after' descriptions of the institution's residents or in the contradiction between the prejudice of dismal expectations and the happy, cheerful community represented in the articles. They adopt similar metaphors, including the recurring image of light penetrating darkness and the conceit of the institution as housing a 'family', with its persistent infantilization of the residents of the institution as 'children'. And they develop similar characterizations, with the same individuals being featured in different texts, so that certain residents acquire a literary existence.

These works tread in the path of previous narratives describing visits to facilities for people identified as being 'idiots', including William Twining's account of Johann Jacob Guggenbühl's institution at Abendberg in Switzerland, two unsigned articles recounting a visit to the Bicêtre in Paris and elaborating on Voisin's approach to the education of idiots that appeared in consecutive issues of *Chambers's Edinburgh Journal*, and articles by John Conolly and Samuel Gaskell – superintendents of the Middlesex and Lancaster Lunatic Asylums, respectively – who also journeyed to Paris to report on the education of 'idiots' at the Bicêtre.[8] Following these examples, which argued for the benefits of the pedagogical and social education provided in these institutions, accounts of visits to Earlswood regularly lauded the peaceful and benevolent community established there.[9]

In this chapter I anatomize these Earlswood travel narratives, focusing on their shared thematic concerns and their representational strategies; to do so, I explore narrative similarities including the journey to Earlswood, common rhetorical strategies, overviews of daily life in the institutions, the role of Christian faith and philanthropy, and the portraiture of characters (recurring or otherwise) in the narratives. The travelogues also share a common narrative arc, from the arrival at Earlswood and the brisk dispelling of popular misconceptions about idiocy, to the representation of a smoothly functioning society, often culminating in the observation that the asylum represents a model society of committed Christian leaders governing a pliant, respectful community, and an exhortation for readers to visit Earlswood or direct financial support towards the Earlswood Charity, established by its co-founder the Reverend Andrew Reed.[10] My goal in anatomizing the travelogues in this way is to illuminate the impact this kind of complex representation might have had on a popular understanding of what characterized idiocy and its treatment, as well as on the eventual development of conceptions of idiocy as more threatening to the nation's social and political body.

Going to Earlswood

The journey to Earlswood is one of the first features to appear in many of these writings and immediately marks them as travelogues. Asylums were constructed as environments standing apart from the bustle of English life, according to the guidelines proposed by John Conolly, the established authority on the subject, who had written that

> the best site is a gentle eminence, of which the soil is naturally dry, and in a fertile and agreeable country, near enough to high roads, a railroad, or a canal, and a town, to facilitate the supply of stores, and the occasional visits of friends of the patients, and to diversify the scene without causing disturbance.[11]

Earlswood fulfilled all of these criteria, being 'delightfully situated about a mile and half from the Redhill station of the London to Brighton Railway',[12] which could deliver passengers from London in less than two hours.

The Reverend Edwin Sidney was a frequent passenger on this railway. Sidney, the Anglican rector at Cornard Parva, Suffolk, from 1846 to 1872, a writer on science (especially agriculture) and a vigorous supporter of Earlswood, published four pamphlets on the institution and delivered lectures around England in its aid.[13] We have already read the introductory paragraph to his first Earlswood travelogue. His 1861 *Second Visit to Earlswood* begins with him launching a surprise visit to the institution, and shares similar features with the 1860 article's introduction:

> in about half-an-hour we were in the train. The sun shone brightly on the highly-cultivated scenes through which we were carried rapidly along, and in the midst of which are so conspicuous those striking edifices that are such exemplary monuments of English science, art, and charity. I could not help exulting in the thought of the favourable impression they must make on foreigners travelling from the Continent to London. We soon reached Red Hill [*sic*], and one of

the first persons we saw on our way through the village, was a pupil of the Idiot
Asylum, who acts as a postman.[14]

In 1864 he published *A Fête Day at Earlswood*, opening with the observation
that

> It is characteristic of the principal achievements of the present day, that they are
> such as would have been pronounced the wildest dreaming if they had been pre-
> dicted to those who lived only a half-century ago. Who could then have believed
> that London, or any part of it, would be traversed by one railway underneath
> its buildings, and by another crossing the Thames and running over their tops?
> Still more strange would it have seemed had it been foretold that any of the
> passengers by either of them would be on their way to London Bridge, to go by
> another line of railway to one of the most agreeable of holidays, the attraction to
> a company of its generous and kind citizens, being a summer fête for the pleasure
> and the benefit of an assemblage of poor Idiots! He that prophesied of such a
> day, would be lucky if he escaped by being regarded only as a harmless madman,
> and avoided confinement.[15]

The common thread in Sidney's three introductory paragraphs is the
railway, functioning not only as a means of undertaking a journey but also as
an emblem of scientific progress. Sidney's consistent foregrounding of the
accomplishments of the age imply that the practices followed at Earlswood
are also accomplishments – scientific, intellectual, and moral – comparable
to the others singled out on his various journeys to the institution. As with
the introductory paragraph to the first visit, these passages also mark border
crossings: in the 1861 article Sidney imagines himself a continental foreigner
marvelling at the countryside's 'monuments of English science, art, and
charity', and in the 1864 piece as a time-travelling Englishman of 'a half-
century ago' astonished by both the engineering and the moral advances of
the new age.

Other writers, while less overt in their evocations of such intellectual, scientific, and moral progress, also use rail travel to place their narratives within the
travelogue genre. Joseph Charles Parkinson observes in his *A Day at Earlswood*
that 'Travellers by the South-Eastern Railway are attracted by the sight of
a palatial building near Redhill; and perhaps read its uses from an adjacent
board',[16] and notes that

> from time to time it is visited by the representatives of the press, and accounts
> are published of what the idiots said and did, and how they looked at a repre-
> sentation of private theatricals, or during an amateur concert got up for their
> amusement. But these occasions are purely exceptional, and the ordinary inner
> life of this remarkable place is as little known as that of a man who conceals a

secret pride, or ambition, or scorn, beneath a frivolous or jocular exterior, and the result is that scant justice is occasionally done to its remedial discipline, to its scrupulous internal economy, and to the broad spirit of charity in which its good is worked.[17]

In his role as a traveller to Earlswood, Parkinson intends to remedy these more superficial visitors' accounts of the institution, presenting it to his readers in its everyday attire. His evocation of the train passenger observing Earlswood situates his piece as a travelogue, as our narrator crosses a border into unknown (or avoided) territories, and it positions the author as the guide to this unusual world.[18]

Some Earlswood travelogues employ other strategies to create physical and psychological distance. 'Born Idiots Bred Sane', an unsigned article in *Chambers's Journal* in 1859, claims that 'it was in Pennsylvania that attention was first paid upon a public scale to the care and mental improvement of idiots' and that 'travellers saw and brought home accounts of the wonderful cures effected by constant medical attendance, combined with a gradual development of the various powers of the mind'.[19] While this observation documents the inspiration for institutions like Earlswood, it also renders them exotic foreign imports originating on the other side of the Atlantic Ocean.

The writer's rhetoric could displace the asylum in time as well as space. When Charles Dickens wrote of his visit to Park House, Highgate, Earlswood's forerunner as the National Asylum for Idiots, he observed that it was

> a fine detached house, beautifully situated at a considerable elevation above the metropolis … and looking down upon the spot where Richard Whittington heard the bells summoning him to his glorious destiny of being thrice Lord Mayor of London.[20]

Dickens stresses the institution's location on a hill overlooking the metropolis and links it with a semi-mythical moment in London's history, placing it at both a physical and a temporal distance, while at the same time asserting a historical connection to the city.

The journey, and comparable distancing methods, form a crucial part of the opening sections of visitors' narratives of Earlswood. The asylum, wherever it may be, must be understood as both English – as an instance of the reforming genius and philanthropic generosity of the nation – and separate from the rest of the English world. The land of 'Idiocy' became, in effect, a colony that lay within the asylum's borders, governed by benevolent Englishmen.

The rhetoric of Earlswood visits

While the institution itself may exist in a world foreign to most English men and women, the rhetorical approaches used to introduce readers to that strange land draw upon familiar images and ideas. These well-worn rhetorical strategies, tropes, and images provided a shortcut that enabled Earlswood's travelogue writers to define their experiences in ways their readers were already conceptually equipped to accept, if not to fully understand.

One of the most frequently used approaches in these narratives was to posit an initial contrast between one's expectation of 'idiots' and the reality greeting the visitor upon touring Earlswood. Parkinson offers a good example: he alludes to the 'unfounded and unjust' popular notions of 'the helpless gibbering wretch, loathsome to others and a torment to himself; the scarcely human object, to be passed by with a shudder, and forgotten as speedily as possible; the shrieks, and groans, and cries associated with the idiot of the past'. But these, he tells us, 'are not to be found. In their place is a happy united family, proud of its occupations, attached to its instructors and friends, harmonious in its relations, and quiet and peaceful in its life'.[21]

Indeed, some Earlswood travelogues go beyond simply rejecting the 'repulsive', instead presenting the asylum in a manner that recalls utopian narratives, reporting to the populace on the organization of an unusual and surprisingly efficient society. As Ruth Levitas notes, the idea of utopia, whether literary or political, can be broadly defined as 'the expression of the desire for a better way of being',[22] and this is certainly the Christian humanist impulse driving most of these Earlswood travelogues. They describe not simply a charitable institution, but an insulated society of pliant and grateful individuals governed by benevolent leaders; John Langdon Down and Earlswood's philanthropic co-founder the Reverend Andrew Reed especially stand out in the narratives as heroic characters. Further, Down's 'rule of kindness' at Earlswood, and the apparent kindness and generosity of the asylum's inmates, can provide a satirical commentary on the distinctly less kind world outside of the asylum, as it does in Parkinson's concluding observation that one leaves Earlswood with 'a shrewd suspicion that lower moral natures may be found among the weak and selfish of the sane'.[23] The utopian tone is heightened by the frequent juxtaposition of the anticipation of dismal or despairing scenes with the 'reality' of the institution as represented in the writings. Parkinson describes Earlswood as an 'eminently happy place', but the 'utopian' features of this narrative are also infused with pathos; its residents also form 'a class apart, ... never ... lightened by any of the ordinary enjoyments of human life'.[24]

Charles Dickens establishes a similar set of contrasts when he opens

'Idiots', the article describing his 1853 visit to Park House, with the observation that, regardless of time or geography,

> the main idea of an idiot would be of a hopeless, irreclaimable, unimprovable
> being. And if he be further recalled as under restraint in a workhouse or lunatic
> asylum, he will still come upon the imagination as wallowing in the lowest
> depths of degradation and neglect: a miserable monster, whom nobody may put
> to death, but whom every one must wish dead, and be distressed to see alive.[25]

However, after establishing this expectation, he quickly refutes it:

> the cultivation of such senses and instincts as the idiot is seen to possess, will,
> besides frequently developing others that are latent in him but obscured, so
> brighten those glimmering lights, as immensely to improve his condition, both
> with reference to himself and to society.[26]

Such comparisons – they are numerous in these travelogues – establish two
orders of 'idiots': those who benefit from the practices occurring at Earlswood
and similar institutions, and those who are not within the institution and
remain 'unreclaimed' for humanity. The 'helpless gibbering wretch' described
by Parkinson does not disappear; he remains part of the world precisely
because he is not within the ameliorating environment of the asylum. As
Sidney notes at the end of his 1864 fête-day visit to Earlswood,

> If all the idiots that have never been subjected to such methods for their ame-
> lioration, could be collected from any considerable area where such might
> be found, for a fête, it is too easy to conceive what a day of misery and confu-
> sion it must prove. But here were order, obedience, regularity, cheerfulness,
> mingled with drollery, eccentric sayings and doings, emulation without seeming
> envy, decent enjoyment of the good things provided, and displays of skill
> and intelligence, combined with the most encouraging symptoms of genuine
> gratification.[27]

The difference between the two types of idiots is not temporal, but spatial
– it rests upon whether or not the individual resides in the asylum and has
benefited from this enlightened education. Sidney presents this image in
advocating for support for Earlswood and similar efforts; however, at the same
time this rhetoric works by generating anxiety about those 'idiots' not within
asylum. While this was only a faint concern in 1864, by the end of the nineteenth century English society would be much more fearful of the unconfined
idiot, as historians such as Mark Jackson and Mathew Thomson have ably
documented.[28]

Another commonly used conceit was that instruction practised within
the asylum brought light into darkness. Dickens, for instance, refers to the

'brighten[ing]' of the 'glimmering lights' of the idiot intellect. In 1862, when Eliza Grove edited a collection of poetry and fiction to raise funds for 'The Idiot and his Institution', she gave it the title *A Beam for Mental Darkness*. Parkinson refers casually to the 'dimmed or partial intelligence' of Earlswood's inmates.[29] Sidney repeats this image in observing of Earlswood that 'the Christian philanthropist may note the efficacy of the plain and verifying truths of the Gospel, as it causes light to beam forth from Darkness',[30] while an article in *Punch*, inspired by Sidney's 1859 narrative, notes that Earlswood aims at 'blowing the faint spark of mind into as great as blaze as possible'.[31] The article in *The Quiver*, 'A Visit to an Idiot Asylum, or, Light in Darkness', opens with the observation that

> Men of scientific pursuits assert that throughout the vast regions of space absolute darkness prevails; and men whose lives are devoted to the healing art present to us a similar assurance in reference to the human intellect. These benefactors to our race prove, by the combined exercise of skill, patience and kindness, that dawns of light may be discovered in the darkest mind.[32]

As these examples suggest, the 'light in darkness' image functions in multiple ways, connecting intrepid explorers mapping new lands, scientists discovering new knowledge, and asylum staff 'enlightening' their charges. As such, this language also recalls that used to describe the activities of those agents of the empire – explorers, missionaries, and colonial administrators – engaged in extending its reach and bringing the 'light' of British civilization and Christianity to the darkness of primitive heathens.

Perhaps the strongest instance of this multiplicity of metaphorical possibilities, including analogies with British imperialism, appears not in an asylum travelogue but in an 1868 article by poet and asylum advocate Dora Greenwell, who brings together scientific research, geographical exploration, philosophy, and theology to introduce her theme: the 'education of imbeciles'. She observes in opening her article that 'In every human being, be he the mightiest or the meanest among the family of Adam, there exists a vast dimly lighted region of unknown extent and unascertained resources'. After elaborating upon this point, she states that 'All that we know of our own nature tends to awaken surmises as vague and wild as were those of Cortez when he gazed "Silent upon a peak of Darien"'[33] This allusion to John Keats's poem 'Upon First Looking into Chapman's Homer' (one of many literary references in her piece) reinforces her own conceit of the growth of the intellect as comparable to the exploration of foreign lands; notably, at this point in the nineteenth century such explorers 'came to be regarded as emblematic figures, ideal types of imperial masculinity who embodied the highest ideals of science and

Christian civilisation'.[34] The image of the hero on his intellectual quest recurs later in Greenwell's article:

> Not that adept watching his crucible, nor Newton pondering over the mighty problem of the universe, ever brought more zeal and patient devotion to bear upon his task than is here given to quicken the dormant intellect of an idiot, to aid the obscure travail of some poor feeble and fettered soul, to send a ray of light glimmering down the deep sunken shaft of the pit where humanity lies bound like Joseph, and forgotten of his brethren.[35]

The labours of the intrepid explorers of idiocy illuminate the dark places of the 'idiot mind' as other explorers have brought to light and civilization other unknown regions of the world; or, perhaps with equal accuracy, the asylum physician can be seen an analogous to British imperial forces colonizing other cultures. In either case, Greenwell's narrative creates heroes of the asylum movement's leaders, a feature shared, in a less emphatic manner, by most asylum travelogues.

'... the ordinary inner life of this remarkable place ...'

The space of the 'idiot asylum' is a parallel world, demarcated from but mirroring the society that erected it. Most visitors' narratives, upon bringing the reader to the asylum, focus initially on the exterior and physical characteristics of the institution, and then travel within to explore its interior.

The institution's facade provides the focus of a series of *Illustrated London News* articles on the various homes of the National Asylum for Idiots between 1849 and 1854: the buildings at Park House, Highgate,[36] Essex Hall, Colchester,[37] and, finally, the Royal Earlswood Asylum,[38] provide the visual anchors for three short articles on the 'asylum for idiots', while a fourth represents Prince Albert at the stone-laying ceremony for the Earlswood Asylum.[39] This architectural emphasis is a function of the magazine's format, which (as its name implies) stressed the visual. However, some of the articles also foregrounded royal visitors to the asylums, including the Duke of Cambridge and Prince Albert to Park House, and noted Prince Albert's patronage of Earlswood (unfortunately, neither the Duke nor the Prince recorded their visits for publication or posterity).

Most other narratives describing the institution move from the exterior to the entrance hall (perhaps noting the reception room), then travel through the institution's various facilities: dining hall, playrooms, gymnasium, workshops, garden, and livestock area. In the process, they document not only the physical layout of the institution but also a pedagogical and moral geography that seeks to inculcate in residents the basic skills and behaviours appropriate to mid-nineteenth-century English society. Cheyne Brady, a Dublin solicitor and philanthropist whose visit forms a part of his 36-page pamphlet *The Training of Idiotic and Feeble-Minded Children*, published in 1864, and then slightly condensed and republished in the *Golden Hours* article 'A Visit to Earlswood', begins by noting 'an extensive pile of building, handsomely ornamented, and bearing more the appearance of a palace than an asylum'. He then enters 'a large and spacious hall' before being shown to dormitories – 'spacious, clean and well-ventilated' – and the wardrobe. While being escorted by the medical superintendent Dr John Langdon Down in an upper corridor, he is able to look down over the dining hall at meal time. 'On this our first sight of the idiots, we were greatly surprised to see them behaving with perfect propriety', he writes. 'Order reigned throughout'. From this point Brady visits the kitchen, the laundry, the workshops where 'the children ... are picking cocoa-fibre for mats, splitting rods for baskets, or preparing horsehair for mattresses', the tailors' shop, a shoemaking department, a basket room, a carpentry shop, and schoolrooms. From here he passes to the 'girls' department', which 'is quite distinct from the boys', and describes activities in their playrooms and classrooms, before returning to the boys' section, where he witnesses the 'shopkeeping' lessons; finally he visits the nursery for the very young and the infirmary. Leaving the main building, he investigates the garden and livestock facilities, where he observes 'nearly thirty of the pupils ... engaged in farming operations'.[40] Brady's progress through the institution is orderly, and his descriptions objective and matter-of-fact.

This cataloguing is characteristic of Earlswood travelogues, and forms the largest part of many of them, including Brady's. Sidney's first visit to Earlswood follows a similar trajectory, including the brief detour through the facilities for girls, but providing more detail and placing greater emphasis on individual residents. These reiterated catalogues form a compelling feature of the Earlswood narratives, and can be explained in part by noting that visitors were simply describing what they saw: for instance, they were presented with a series of separate workshops, each attending to the development of different skills, and so they described this arrangement. But the writers do more than this: they shape narrative, they add judgement, they interpret and they extrapolate. These similarities might also be attributed to the fact that in most instances the tour is escorted at least in part by Dr John Langdon Down, and that Down's tours followed a regular course;[41] indeed, Parkinson's narrative, taken after Down had left Earlswood, follows a different trajectory and builds a narrative around characters rather than the internal geography of the asylum. In all cases, though, there is a genre imperative at work: as travelogues documenting life in an unusual and isolated society, some sociological and ethnographic description is called for. These narratives are expected, if not actually compelled, to report upon Earlswood's physical layout, its means of functioning, and even its social structures, hierarchies, and personalities, in a manner that reinforces the impression that it constitutes a separate society, a separate world.

Visitors' accounts portray the institution at different times replicating the structures of the family, the hospital, the school, and even the village, with its division of labour and class system. As Andrew Halliday, the uncredited author of 'Happy Idiots', points out, 'The Asylum is at once a hospital, a school, and a workshop within; without, a gymnasium, a garden and a farm'.[42] Residents are variously referred to as pupils, inmates, and patients, often all three in the same article (as is the case with Sidney's narratives). Articles dwell on the range of workshops, gardens, and livestock facilities that enabled the asylum, without actually being self-sustaining, to model the labour contributing to the English economy, or at least those cottage economies of previous genera-tions that had been vanishing with the country's industrialization. In this, the asylum also expresses a simpler society, a more primal and communal version of the England that by the 1850s had been irrevocably replaced by a modern industrialized nation. But education at Earlswood was not lacking reference to the world of commerce. The pioneering pedagogue Édouard Séguin, who visited Earlswood at least twice in the 1870s, was particularly struck by 'the TEACHING OF BUYING AND SELLING in a store-class-room, where the students are alternately buyers and sellers' (emphasis in original).[43]

Earlswood's social organization follows English class stratifications, with separate services and privileges for residents according to their means. 'The Earlswood inmates may be divided in three classes', observes Parkinson. 'those who are elected on the charity, and who pay nothing; those whose friends can partly pay for their cost, and who are admitted at a commuted rate fixed by the Board of Management, and those who are the children of prosperous parents, who are able and willing to pay the full sum charged'. Of these latter, some enjoyed private sitting rooms and personal attendants, and dined in seclusion.

So while Earlswood contained a separate society, it was modeled on that to be found – ideally, at any rate – in the England beyond its walls. Visitors con-sistently dwell on the institution's productivity, with much emphasis on how the food is furnished by the asylum gardens and the residents' outfits made in the institution. Describing an Earlswood fête-day, Sidney refers the reader to 'five or six ample tents … [and] Flags innumerable … waving in the breeze', and then marvels at how 'every tent, every pole and nearly every flag was made in the establishment'.[44] Notably, however, there were excursions beyond a closed system: forms of trade, exchange, or even entry into the British society that lay beyond Earlswood's sequestered gardens, fields, and 'manor house'. Parkinson describes an 'idiot carrier ... [who] drives his donkey-cart down to the railway station daily, and brings all parcels safely back' and 'an idiot postman who conveys all letters to and from the post without a single error';[45] the postman also appears at the opening of Sidney's *Second Visit to Earlswood* and in his *Fête-Day at Earlswood*. Such forays into the world beyond the asylum are not surprising; after all, the institution's role in these early years was to educate and prepare its residents as much as possible for a return to their families and communities.

The Christian institution and the asylum family

'The dream of the monks and hospitallers of old has been realised – alms-giving has become an art', writes Halliday in opening 'Happy Idiots'.[46] The asylum was an expression of Christian charity that 'triumphed' through 'science, patience, love and prayer',[47] and aimed to nurture Christian senti-ment in the bosoms of its inmates, preparing them for the afterlife. As Sidney writes, 'It is a remarkable circumstance that many of the idiots are more capable of religious than of any other instruction. Every ray of light communi-cated to them seems to converge to this focus'.[48] He then provides examples of this phenomenon and draws morals from it; for instance, when Sidney ques-tions an ill Earlswood inmate on religious matters in an impromptu catechism, he notes that the boy's responses demonstrate 'what a gracious compensation God had given him for the defects in his bodily powers and mental abilities, and the illness that was now wasting his feeble constitution'.[49] This point was repeated in a 1865 article in the *Edinburgh Review*, the anonymous writer noting that 'Nothing is more striking in many idiots than their susceptibility of religious impression and instruction, happily verifying the beatitude uttered by the Saviour in reference to the poor in spirit'.[50] Such observations echo the older notion of the 'idiot' as 'innocent', albeit now within the narrow confines of the institution, which educates the 'idiot' to embrace his Christian soul. The asylum, a philanthropic Christian effort, was founded by the Reverend Andrew Reed, a non-conformist minister, and Dr John Conolly, superinten-dent of the Middlesex County Lunatic Asylum; both were committed to the idea of charity as a responsibility of the devout Christian.[51] As Reed, speaking at the 1849 Annual General Meeting of the National Asylum for Idiots, noted,

We owe a long and heavy debt to the poor Idiot for past abuse, neglect and cruelty. ... That which should have been first in our sympathies is last ... . We are supplying the last link to the golden chain of Charity, – of all ornaments, the fairest that ever rested on the breast of a noble people.[52]

Significantly, the golden chain of Charity is here presented as a feature of an advanced society, the 'noble people' of the UK. Similarly, Sidney, writing of the fête-day at Earlswood, asserts that Earlswood is an

> enterprise in the truest spirit of the injunction of our Divine Lord and Master, when he commanded those who made a feast to call the poor, the maimed, the halt, and the blind. In the capabilities of enjoyment manifested by the poor imbeciles, we have the most valuable proof of the possibility of ameliorating the condition of those lowest in the human scale, and the consequent duty of aiding in such a truly Christian work.[53]

Often, the 'idiot' figures as a member of a larger human or Christian 'family': for example, the 1853 *Illustrated London News* article refers to 'these most helpless members of the human family',[54] while Greenwell observes that 'among the family of Adam, there exists a vast dimly lighted region of unknown extent and unascertained resources' – that is, the world of the 'idiot' – and then narrows her focus to rest upon the 'Christian nation', concluding that

> in the idiot, and *in those most nearly connected with him* [i.e., family members; emphasis in original], are to be found ... the persons who need all the help and support and comfort which the stronger members of the Christian family are bound to furnish to the weak and heavily burdened ones ... . Each circumstance connected with the human nature in which we share cannot but appear to us in the light of a family consideration.[55]

As these passages suggest, in the minds of asylum advocates Christianity provided both a rationale and a tool for redressing some of the ills of idiocy and reclaiming the 'idiot' for the Christian family.

Indeed, the image of the family was potent: the notion that the staff and residents of the institution constituted a 'family' was a frequent conceit perpetuated by asylums of the day.[56] For 'idiot asylums' specifically, the metaphor first appears in the 1849 *Annual Report* of the Park House asylum, which observed that 'the first gathering of the idiotic family' was 'a spectacle, unique in itself, sufficiently discouraging to the most resolved, and not to be forgotten in time after by any'. After dwelling on this initial 'period of distraction, disorder, and noise of the most unnatural character', the report noted that 'it seemed as though nothing less than the accommodations of a prison would meet the wants of such a family'. However, after a year the asylum residents form 'not only an improving, but a happy family. And all this is secured without the aid of correction or coercion. The principle which rules in the house is

Love – Charity – Divine Charity!'[57] The 1851 *Annual Report* reiterates that 'so helpless and unpromising a family perhaps was never brought together', before describing the institution's successes in the face of this unpromising initial prognosis.[58]

Not surprisingly, the 'family' analogy also appears in the writings of many of Earlswood's visitors. Sidney asserts at the end of *A Visit to Earlswood*, which he calls a 'simple description of a day spent among the unfortunates of the human family', that 'nowhere will [readers] find a better regulated family';[59] in recounting his second visit he recalls being told by Dr Down 'that the family were assembling in the dining-hall for morning prayers'.[60] An 1863 article in *The Quiver*, built largely upon Sidney's observations in *Earlswood and its Inmates*,[61] refers to 'poor, afflicted sons and daughters of the human family',[62] while Parkinson describes 'a happy united family, proud of its occupations, attached to its instructors and friends, harmonious in its relations, and quiet and peaceful in its life'.[63] The institution's masters serve as parental figures, even supplanting the mother, as suggested in a passage in an unsigned 1865 *Edinburgh Review* article noting that the 'gentle treatment of invalids ... caused a youth at Earlswood to say, "I love the doctor better than my mother"'.[64]

Family eccentrics and others

Most families have their eccentric members, and the writers of Earlswood travelogues were keen to foreground the quirks and idiosyncrasies of the asylum's inhabitants. Characterization becomes especially important in the longer narratives, usually foregrounding the good humour and wit of the residents as a sign of the care and training they have received. In some instances, the particular skills of certain residents are also emphasized, and these come to represent the unusual, unfathomable nature of idiocy.[65]

In his first visit, Sidney identifies 'a youth whose manner indicated unmistakably what he was ... yet he has a truly surprising memory for historical facts, and how he picked them up is a mystery'; after giving instances of this person's knowledge, Sidney writes that 'imbecile human nature is seen here in strange forms indeed'.[66] Nicknamed 'the historical cook'[67] by Sidney, he reappears as 'the whimsical historical cook'[68] in Sidney's second visit and as 'the droll creature ... the history-loving cook'[69] in his fête-day report. He is also described in the unsigned 'Born Idiots Bred Sane', as 'the historical cook' in Cheyne Brady's narrative (where he is asked several questions, 'nearly all of which he answered with marvelous accuracy'[70]), and, in Parkinson's narrative, as the 'historical idiot ... a curiosity... [with] a prodigious memory [who] can, and does, answer recondite questions in history with extreme exactitude'.[71]

The article in the *Edinburgh Review* reiterates Sidney's representations of the 'historical cook',[72] as does the one in *The Quiver*.[73] Indeed, an unsigned 1865 article in the professional *Journal of Mental Science* notes that 'Everyone in this country is familiar with the achievements of the historical idiot'.[74]

But the 'historical cook', renowned as he was, could not claim to be the most famous of Earlswood's residents. Even more frequently described was the 'excellent draughtsman who can now dispose of his drawings at a good price', who had 'also shewn great skill in making a model of a man-of-war, every part of which is in just proportion'.[75] While never named in these narratives, the 'excellent draughtsman' was James Henry Pullen, sometimes known as 'the genius of Earlswood', and the individual for whom Down coined the term 'idiot savant'.[76] Pullen's accomplishments in drawing and construction were described in nearly every Earlswood travelogue, including each of Sidney's, *The Quiver's* article, Cheyne Brady's narrative in *Golden Hours*, and Parkinson's pamphlet. The *Journal of Mental Science* also described 'the constructive idiot' whose drawings 'are so excellent and curious as to form ornaments of the Palace'.[77] Indeed, one of Pullen's model ships was exhibited at the 1862 Paris Exhibition,[78] and today visiters can still wonder at his model of the *SS Great Eastern* at the Langdon Down Museum at Normansfield in Middlesex.

While Pullen and the 'historical cook' are ubiquitous, other individuals make one-time appearances. For instance, Parkinson's tour through the mat-making and carpentry shops is enlivened with tales of the individuals labouring to learn these trades, such as the 'stout man of five and twenty' who 'tickle[s] with his fat forefinger the palm of the hand you hold behind your back' and 'nods his broad good-humoured face like a grotesque Chinese monster and grins at your surprise'.[79] In addition, some anecdotes reappear across articles. 'Born Idiots Bred Sane' tells how 'one of the boys, who had never spoken, and was supposed to be dumb, became very ill, and while confined to his bed, suddenly exclaimed: "Why do I suffer thus?"'[80] The same story appears in Sidney's first Earlswood travelogue[81] and in Cheyne Brady's narrative,[82] suggesting that it may have been a stock feature of Down's expositions of Earlswood life.

These literary portraits of Earlswood's inmates, whether the subject is a 'historical cook', an 'excellent draughtsman', or one of the numerous other characters to enliven the travelogues, convey a sense of a cohesive community. The features shared by the residents dominate over individual traits, as each narrative stresses that the inmates are indeed idiots, even if endowed with specific capacities or winning personalities. As Parkinson asserts in his account, which is particularly reliant on character sketches, Earlswood's inhabitants form 'a class apart, and ... would never be lightened by any of the ordinary enjoyments of human life'.[83] In these literary portraits, the engaging identities of Earlswood's inmates remain subsumed under this defining characteristic.

If residents appeared in Earlswood travelogues, so did the medical super-intendent, Dr John Langdon Down. He is an omnipresent figure in Sidney's writings, capably managing the asylum and acting as a visitors guide. Sidney remarks upon the asylum residents' 'manifestation of regard' for Down, con-cluding that he has 'disciplined them well without losing their affection';[84] he recounts grateful letters from parents to Down;[85] he notes how Down's 'able treatment' transformed a boy, 'troublesome and mischievous as an ape', into 'a boy of a quiet, tractable, and pleasing demeanour'.[86] Brady also foregrounds Down's role, describing him as the 'able and intelligent superintendent' who guides him through the asylum.[87] The *Edinburgh Review* article 'Idiot Asylums', which draws on these narratives, refers to Dr Down's 'ingenious and intelligent mind'.[88] Other staff members make occasional appearances: Sidney refers to the 'worthy and intelligent matron, Mrs. Grimshaw', in each of his narratives, noting that on fête-day she 'was almost as ubiquitous among the pupils' as Dr Down.[89] These portraits of the superintendent and his most prominent staff members further the heroic narrative of intrepid explorers bringing light to darkness. If 'idiocy' is analogous to a colonized state, then Down is the most active representative of the world of benevolent intelligence that seeks to bring civilization to his primitive charges. By the time of Parkinson's visit, Down had been replaced as medical superintendent by Dr George Grabham, whose literary appearances in the writings of asylum tourists are much more subdued.

Interpreting travellers' tales

These writings represent a new form of discourse surrounding ideas of idiocy and imbecility in the middle of the nineteenth century. Indeed, the circum-stances were new: asylums were a recent phenomenon, creating unprec-edented gatherings of people identified as 'idiots'. A community characterized by 'idiocy' did not exist before these asylums, and was not described before these travelogues. Reports of what passed in asylums thus shaped a new image of idiocy, one in which the condition is not isolated within a few individuals in families or communities, but exists as a feature shared in an enclosed society representing a significant portion of humanity; as I suggest earlier, the asylum, and idiocy itself, becomes analogous to a colonized territory. This new narra-tive of 'idiocy' took the pathos traditionally embodied by the 'poor idiot' and applied it to a separate society of 'idiots' governed by heroic characters such as Down and underpinned by a philosophy of Christian philanthropy.

In these narratives the asylum inhabitants remain consistently 'other';

their humanity, while repeatedly being affirmed (this is a primary objective of the narratives, after all) is also allotted a peculiar morphology, making them humans of a different order. This 'othering' of Earlswood's inhabitants is most evident in the very use of the terms 'idiot' and 'imbecile', which assign individuals an identity based primarily on only one of their features – their apparent mental incapacities. Consider a short anecdote recounted by Sidney:

> There is one boy who has little or no appearance of his unfortunate condition, who was met by a visitor who asked, not very wisely, perhaps, 'What, are you an idiot?' 'O, no,' he answered, 'I am an *individual*' (emphasis in original).[90]

We are told no more about this boy, and the humour and pathos of this anecdote is that, in the schema of Sidney's narrative, the boy is not an individual but an idiot, and representative of that class.

The unique status – intellectual, moral, and physical – of the 'idiot' and the institution occupies these narratives, which work to discern just what distinguishes and defines the inhabitants of Earlswood. The shared features of the Earlswood travelogues anatomized in this chapter also function as tools for 'othering' its residents. The journey to Earlswood that places it at a distance from London, the 'darkness' that is enlightened by inspired physicians and teachers, the independent structure of this separate realm, and the notion of this world as inhabited by a family replete with idiosyncratic and eccentric characters are all strategies for affirming Earlswood as an unusual and largely self-contained world, and its denizens as forming a strange and distinct, but, ultimately, human society.

As many of these narratives were petitions to the philanthropic impulses of their readers, they also aimed to strengthen a connection between the people of Earlswood and those of England, while maintaining the crucial distinction. Parkinson adopts an interesting strategy: 'A general air of mental weakness and stupidity is over them all', he writes of Earlswood's residents. 'They laugh consumedly at trifles, have little self-control, are obtuse in catching your meaning, and sometimes seem perversely obstinate in refusing to understand. But who has not suffered from these very deficiencies in his acquaintances outside?'[91] He reiterates this observation – that the people inside Earlswood are not so different from some with whom his readers are familiar – throughout his travelogue, which follows the assertion that 'Idiocy cannot be defined' with the claim that

> many of the weaknesses and defects of [Earlswood's] inmates are shared in a greater or lesser degree by the outside world, and one of the most startling conclusions to be drawn from a quiet day spent with these unfortunates, is the narrowness of the border-line between idiocy and what vain man calls sense.

If the most stupid of one's acquaintances and friends were selected on the one hand, and the most intelligent of the idiots picked out on the other, an astute jury would be puzzled to decide which were the most capable of taking care of themselves, which the least like to be injurious to the community.[92]

Indeed, he says, 'You have constantly to ask which are inmates and which attendants as you progress through the house and grounds',[93] questions that ultimately prompt his observation, lifted from *Hamlet*, that 'In the course of a day at Earlswood you become acquainted with many things not previously included in your philosophy'.[94] According to Parkinson, Earlswood poses a moral and intellectual challenge to its visitors: it unsettles one's expectations of idiocy, leading not only to a re-evaluation of that condition but also a transformation of one's 'philosophy'. Yet at the same time, as previously noted, Parkinson explicitly assigns Earlswood's residents to a distinct and separate realm.[95]

It is useful at this point to consider the authors themselves, and what they share. Not surprisingly, many are concerned with social welfare, part of a larger mid-Victorian movement to address the afflictions of the less fortunate. Some, such as the Reverend Sidney, are overt advocates of Christian philanthropy. And, notably, all are men. Women were certainly involved in supporting Earlswood – indeed, they played a central role in fundraising and organizing fêtes and bazaars;[96] there were also many female staff members, including Mrs Grimshaw and the woman who surprised one narrator, causing him to write 'I was certainly not prepared for the statement of one of the female attendants – that she was happy at Earlswood, that she had been there three years, and that she should not like to go to another place'.[97] And there were many literary responses to the education of 'idiots' by female writers: Dora Greenwell and Eliza Grove are only two of many women who supported the work of these institutions in their writings.

But in the nineteenth century, the travel narrative genre was primarily a male domain. Exploration was, for the Victorians, a masculine, usually Christian act, requiring a certain muscular fortitude. Charles Dickens provides an interesting perspective of the role of gender in his Park House travelogue. He imagines a reluctant reader from 'that class of person ... who are so desperately careful to receive no uncomfortable emotions from sad realities or pictures of sad realities'; this reader, in Dickens's fanciful rendition, responds to his narrative by exclaiming '"O, but all this must be excessively painful"', to which Dickens in turn exclaims: 'Madam, you are a lady of very fine feelings, you are very easily shocked, you "Can't bear" a great deal ... you will excuse my saying that I would not have so sensitive a heart in my bosom for the dignity of the whole corporation'.[98] The sensitive reader, the one to be 'put off' by descriptions of 'idiot' humanity, is for Dickens a woman of delicate sensibility; her opposite, the intrepid traveller venturing into the apparently dark realm of the asylum, was very much a man. 'I fully expected that the sight of so many idiotic creatures in a body would be exceedingly painful. It certainly was painful, but far less than I imagined', writes Halliday in 'Happy Idiots',[99] plunging fearlessly – perhaps manfully? – into Earlswood on the same 1864 fête-day celebrations as those described by Sidney. The role of the male guide, in each narrative, is to ascertain and assert the suitability of Earlswood as a destination to visit; although the institution threatens to be a realm of darkness and despair, readers discover that it is, in fact, enlightened, first by its dedicated staff and then by its visitors, the men who, in writing about their travels, illuminate the asylum for future travellers. Sidney closes his first travelogue observing that

> I have been induced to write this simple description ... hoping that some who kindly read it may be led to devote a few hours to a like inspection, with a view to its benefit ... go, the first fine morning that can be spared, take a return ticket to Red Hill [sic] by the Brighton Railway, and walk or drive to Earlswood.[100]

His second travelogue ends with a similar exhortation, as he urges the 'wealthy and charitable of this great nation' to 'have one day's bright holiday within its walls, and its gardens, farm, and gymnasium'.[101] And, as we have seen, his third travelogue opens with the 'generous and kind citizens' on their way to an Earlswood fête-day.[102] Brady completes his account with the blunt assertion that 'The asylum is open daily to visitors'.[103] And Parkinson closes with a distant echo of Dickens, observing that 'Earlswood should be visited freely, and without the faintest anticipation of aught shocking or repulsive. Indeed, the strongest impressions it leaves behind are respect and liking for the kindly idiots'.[104] The potentially dangerous, uncertain realm of the idiot asylum is thus made safe for all manner of travellers, who need not fear the 'shocking' or 'repulsive'. Contained in the asylum, the unsettling condition of idiocy is tamed and civilized.

By the end of the 1860s the Earlswood travelogue was appearing less frequently, and in 1874, *Chambers's Journal* published a retrospective piece glancing back upon that journal's role in establishing Earlswood, noting that 'in Paris, thirty-one years ago, we took the opportunity of visiting ... the Bicêtre' to examine the education of some two hundred 'natural idiots' housed there. According to 'WC' (likely William Chambers, the journal's editor), this 1843 visit recounted in an article of November that year,[105] inspired the creation of Earlswood – a powerful claim for the impact of asylum travelogues.[106] 'What a blessing it must be to many parents that there exist institutions such as those we have specified', the article concludes.[107] As early as 1849, the first annual report of the National Asylum for Idiots was able to claim that 'The benefit has already extended beyond the sphere of our exertions. The tone of public feeling in relation to the poor Idiot has been raised. He can never again be the forlorn abandoned, scorned, imprisoned creature he once was'.[108] Twenty years later the 'idiot institution' had become established as a medical and pedagogical enterprise in England, with Earlswood being joined by institutions in other parts of the country. Visitors would continue to publish asylum travelogues, but they would be fewer as the novelty of the enterprise diminished. Indeed, the travelogues of these early years of Earlswood had already performed their function: placing the institution in the public eye, soliciting for funds and sympathy, and, most profoundly, creating a new image of the 'idiot', an image that would resonate for the remaining decades of the nineteenth century and into the twentieth.

The mid-nineteenth century saw a dramatic shift in the understanding of idiocy. Previously a condition associated with individuals, idiocy was transformed into the defining characteristic of a particular community, one needing the guidance, discipline, and enlightening pedagogy of committed Christian philanthropists in order to be lifted into humanity. Earlswood travelogues functioned as an important tool for transforming ideas of idiocy. In the 1850s and 1860s, the most common tone of these travelogues was more than optimistic; it was laudatory, praising the institution's efforts in taming idiocy and improving the lot of the 'idiots'. But at the same time they developed the idea of the idiot as profiting when situated within a separate environment peopled by similar individuals. In the asylum, although the inhabitants of the institution retained their fundamental limitations, their government by Down and others had created a well-organized, functional, but separate community.

Of course, this vision of the asylum as a functional, occasionally even idealized society that can be visited by well-meaning tourists was short-lived. The early objective of the asylum to educate its residents and eventually return them to their home communities was eventually abandoned, and the institution became instead a permanent home for its inmates – the promise of education was unrealized, and many families were unable, for financial or other reasons,[109] to receive their offspring back into their homes. By the final two decades of the nineteenth century, with the rise of degeneration theory and anxieties over immigration, poverty and crime, idiocy was reconstructed as a social threat – a symptom of moral and physical decline that needed to be isolated for the good of the community.[110] In a diary entry for 9 January, 1915, in the first years of eugenic enthusiasm in England, Virginia Woolf tells of how, while out on a walk,

on the towpath we met & had to pass a long line of imbeciles. The first was a
very tall young man, just queer enough to look at twice, but no more; the second
shuffled, & looked aside; & then one realized that every one in that long line was
a miserable ineffective shuffling idiotic creature, with no forehead, or no chin, &
an imbecile grin, or a wild suspicious stare. It was perfectly horrible. They should
certainly be killed.[111]

The 'long line' of idiots proves unsettling for Woolf, in a way that single individuals would not be – the first young man was, after all, 'just queer enough
to look at twice, but no more'. By the time Woolf is writing – over fifty years
after the Earlswood travelogues – the idiot has come to represent a large class
of threatening individuals who must be contained. While this understanding
of idiocy is associated most strongly with the later nineteenth and first half of
the twentieth centuries, the process of creating this class of socially exiled and
denigrated individuals began unwittingly in the 1850s, with the Earlswood
travelogues as its most prominent literary engine. The asylum pupils whose
lives were documented, and whose humanity was praised, by Sidney, Brady,
Parkinson, Dickens and others, would metamorphose, by virtue of being
constituted in these writings as inhabitants of a separate world, into the collection of 'horrible' idiots that so disturbed the early twentieth century. The
legacy of these representations remains powerful, their impact still resonat-
ing today in policies and practices that marginalize and denigrate people
identified as having intellectual or learning disabilities.

Notes

1 Edwin Sidney, *A Visit to Earlswood (The Asylum for Idiots), May 19, 1859* (London,
1860), 1.
2 Earlswood grew out of the first large British institution for those identified as
'idiots', Park House, Highgate, in London, which opened in April 1848. In 1850,
Park House, by now also known as the National Asylum for Idiots, expanded to
include Essex Hall in Colchester. An ever-growing number of applicants encour-
aged the asylum's supporters to build a new facility especially as an institution for
idiots, which led to the creation of Earlswood.
3 See, especially, David Wright's *Mental Disability in Victorian England: The
Earlswood Asylum 1847–1901* (Oxford: Clarendon, 2001). This is not to overlook
Mark Jackson's work on Mary Dendy's Sandlebridge school and colony in his *The
Borderland of Imbecility: Medicine, Society and the Fabrication of the Feeble Mind
in Late Victorian and Edwardian England* (Manchester: Manchester University
Press, 2000); however, Jackson's focus falls very much on the late Victorian and
Edwardian period, a later era than that of this chapter.

4 Murray K. Simpson, *Modernity and the Appearance of Idiocy* (Lewiston: Edwin Mellon, 2014), 117.

5 Barbara Korte, *English Travel Writing From Pilgrimages to Postcolonial Explorations*, translated by Catherine Matthias (London: Macmillan, 2000), 9.

6 Carl Thompson, *Travel Writing* (London: Routledge, 2011), 10.

7 See, for instance, Edward Said, *Culture and Imperialism* (New York: Knopf, 1993), 10.

8 William Twining, *Some Accounts of Cretinism, and the Institution for its Cure, on the Abendberg, Near Interlachen, in Switzerland* (London: John W. Parker, 1843); 'Summer Loiterings in France: Gossip about Paris', *Chambers's Edinburgh Journal* 12 (4 November, 1843), 333–335; 'Voisin on Idiocy', *Chambers's Edinburgh Journal* 12 (11 November, 1843), 338–339; John Conolly, 'Notices of the Lunatic Asylums of Paris', *British and Foreign Medical Review* 19 (1845), 281–298. Samuel Gaskell's visit was documented over three pieces: 'A Visit to the Bicetre', *Chambers's Edinburgh Journal* 17 (9 January, 1847), 20–22; 'Education of Idiots at the Bicetre', *Chambers's Edinburgh Journal* 17 (30 January, 1847), 71–73; and 'Education of Idiots at the Bicetre', *Chambers's Edinburgh Journal* 17 (13 February, 1847), 105–107.

9 Reports by Earlswood's visitors in the 1850s and 1860s were, in this respect, quite different from the more famous 'bedlam' narratives of the seventeenth and eighteenth centuries, in which visitors to lunatic asylums observed not instances of philanthropic benevolence and enlightened instruction but examples of human folly, despair, and vice.

10 Wright, *Mental Disability in Victorian England*, 120.

11 John Conolly, *The Construction and Government of Lunatic Asylums and Hospitals for the Insane* (London: John Churchill, 1847), 8.

12 Cheyne Brady, *The Training of Idiotic and Feeble-Minded Children* (Dublin: Hodges, Smith and Co., 1865), 17.

13 For more information on the Reverend Sidney (1798–1872), see Aileen Fyfe's *Science and Salvation: Evangelical Popular Science Publishing in Victorian England* (Chicago: University of Chicago Press, 2004), or P. H. M. Cooper's *Fossils, Faith and Farming: Newspaper Portraits of Little Cornard in the Darwinian Age Together with some Account of the Reverend Edwin Sidney, A. M.* (Great Cornard: Little Cornard Conservation Society, 1999).

14 Edwin Sidney, *Second Visit to Earlswood (The Asylum for Idiots), May 17, adjourned to June 8, 1861* (London, 1861), 3.

15 Edwin Sidney, *A Fête-Day at Earlswood, June 16, 1864* (London, 1864), 3.

16 J. C. Parkinson, *A Day at Earlswood* (London, Stahan & Co., 1869), 4. This narrative was first published in the *London Daily News* before being reprinted as a pamphlet to raise funds for the Royal Albert Idiot Asylum in Lancaster.

17 Ibid., 4.

18 A regular contributor of articles on social issues to popular periodicals, which included *Temple Bar* as well as Dickens's *Household Words* and *All the Year Round*,

Parkinson was also familiar with the increasingly common 'urban travelogue'. Indeed, he had engaged with the form in his capacity as a minor civil servant having 'investigated and reported upon abuses in the administration of the Houseless Poor Act and on conditions in workhouses'; he had also published 'travelogues' into the 'blind alleys and dark courts' of London's underworld. Seth Koven quotes from Parkinson's urban travelogue 'On Duty with the Inspector', published in *Temple Bar* in June 1856, in his *Slumming: Sexual and Social Politics in Victorian London* (Princeton: Princeton University Press, 2004), 66.

19 'Born Idiots Bred Sane', *Chambers's Journal of Popular Literature, Science and Arts*, 307 (19 November, 1859), 324.

20 Charles Dickens and William Henry Wells, 'Idiots', *Household Words*, Vol. 7, No. 167 (4 June, 1853), 316.

21 Parkinson, *A Day at Earlswood*, 5.

22 Ruth Levitas, *The Concept of Utopia* (Oxford: Peter Lang, 2010), 9. Notably, Edouard Séguin's pioneering work in educating the 'idiot' in France was inspired philosophically by the writings of the socialist-utopian Saint-Simon.

23 Parkinson, *A Day at Earlswood*, 20.

24 Ibid., 15–16.

25 Dickens and Wills, 'Idiots', 313.

26 Ibid.

27 Sidney, *A Fête-Day at Earlswood*, 19.

28 Jackson, *The Borderland of Imbecility*; Mathew Thomson, *The Problem of Mental Deficiency: Eugenics, Democracy and Social Policy in Britain c. 1870–1959*, Oxford: Oxford University Press, 1998.

29 Parkinson, *A Day at Earlswood*, 10.

30 Sidney, *Second Visit to Earlswood*, 29.

31 'An Epicurean in an Asylum', *Punch* 37 (27 August, 1859), 83.

32 'A Visit to an Idiot Asylum: or, Light in Darkness', *The Quiver* (23 February, 1863), 381.

33 Dora Greenwell, 'On the Education of the Imbecile', *North British Review* 49 (1868), 73.

34 Thompson, *Travel Writing*, 53. Note that Henry Morton Stanley's *Through the Dark Continent*, about his African quest to find Dr Livingstone, was published in 1878.

35 Greenwell, 'On the Education of the Imbecile', 91.

36 'The Asylum for Idiots', *Illustrated London News* (31 March, 1849), 211–212.

37 'The Asylum for Idiots', *Illustrated London News* (22 March, 1851), 235–236.

38 'The New Asylum for Idiots', *Illustrated London News* (11 March, 1854), 213–214.

39 'The Asylum for Idiots', *Illustrated London News* (25 June, 1853), 509–510.

40 Brady, *The Training of Idiotic and Feeble-Minded Children*, 18–22.

41 Down was the medical superintendent of Earlswood from 1858 to 1868, when he left to establish a private institution at Normansfield.

42 Andrew Halliday, 'Happy Idiots', *All the Year Round* (23 July, 1864), 567;

while the article is unsigned in the journal, the author is identified by Ella Anne Oppenlander as Andrew Halliday, a regular journalist and, briefly, sub-editor of the journal *All the Year Round*, edited by Charles Dickens. See Ella Anne Oppenlander, *Dickens'* All the Year Round: *Descriptive Index and Contributor List* (Troy, NY: Winston, 1984).

43 Edward Seguin, *Report on Education* [1875] (Delmar, NY: Scholars Facsimiles and Reprints, 1976), 94. Interestingly, Séguin goes on to note that 'this teaching is rendered the more necessary, as the institutions for idiots become larger and more separated from the world. For ... the street-abandoned idiot, or the one cared for ... at home, or the one free in his movements between school-hours ... meets ... with opportunities of witnessing many transactions – and particularly of comprehending the commercial characters of exchange – impossible to enumerate ... . The idiot shut up in a perfectly organized, self-feeding machine, has no opportunity of conceiving the reciprocities of life; he cannot help feeling that the world – the only world he knows – is made for him, and that it is for him to receive without rendering compensation'. Séguin's observations present a critique of large institutions that remove the individual from practical education in a larger society, and provide a counterpoint to the 'before' and 'after' imagery that writers such as Sidney, Dickens, and Parkinson employ in describing the benefits of Earlswood. Note that Séguin anglicized his name in his publications after he emigrated to the US following the failed European revolutions of 1848.

44 Sidney, *A Fête-Day at Earlswood*, 5.

45 Parkinson, *A Day at Earlswood*, 17.

46 Halliday, 'Happy Idiots', 564.

47 'A Visit to Earlswood', *Golden Hours: A Monthly Magazine for Sunday Reading* 26 (February, 1866), 28.

48 Sidney, *A Visit to Earlswood*, 17.

49 Ibid., 18.

50 'Idiot Asylums', *Edinburgh Review* 122 (July 1865), 54.

51 For more on Reed's and Conolly's roles in the creation of Earlswood, see David Wright's *Mental Disability in Victorian England*, especially 30–34.

52 *Annual Report 1849*, Royal Earlswood Hospital Archives, 392/1/2/1, Surrey Record Office.

53 Sidney, *A Fête-Day at Earlswood*, 20–21.

54 'The Asylum for Idiots', *Illustrated London News* (25 June, 1853), 510.

55 Greenwell, 'On the Education of the Imbecile', 73, 100.

56 Wright, *Mental Disability in Victorian England*, 143.

57 *Annual Report 1849*, Royal Earlswood Hospital Archives, 392/1/2/1, Surrey Record Office.

58 *Annual Report 1851*, Royal Earlswood Hospital Archives, 392/1/2/1, Surrey Record Office.

59 Sidney, *A Visit to Earlswood*, 26.

60 Sidney, *Second Visit to Earlswood*, p. 21.

61 Sidney, *Earlswood and Its Inmates: A Lecture Delivered at the Literary and Scientific Institution, Croyden, Surrey, on Monday, Dec. 22, 1862* (Croydon, 1863).

62 'A Visit to an Idiot Asylum, or Light in Darkness', *The Quiver* 29 February, 1863: 383.

63 Parkinson, *A Day at Earlswood*, 5.

64 'Idiot Asylums', *Edinburgh Review* 122 (July 1865), 48.

65 Séguin criticized Earlswood's showcasing of exceptional residents, writing that the public appetite 'must be served by the idiots with all kinds of sauces – musical, arithmetical, architectural &c. with more money, and time stolen from the legitimate training of all the pupils, it is easy to find among them some one with a gift salient over the wreck of the other faculties, and to set them up as the great attraction for idlers and a living prospectus for the school. They are, and will be, nothing else. The gift thus developed, at the expense of their own, and of the general training, will never serve the gifted; it can be but wondered at, and they, being the more pitied for it. This evil practice is not confined to Earlswood; other schools for idiots have their pet mathematicians, &c; good-for-nothing, ordinary schools and universities, too, cultivate these unhealthy products. Once used for show, the child is used up for life: This is not education, but holocaust'. Séguin, *Report on Education*, 95.

66 Sidney, *A Visit to Earlswood*, 9.

67 Ibid., 12.

68 Sidney, *Second Visit to Earlswood*, 22.

69 Sidney, *A Fête-Day at Earlswood*, 6.

70 Brady, *The Training of Idiotic and Feeble-Minded Children*, 20.

71 J. C. Parkinson, *A Day at Earlswood*, 6–7.

72 'Idiot Asylums', *Edinburgh Review*, 60.

73 'A Visit to an Idiot Asylum', *The Quiver*, 382.

74 'The Psychology of Idiocy', *Journal of Mental Science* 11 (1865), 11.

75 'Born Idiots Bred Sane', *Chambers's Journal*, 325.

76 F. Sano, 'James Henry Pullen, the Genius of Earlswood', *Journal of Mental Science* 64 (July 1918).

77 'The Psychology of Idiocy', *Journal of Mental Science* 11 (1865), 13.

78 Parkinson, *A Day at Earlswood*, 11.

79 Ibid., 6.

80 'Born Idiots Bred Sane', *Chambers's Journal*, 325.

81 Sidney, *A Visit to Earlswood*, 18.

82 'A Visit to Earlswood', *Golden Hours*, 30.

83 Parkinson, *A Day at Earlswood*, 15–16.

84 Sidney, *A Visit to Earlswood*, 9.

85 Sidney, *Second Visit to Earlswood*, 16, 28.

86 Sidney, *A Fête-Day at Earlswood*, 8.

87 'A Visit to Earlswood', *Golden Hours*, 28.

88 'Idiot Asylums', *Edinburgh Review* 53.

89   Sidney, *A Fête-Day at Earlswood*, 18.

90   Sidney, *Second Visit to Earlswood*, 16.

91   Parkinson, *A Day at Earlswood*, 6.

92   Ibid., 3–4.

93   Ibid., 5.

94   Ibid., 17.

95   Ibid., 15–16.

96   Wright, *Mental Disability in Victorian England*, 132.

97   Halliday, 'Happy Idiots', 568.

98   Dickens and Wills, 'Idiots', 316.

99   Halliday, 'Happy Idiots', 566.

100   Sidney, *A Visit to Earlswood*, 26.

101   Sidney, *Second Visit to Earlswood*, 30.

102   Sidney, *A Fête-Day at Earlswood*, 3.

103   'A Visit to Earlswood', *Golden Hours*, 31.

104   Parkinson, *A Day at Earlswood*, 20.

105   See Korte, *English Travel Writing*.

106   WC, 'Improved Treatment of Imbeciles', *Chambers's Journal of Popular Literature, Science and Arts* (29 August, 1874), 553.

107   Ibid., 554.

108   *Annual Report 1849*, Royal Earlswood Hospital Archives, 392/1/2/1, Surrey Record Office.

109   Wright, *Mental Disability in Victorian England*, 94–96.

110   See Jackson's *The Borderland of Imbecility* and Thomson's *The Problem of Mental Deficiency* for more on the late nineteenth/early twentieth-century anxiety about idiocy.

111   Virginia Woolf, *The Diary of Virginia Woolf Vol 1: 1915–1919*, edited by Anne Olivier Bell (London: Hogarth 1977), 13.

Select bibliography

Primary sources

Amos, A. 'Lectures in medical jurisprudence delivered in the University of London: on insanity'. *London Medical Gazette* 8 (July, 1831): 417–425.

Anon. *The case of Henry Roberts, Esq, a gentleman who by unparalleled cruelty was deprived of his estate under the pretence of idiocy.* London, 1767.

Anon. 'Commission of Lunacy, Bagster v Newton'. *London Medical Gazette* 10 (21 July, 1832): 519–528.

Anon. 'Editorial', *London Medical Gazette* 10 (28 July, 1832): 553–558.

Archenholz, Johann. *A picture of England: containing a description of the laws, customs, and manners of Wilhelm von England.* Vol. 1. London, 1789.

Arnold, Thomas. *Observations on the Nature, Kinds, Causes, and Prevention of Insanity, Lunacy, or Madness.* 2 vols. Leicester: Robinson & Cadell, 1782–86.

'The Asylum for Idiots'. *Illustrated London News* (31 March, 1849): 211–212.

'The Asylum for Idiots'. *Illustrated London News* (22 March, 1851): 235–236.

'The Asylum for Idiots'. *Illustrated London News* (25 June, 1853): 509–510.

Augustine. *On Christian Teaching* [397/426]. Translated and introduced by R. P. H. Green. Oxford: Oxford University Press, 1997.

Augustine: De Doctrina Christiana [397/426]. Edited by R. P. H. Green. Oxford Early Christian Texts. Oxford: Oxford University Press, 1995.

Bartholomaeus Anglicus. *De proprietatibus rerum*, edited by John de Trevisa. London: Berthelet, 1535.

Battie, William. *A Treatise on Madness.* London: J. Whiston and B. White, 1758.

Baxter, Richard. *Certain Disputations of Right to Sacraments.* London: Thomas Johnson, 1657.

Baxter, Richard. *The Universal Redemption of Mankind.* London: John Salusbury, 1694.

B. E. (Gent.) *A new dictionary of the terms ancient and modern of the canting crew in its several tribes, of gypsies, beggers, thieves, cheats & c.* London, 1699.

Beck, Theodric. *Elements of medical jurisprudence.* London, 1836.

Blake, Thomas. *The Covenant Sealed.* London: Roper, 1655.

Boissier de Sauvages de la Croix, François. *Nosologia methodica.* Vol. 2. Amsterdam: Fratrum de Tournes, 1768.

Bourneville, Désiré-Magloire. *Recherches cliniques et thérapeutiques sur l'épilepsie, l'hystérie et l'idiotie.* 26 vols. Paris: Bureaux de Progrés Médical and Felix Alcan, 1872–1907.

Bracton, Henry de. *Bracton's Notebook.* Edited by Frederic W. Maitland. 3 vols. London: Clay, 1887.

Bracton, Henry de (attributed). *De legibus et consuetudinibus Angliae: On the Laws and Customs of England* [c.1220–50]. Edited by George E. Woodbine and translated by Samuel E. Thorne. 4 vols. Cambridge, MA: Harvard University Press, 1968–77.

Brant, Sebastian. *Das Narrenschiff. Nach der Erstausgabe (Basel 1494) mit den Zusätzen der Ausgaben von 1495 und 1499 sowie den Holzschnitten der deutschen Originalausgaben* [1494], edited by Manfred Lemmer. Tübingen: Max Niemeyer Verlag, 1986.

Britton. Edited and translated by Francis M. Nichols. 2 vols. Oxford: Clarendon Press, 1865.

Brady, Cheyne. *The Training of Idiotic and Feeble-Minded Children.* 2nd edn. Dublin: Hodges, Smith & Co., 1865.

Brydall, John. *Non compos mentis: or the law relating to natural fools, mad folks and lunatic persons inquisited and explained for the common benefit.* London, 1700.

Cawdrey, Daniel. *A Sober Answer to a Serious Question.* London: Christopher Meredith, 1652.

C[hambers], W[illiam]. 'Improved Treatment of Imbeciles'. *Chambers's Journal of Popular Literature, Science and Arts* (29 August, 1874): 553–554.

Chitty, J. *A practical treatise on medical jurisprudence.* London, 1834.

Coke, Sir Edward. *Institutes of the laws of England.* London, 1628.

Collinges, John. *The Preacher (Pretendly) Sent, Sent Back.* London: Livewell Chapman, 1658.

Collinges, John. *Responsaria Bipartita.* London: H. Hills, 1654.

Collinson, George Dale. *A treatise on the law concerning idiots, lunatics, and other persons non compotes mentis.* London, 1812.

Condillac, Etienne Bonnot de. *An Essay on the Origin of Human Knowledge: Being a Supplement to Mr. Locke's Essay on the Human Understanding* [1756]. Translated by Thomas Nugent. Gainsville: Scholar Facsimiles and Reprints, 1971.

Condillac, Etienne Bonnot de. 'Treatise on Sensations'. In *Philosophical Writings of Etienne Bonnot, Abbé de Condillac* [1754]. Translated by Franklin Phillips in collaboration with Harlan Lane. Hillsdale NJ: Lawrence Erlbaum Associates, 1982: 155–339.

Conolly, John. *The Construction and Government of Lunatic Asylums and Hospitals for the Insane.* London: John Churchill, 1847.

Conolly, John. *The Treatment of the Insane Without Mechanical Restraints.* London: Smith, Elder & Co., 1856.

Crichton, Alexander. *An Inquiry into the Nature and Origin of Mental Derangement.* London: T. Cadell, Junior and W. Davies, 1798.

Cullen, William. *First Lines of the Practice of Physic.* Vols I–IV. Edinburgh: C. Elliot, 1789.

Cullen, William. *Nosology: Or, A Systematic Arrangement of Diseases by Classes, Orders, Genera, and Species.* Edinburgh: C. Stewart and Co., 1800.

Defoe, Daniel. *Mere nature delineated: or, A body without a soul. Being observations upon the young forester lately brought to town from Germany. With suitable applications. Also, a brief dissertation upon the usefulness and necessity of fools, whether political or natural*. London: T. Warner, 1726.

'Des Mönches Not' [c.1290]. In *Novellistik des Mittelalters. Märendichtung*, edited by Klaus Grubmüller, 591–617. Frankfurt a.M.: Bibliothek des Mittelalters, 2011.

Diagnostic and Statistical Manual of Mental Disorders, Fifth Edition (DSM-5). Arlington, VA: American Psychiatric Association, 2013.

Dickens, Charles and William Henry Wells. 'Idiots'. *Household Words*. Vol. 7, No. 167 (4 June, 1853): 313–317.

'Die Halbe Birne' [1300]. In *Novellistik des Mittelalters. Märendichtung*, edited by Klaus Grubmüller, 178–207. Frankfurt a.M.: Bibliothek des Mittelalters, 2011.

Down, John Langdon. 'Observations on an ethnic classification of idiots'. *Clinical Lecture Reports of the London Hospital* 3 (1866): 259–62.

Down, John Langdon. *On some of the mental afflictions of childhood and youth, being the Lettsomian lectures delivered before the Medical Society of London in 1887*. London, 1887.

Drake, Roger. *The Bar Against Free Admission to the Lord's Supper Fixed*. London: Philip Chetwind, 1656.

Drake, Roger. *A Boundary to the Holy Mount*. London: S. Bowtell, 1653.

Duncan, P. Martin, M. B. Lond, et al. 'Notes on Idiocy'. *Journal of Mental Science* 7 (1861): 232–252.

Duncan, P. Martin and William Millard. *A Manual for the Classification, Training, and Education of the Feeble-Minded, Imbecile, and Idiotic*. London: Longmans, Green and Co., 1866.

Edgeworth, Maria and Richard Lovell Edgeworth. *Practical Education. In Two Volumes*. [1798] New York and London, 1974.

'An Epicurean in an Asylum'. *Punch* 37 (27 August, 1859): 83.

Esquirol, Jean-Étienne Dominique. *Mental Maladies: A Treatise on Insanity* [1854]. Translated by E. K. Hunt. New York: Hafner Publishing Company, 1965.

Fleta [c.1290], edited and translated by Henry G. Richardson and George O. Sayles. 3 vols. Selden Society Publications 72, 79, 99. London, 1955, 1972, 1984.

Fodéré, F. E. *Traité de médecine légale et d'hygiène publique ou de police de santé: tome premier*. 2nd edn. Paris, 1813.

Freud, Sigmund. *General Introduction to Psychoanalysis* [1916–17]. Translated by G. Staneley Hall. New York: Horace Liverwright, 1920.

Frugard, Roger. *Chirurgia* [c.1180]. In *Anglo-Norman Medicine*, edited by Tony Hunt. 2 vols. Cambridge: D. S. Brewer, 1994.

Georget, Etienne-Jean. *De la folie: considerations sur cette maladie*. Paris, 1820.

Georget, Etienne-Jean. *Discussion médico-legale sur la folie ou alienation mentale*. Paris, 1826.

Gilbertus Anglicus. *Healing and Society in Medieval England: A Middle English Translation of the Pharmaceutical Writings of Gilbertus Anglicus* [c.1230–50], edited by Faye Marie Getz. Madison: University of Wisconsin Press, 1991.

Glanville, Ranulf. *De Legibus et Consuetudinibus Regni Angliae* [1187–89], edited by George E. Woodbine. New Haven: Yale University Press, 1932.

Greenwell, Dora. 'On the Education of the Imbecile'. *North British Review* 49 (1868): 73–100.

Grose, Francis. *A dictionary of the vulgar tongue.* London, 1788.

Grove, Eliza. *Narrative Poems, and A Beam for Mental Darkness for the Benefit of the Idiot and his Institution.* London: Dean and Son, 1856.

Guy, William. *Principles of forensic medicine.* 2nd edn. London, 1861.

[Halliday, Andrew]. 'Happy Idiots'. *All the Year Round* 11 (23 July, 1864): 564–569.

Haslam, John. *Medical jurisprudence as it relates to insanity according to the law of England.* London, 1817.

Heinrich von Freiberg. *Tristan: der willetôre Tristan* [c.1290], edited by Karl Bartsch. Amsterdam: RODOPI, 1966.

Hicks, William. 'Selections from *Oxford Jests*' [1671]. In *A Nest of Ninnies and Other English Jestbooks of the Seventeenth Century,* edited by P. M. Zall, 235–247. Lincoln: University of Nebraska Press, 1970.

Highmore, A. *A treatise on the law of idiocy and lunacy.* London, 1807.

Hobbes, Thomas. *Leviathan* [1651]. Corvallis: Oregon State University. http://ore gonstate.edu/instruct/phl302/texts/hobbes/leviathan-contents.html. Accessed 27 April, 2012.

Howe, Samuel Gridley. *On the Causes of Idiocy* [1848]. New York: Arno Press and The New York Times, 1972.

Hugh of St Victor. *The Didascalion of Hugh of St. Victor* [c.1130]. Translated and introduced by Jerome Taylor. New York: Columbia University Press, 1991.

Hugo von Sankt Viktor. *Didascalion de studio legend* [c.1130]. Fontes Christiani 27. Freiburg: Herder, 1997.

Humfrey, John. *An Humble Vindication of a Free Admission unto the Lord's Supper.* London: Edward Blackmore, 1651.

Humfrey, John. *A Rejoynder to Mr Drake.* London: Edward Blackmore, 1654.

Humfrey, John. *A Second Vindication of a Disciplinary, Anti-Erastian, Orthodox Free Admission to the Lord's Supper.* London: Edward Blackmore, 1656.

'Idiot Asylums'. *Edinburgh Review* 122 (July 1865): 37–74.

Ireland, William Wotherspoon. *On Idiocy and Imbecility.* London: J. & A. Churchill, 1877.

Itard, Jean-Marc-Gaspard. *The Wild Boy of Aveyron* [1801/1806]. Foreword by the Author. Translated by George and Muriel Humphrey. New York: Appleton Century Crofts, 1962.

Konrad von Megenberg. *Buch der Natur* [c.1349–50], edited by Robert Luff and George Steer. Tübingen: Max Niemeyer Verlag, 2003.

Krafft-Ebing, Richard von. *Lehrbuch der Psychiatrie auf Klinischer Grundlage für Practische Ärtze und Studirende.* 3 vols, Stuttgart: Verlag von Ferdinand Enke, 1879–80.

Locke, John. *An Essay Concerning Human Understanding* [1689], edited by Peter Nidditch. Oxford: Clarendon Press, 1975.

Locke, John. 'Some Thoughts Concerning Education' [1693]. In *John Locke on Education*. Edited by Peter Gay, 19–176. New York: Teacher College Press, 1964.

Maudsley, Henry. *The Pathology of Mind*. 3rd edn. London: Macmillan & Co., 1879.

Mercier, Charles. *Crime and Insanity*. London: Williams and Northgate, 1911.

Mercier, Charles. *Sanity and Insanity*. London: Walter Scott, 1890.

The Mirror of Justices. Edited by W. J. Whittaker and introduced by F. W. Maitland. Selden Society Publications, no. 7. London: Selden Society, 1893.

Morice, William. *The Common Right to the Lord's Supper Asserted*. London: Richard Roiston, 1657.

'The New Asylum for Idiots'. *Illustrated London News* (11 March, 1854): 213–214.

Pargeter, William. 'Observations on maniacal disorders' [1792]. In *Patterns of Madness in the Eighteenth Century: A Reader*. Edited by Allan Ingram, 179–86. Liverpool: Liverpool University Press, 1998.

Parkinson, J. C. *A Day at Earlswood*. London: Strahan and Co., 1869.

The Parliament Rolls of Medieval England. Edited by C. Given-Wilson et al. CD-ROM. Leicester: Scholarly Digital Editions, 2005.

Perfect, William. *Select Cases in the Different Species of Insanity, Lunacy, or Madness, with the Modes of Practice as Adopted in the Treatment of Each*. Rochester: Gillman, 1787.

Pinel, Philipe. *Medico-philosophical treatise on mental alienation* [1800, 1809]. Translated by Gordon Hickish, David Henly, and Louis C. Charland. Chichester: Wiley-Blackwell, 2008.

Pinel, Phillipe. *A Treatise on Insanity* [1806]. Translated by D. D. Davis. New York: Hafner Publishing Co., 1962.

Powell, Thomas. *The attourney's academy, or the manner and forme of proceeding practically upon any suite, plaint or action whatsoever, within this kingdome: especially in the great courts at Westminster*. London, 1623.

Quintilian. *The Institutio oratoria of Quintilian* [c.95], Vol. I. Translated by H. E. Butler. Loeb Classical Library 124. Cambridge, MA and London: Harvard University Press/Heinemann, 1980.

Ray, I. *A treatise on the medical jurisprudence of insanity*. London, 1839.

The Roll and Writ File of the Berkshire Eyre of 1248. Edited by M. T. Clanchy. Selden Society 90. London: Selden Society Publications, 1973.

Rotuli Parliamentorum, ut et Petitiones, et Placita in Parliamento. 6 vols. London: Record Commission, 1783, reprint 1832.

Rousseau, Jean-Jacques. 'A Discourse upon the origin and foundation of the inequality among mankind' [1755]. In *The Social Contract and Discourse on the Origins of Inequality*. Edited by Lester G. Crocker. New York: Pocket Books, 1967.

Rousseau, Jean-Jacques. *Émile, or On Education*. Edited, translated and introduced by Allan Bloom. London: Penguin, 1991.

Rousseau, Jean-Jacques. *The Social Contract* [1762]. In *The Essential Rousseau*. Translated by Lowell Blair. New York: New American Library, 1974.

Saunders, Humphrey. *An Anti-Diatribe*. London: Thomas Newberry, 1655.

Séguin, Édouard. *Idiocy and its Treatment by the Physiological Method*. New York: William Wood & Co., 1866.

Séguin, Édouard. *Report on Education* [1875]. Delmar, NY: Scholars Facsimiles and Reprints, 1976.

Shelford, L. *A practical treatise on the law concerning lunatics, idiots and persons of unsound mind*. London, 1833.

Sidney, Rev. Edwin. *Earlswood and Its Inmates: A Lecture Delivered at the Literary and Scientific Institution, Croyden, Surrey, on Monday, Dec. 22, 1862*. Croydon, 1863.

Sidney, Rev. Edwin. *A Fête-Day at Earlswood, June 16, 1864*. London: 1865.

Sidney, Rev. Edwin. *A Visit to Earlswood (The Asylum for Idiots), May 19, 1859*. London: 1860.

Sidney, Rev. Edwin. *Second Visit to Earlswood (The Asylum for Idiots), May 17, Adjourned to June 8, 1861*. London: 1861.

Smith, John. 'Distress of mind in old age'. [Extract from *King Solomons Portraiture of Old Age* (1666).] In *Three Hundred Years of Psychiatry, 1535–1860*. Edited by Richard Hunter and Ida Macalpine, 182–183. Oxford: Oxford University Press, 1963.

Smollett, Tobias. *The adventures of Roderick Random* [1748]. London: Everyman, 1975.

Spillan, D. 'Introduction'. In Ray, Isaac, *A treatise on the medical jurisprudence of insanity*. London, 1839.

Spitzka, Edward Charles. *Insanity, its Classification, Diagnosis and Treatment: A Manual for Students and Practitioners of Medicine*. New York: Bermingham and Co., 1883.

The Statutes of the Realm. Vol. I. London: Dawsons of Pall Mall, reprint 1963 of 1810 edn.

Swift, Jonathan. *Gulliver's Travels* [1726/1735], edited by Albert Rivero. New York: Norton, 2002.

Swift, Jonathan. 'To Alexander Pope'. In *The Correspondence of Jonathan Swift* [1725]. Edited by Harold Williams, iii, 103. 5 vols. Oxford: Oxford University Press, 1963–65.

Swinburne, Henry. *A treatise of testaments and last wills* [1590]. 8th edn. London, 1743.

Thrumbo, Hurlo. *The merry thought: or the glass-window and bog-house miscellany*. London, 1731.

Timson, John. *The Bar to Free Admission to the Lord's Supper Removed*. London: Thomas Williams, 1654.

Timson, John. *To Receive the Lord's Supper*. London: Thomas Williams, 1655.

Tredgold, Alfred. *Mental Deficiency (Amentia)*. 2nd edn. New York: William Wood & Co., 1915.

Twining, William. *Some Accounts of Cretinism, and the Institution for its Cure, on the Abendberg, Near Interlachen, in Switzerland*. London: John W. Parker, 1843.

Vincent of Beauvais, *De eruditione filiorum nobilium* [c.1250], edited by Arpad Steiner. Wisconsin: Medieval Academy of America, 1938.

'A Visit to an Idiot Asylum: or, Light in Darkness'. *The Quiver* (23 February, 1863): 381–383.

'A Visit to Earlswood'. *Golden Hours: A Monthly Magazine for Sunday Reading* 26 (February, 1866): 28–31.

Willis, Francis. *A Treatise on Mental Derangement*. London: Longman, Hurst, Rees, Orme, and Brown, 1823.

Wolfram von Eschenbach [c.1200–10]. *Parzival*. 2 vols, edited by Karl Lachmann. Stuttgart: Reclam, 1981.

Year Books of Edward II. Edited by Frederic W. Maitland et al. Selden Society, 29 vols. London: Selden Society, 1903–88.

Secondary sources

Andrews, Jonathan. 'Begging the Question of Idiocy: The Definition and Socio-Cultural Meaning of Idiocy in Early Modern Britain: Part 1'. *History of Psychiatry* 9 (1998): 65–95.

Armstrong, Brian. *Calvin and the Amyraut Heresy: Protestantism and Scholasticism in Seventeenth-Century France*. Madison WI: University of Wisconsin Press, 1969.

Asimov, Issac. *The Annotated Gulliver's Travels*. New York: Clarkson Potter, 1980.

Bartlett, Peter and David Wright, *Outside the Walls of the Asylum: The History of Community Care 1750–2000*. London: Athlone Press, 1999.

Bell, H. E. *An Introduction to the History and Records of the Court of Wards and Liveries*. Cambridge: Cambridge University Press, 1953.

Bellamy, Liz. *Jonathan Swift's Gulliver's Travels*. New York: St. Martin's Press, 1992.

Berrios, German E. 'Jaspers and First Edition of *Allgemeine Psychopathologie* – Reflection'. *British Journal of Psychiatry* 202 (2013): 547–566.

Bloor, David. *Knowledge and Social Imagery*. 2nd edn. Chicago: University of Chicago Press, 1991.

Brown, Laura. *Fables of Modernity: Literature and Culture in the English Eighteenth Century*. Ithaca: Cornell University Press, 2001.

Buhrer, Eliza. '"But What is to be Said of a Fool?" Intellectual Disability in Medieval Thought and Culture'. In *Mental Health, Spirituality, and Religion in the Middle Ages and Early Modern Age*, edited by Albrecht Classen, 314–343. Berlin: De Gruyter, 2014.

Bumke, Joachim. 'Wolfram von Eschenbach'. In *Die deutsche Literatur des Mittelalters. Verfasserlexikon Band 10*, edited by Burkhart Wachinger et al., 1376–1418. Berlin: De Gruyter, 1999.

Bumke, Joachim. *Blutstropfen im Schnee. Über Wahrnehmung und Erkenntnis im 'Parzival' Wolframs von Eschenbach*. Tübingen: Niemeyer, 2001.

Bynum, Caroline Walker. *Holy Feast and Holy Fast: The Religious Significance of Food to Medieval Women*. Berkeley: University of California Press, 1987.

Caciola, Nancy. *Discerning Spirits: Divine and Demonic Possession in the Middle Ages*. Ithaca: Cornell University Press, 2003.

Carbonel, F. 'L'idéologie aliéniste du Dr. B. A. Morel: Christianisme social et médecine sociale, milieu et dégénérescence, psychiatrie et régénération. Partie I'. *Annales Médico-Psychologiques* 168 (2010): 666–671.

Carlson, Licia. 'Cognitive Ableism and Disability Studies: Feminist Reflections on the History of Mental Retardation'. *Hypatia* 16.4 (2001): 124–145.

Carlson, Licia. *The Faces of Intellectual Disability: Philosophical Reflections*. Bloomington: Indiana University Press, 2009.

Carlyle, E. I. 'Shelford, Leonard (1795–1864)'. Rev. Jonathan Harris. *Oxford Dictionary of National Biography*. Oxford: Oxford University Press, 2004.

Carnochan, W. B. *Lemuel Gulliver's Mirror for Man*. Berkeley and Los Angeles: University of California Press, 1968.

Castel, Robert. *The Regulation of Madness: The Origins of Incarceration in France*. Translated by W. D. Halls. Cambridge: Polity Press, 1988.

Castoriadis, Cornelius. *The Imaginary Institution of Society*. Translated by Kathleen Blamey. Cambridge MA: MIT Press, 1987.

Chambers, Paul. *Bedlam: London's Hospital for the Mad*. Hersham: Ian Allan, 2009.

Chesler, Phylis. *Women and Madness*. London: Allen Lane, 1972.

Chrobak, Werner. 'Die Schriften Konrads von Megenberg'. In *Konrad von Megenberg. Regensburger Domherr, Dompfarrer und Gelehrter (1309–1374) zum 700. Geburtstag. Ausstellung in der Bischöflichen Zentralbibliothek Regensburg 27. August bis 25. September 2009*, edited by Paul Mai, 51–78. Regensburg: Schnell & Steiner, 2009.

Clanchy, M. T. *From Memory to Written Record: England 1066–1307*. 3rd edn. Chichester: Wiley-Blackwell, 2013.

Cohen, Deborah. *Family Secrets: Living with Shame from the Victorians to the Present Day*. Oxford: Oxford University Press, 2013.

Collingwood, R. G. *The Idea of History*. Revised edn. Oxford: Oxford University Press, 2005.

Cooper, David. *Psychiatry and Anti-Psychiatry*. Abingdon: Routledge, 1967.

Cooper, P. H. M. *Fossils, Faith and Farming: Newspaper Portraits of Little Cornard in the Darwinian Age Together with some Account of the Reverend Edwin Sidney, A. M.* Great Cornard, Sussex: Little Cornard Conservation Society, 1999.

Cotter, W. *Miracles in Greco-Roman Antiquity: A Sourcebook for the Study of New Testament Miracle Stories*. Abingdon and New York: Routledge, 1999.

Cranefield, Paul F. 'A Seventeenth-Century View of Mental Deficiency and Schizophrenia: Thomas Willis on "Stupidity or Foolishness"'. *Bulletin of the History of Medicine* 35 (1961): 291–316.

Cranefield, Paul F. and Walter Federn. 'The Begetting of Fools: An Annotated Translation of Paracelsus'. *The Bulletin of the History of Medicine* 41 (1967): 56–74; 161–174.

Cremin, Lawrence A. 'Preface'. In *John Locke on Education*, edited by Peter Gay. New York: Teacher College Press, 1964.

Crider, Richard. 'Yahoo (Yahu): Notes on the Name of Swift's Yahoos'. *Names: A Journal of Onomastics* 41.2 (1993): 103–109.

Curtis, S. J. and M. E. A. Boultwood. *A Short History of Educational Ideas*. 5th edn. Slough: University Tutorial Press, 1977.

Davis, Lennard J. 'Constructing Normalcy: The Bell Curve, the Novel and the Invention of the Disabled Body in the Nineteenth Century'. In *Disability Studies Reader*, 2nd edn, edited by Lennard J. Davis, 3–16. New York: Routledge, 2006.

de Leon, Jose. 'One Hundred Years of Limited Impact of Jaspers' *General Psychopathology* on US psychiatry'. *The Journal of Nervous and Mental Disease*, 202 (2014): 79–87.

de Man, Paul. 'The Epistemology of Metaphor'. In *Aesthetic Ideology*, edited by Andrzez Warminski, 34–50. Minneapolis and London: University of Minnesota Press, 1996.

Digby, Anne. 'Contexts and Perspectives'. In *From Idiocy to Mental Deficiency: Historical Perspectives on People with Learning Disabilities*, edited by David Wright and Anne Digby, 1–21. London: Routledge, 1996.

Douthwaite, Julia. *The Wild Girl, Natural Man, and the Monster: Dangerous Experiments in the Age of the Enlightenment*. Chicago: University of Chicago Press, 2002.

Downie, J. A. 'Gulliver's Fourth Voyage and Locke's *Essay Concerning Human Understanding*'. In *Reading Swift: Papers from the Fifth Münster Symposium on Jonathan Swift*, edited by Hermann J. Real, 453–463. Munich: Wilhelm Fink, 2008.

Ehrenpreis, Irvin. 'The Meaning of Gulliver's Last Voyage'. *Review of English Literature* 3.3 (1962): 18–38.

Eigen, J. P. *Witnessing Insanity: Madness and Mad Doctors in the English Court*. New Haven: Yale University Press, 1995.

Evans, G. R. *Getting It Wrong: The Medieval Epistemology of Error*. Studien und Texte zur Geistesgeschichte des Mittelalters 63. Leiden: Brill, 1998.

Ferguson, Philip. *Abandoned to Their Fate: A History of Social Policy and Practice Toward Severely Retarded People in America, 1820–1920*. Philadelphia: Temple University Press, 1994.

Ferruolo, Stephen C. *The Origins of the University: The Schools of Paris and their Critics, 100–1215*. Stanford: Stanford University Press, 1985.

Foucault, Michel. *Madness and Civilization: A History of Insanity in the Age of Reason*. Translated by Richard Howard. London: Routledge, 1967.

Fyfe, Aileen. *Science and Salvation: Evangelical Popular Science Publishing in Victorian Britain*. Chicago: University of Chicago Press, 2004.

Gabbard, D. Christopher. '"What He found Not Monsters, He Made So": The I-Word and the Bathos of Exclusion'. *Journal of Literary and Cultural Disability Studies* 2.1 (2008): 1–9.

Gardiner, Anne Barbeau. 'Jonathan Swift and the Idea of the Fundamental Church'. In *Fundamentalism and Literature*. Edited by Catherine Pesso-Miquel and Klaus Stiertorfer, 21–41. New York: Palgrave Macmillan, 2007.

Garrabé, Jean. 'Nosographie et classifications des maladies mentales dans l'histoire de la psychiatrie'. *L'Évolution psychiatrique* 79 (2014): 5–18.

Gay, Peter. 'Introduction'. In *John Locke on Education*, edited by Peter Gay, 1–17. New York: Teacher College Press, 1964.

Gelb, Steven A. 'Social Deviance and the "Discovery" of the Moron'. *Disability, Handicap and Society* 2 (1987): 247–258.

George, Dorothy. *London Life in the Eighteenth Century*. Penguin, London, 1992.

Goldstein, Jan. 'Bringing the Psyche into Scientific Focus'. In *The Cambridge History of Science, Volume 7, The Modern Social Sciences*, edited by Theodore M. Porter and Dorothy Ross, 131–153. Cambridge: Cambridge University Press, 2003.

Goodey, C. F. *A History of Intelligence and 'Intellectual Disability: The Shaping of Psychology in Early Modern Europe*. Farnham: Ashgate, 2011.

Goodey, C. F. 'The Psychopolitics of Learning and Disability in Seventeenth-Century Thought.' In *From Idiocy to Mental Deficiency: Historical Perspectives on People with Learning Disabilities*, edited by David Wright and Anne Digby, 93–17. London: Routledge, 1996.

Goodey, C. F. 'What is Developmental Disability? The Origin and Nature of Our Conceptual Models'. *Journal on Developmental Disabilities* 8/2 (2001): 1–17.

Goodey, C. F. and M. Lynn Rose. 'Mental States, Bodily Dispositions and Table Manners: A Guide to Reading "Intellectual Disability" from Homer to Late Antiquity'. In *Disabilities in Roman Antiquity: Disparate Bodies a Capite ad Calcem*, edited by C. Laes, C. F. Goodey, and M. Lynn Rose, 17–44. Leiden: Brill, 2013.

Goodey, C. F. and Tim Stainton. 'Intellectual Disability and the Myth of the Changeling Myth'. *Journal of the History of the Behavioral Sciences* 37 (2001): 223–240.

Goodich, Michael. *From Birth to Old Age: The Human Life Cycle in Medieval Thought, 1250–1350*. Lanham: University Press of America, 1989.

Goodley, Dan. 'Learning Difficulties, the Social Model of Disability and Impairment: Challenging Epistemologies'. *Disability and Society* 16 (2001): 207–231.

Graves, Lila V. 'Locke's Changeling and the Shandy Bull'. *Philological Quarterly* 60.2 (1981): 257–264.

Grübmüller, Klaus. 'Kommentar'. *Novellistik des Mittelalters*, 1005–1348. Frankfurt a.M.: Bibliothek des Mittelalters, 2011.

Grundmann, Herbert. *Religiöse Bewegungen im Mittelalter*. 2nd edn. Hildesheim: Georg Olms. 1961.

Haase, Nikolaus. 'Das Lehrstück von den vier Intellekten in der Scholastik: von den arabischen Quellen bis zu Albertus Magnus'. *Recherches de Théologie et Philosophie Médiévales* (1999): 21–77.

Halliwell, Martin. *Images of Idiocy: The Idiot Figure in Modern Fiction and Film*. Aldershot: Ashgate, 2004.

Hansen, Bert. *Nicole Oresme and the Marvels of Nature: A Study of his De causis mirabilium with Critical Edition, Translation, and Commentary*. Toronto: Pontifical Institute of Medieval Studies, 1985.

Herzog, Don. *Happy Slaves: A Critique of Consent Theory*. Chicago: University of Chicago Press, 1989.

Hess, Volker and J. Andrew Mendelsohn. 'Sauvages' Paperwork: How Disease Classification Arose From Scholarly Note-Taking'. *Early Science and Medicine* 19 (2014): 471–503.

Higgins, Ian. *Jonathan Swift*. Tavistock: Northcote House, 2004.

Hudson, Nicholas. '*Gulliver's Travels* and Locke's Radical Nominalism'. In *1650–1850: Ideas, Aesthetics, and Inquiries in the Early Modern Era* 1 (1994): 247–266.

Hunter, J. Paul. '*Gulliver's Travels* and the Later Writings'. In *Cambridge Companion to Jonathan Swift*, edited by Christopher Fox, 216–240. Cambridge/New York: Cambridge University Press, 2003.

Jackson, Mark. *The Borderland of Imbecility: Medicine, Society and the Fabrication of the Feeble Mind in Late Victorian and Edwardian England*. Manchester: Manchester University Press, 2000.

Jackson, Mark. '"It Begins with the Goose and Ends with the Goose": Medical, Legal and Lay Understandings of Imbecility in *Ingram v Wyatt*, 1824–1832'. *Social History of Medicine* 11 (1998): 361–380.

Jarrett, S. 'The Moral Economy of Idiocy in the Old Bailey 1690–1834'. MA thesis, University of London, 2013.

Johnson, Michael, ed. *A Critical Edition of the Commentary by William of Wheteley on the Pseudo-Boethian Treatise De Disciplina Scolarium*. PhD thesis, State University of New York at Buffalo, 1982.

Kanner, Leo. *A History of the Care and Study of the Mentally Retarded*, Springfield: C.C. Thomas, 1964.

Kellenberger, Edgar. *Der Schutz der Einfältigen. Menschen mit einer geistigen Behinderung in der Bibel und in weiteren Quellen*. Zurich: Theologischer Verlag Zürich, 2011.

Kemp, Simon. *Medieval Psychology*. New York: Greenwood Press, 1990.

Kendler, K. S. 'An Historical Framework for Psychiatric Nosology'. *Psychological Medicine* 39 (2009): 1935–41.

Kennedy, Maev. 'Peter the Wild Boy's Condition Revealed 200 Years After his Death'. *Guardian*. 20 March, 2011. Accessed 15 March, 2017, www.theguardian.com/artanddesign/2011/mar/20/peter-wild-boy-condition-revealed.

Kittay, Eva Feder. 'The Personal is Philosophical is Political: A Philosopher and Mother of a Cognitively Disabled Person Sends Notes from the Battlefield'. In *Cognitive Disability and Its Challenge to Moral Philosophy*, edited by Eva Feder Kittay and Licia Carlson, 393–413. Malden MA: Wiley-Blackwell, 2010.

Korte, Barbara. *English Travel Writing From Pilgrimages to Postcolonial Explorations*. Translated by Catherine Matthias. London: Macmillan, 2000.

Koselleck, Reinhart. *The Practice of Conceptual History: Timing History, Spacing Concepts*. Stanford, CA: Stanford University Press, 2002.

Küster, A. *Blinde und Taubstumme im römischen Recht*. Cologne: Böhlau Verlag, 1991.

Laing, R. D. *The Divided Self*. London: Tavistock, 1960.

Laing, R. D. and Esterson, Aaron. *Sanity, Madness and the Family*. London: Tavistock, 1964.

Lamont, William. *Richard Baxter of the Millennium: Protestant Imperialism and the English Revolution*. London: Croom Helm, 1979.

Lane, Harlan. *The Wild Boy of Aveyron*. London: George Allen & Unwin, 1977.

Leafe, David. 'The Child Savage Kept as a Pet by King George'. *Daily Mail*. 24 March,

2011. Accessed 15 March, 2017, www.dailymail.co.uk/news/article-1369387/The-child-savage-kept-pet-King-George.html.

Legg, Thomas S. 'Amos, Andrew (1791–1860)'. *Oxford Dictionary of National Biography*. Oxford: Oxford University Press, 2004.

Levitas, Ruth. *The Concept of Utopia*. Oxford: Peter Lang, 2010.

Lexer, Matthias. *Mittelhochdeutsches Handwörterbuch. Erster Band A–M*. Stuttgart: Hirzel, 1979.

'Life Stories', The Social History of Learning Disability – The Open University. www.open.ac.uk/health-and-social-care/research/shld/resources-and-publications/life-stories. Accessed 8 March, 2017.

Lindberg, D. C. 'Alhazen's Theory of Vision and Its Reception in the West'. *Isis* 58 (1967): 321–341.

Lund, Roger. 'Laughing at Cripples: Ridicule, Deformity and the Argument from Design'. *Eighteenth-Century Studies* 39.1 (2005): 91–114.

Lupton, Daniel. 'Swift's Idea of Christian Community'. In *Swift as Priest and Satirist*, edited by Todd C. Parker, 164–181. Newark: University of Delaware Press, 2009.

Mack, Maynard. 'Gulliver's Travels'. In *Swift: A Collection of Critical Essays*, edited by Ernest Tuveson, 111–114. Englewood Cliffs NJ: Prentice-Hall, 1964.

MacLehose, William F. 'A Tender Age': Cultural Anxieties Over the Child in the Twelfth and Thirteenth Centuries. New York: Columbia University Press, 2008.

Manousos, Anthony. 'Swiftian Scatology and Lockean Psychology'. *The Gypsy Scholar* 7 (1980): 15–25.

Marková, Ivana S. and German E. Berrios. 'Epistemology of Psychiatry'. *Psychopathology* 45 (2012): 220–227.

McDonagh, Patrick. *Idiocy: A Cultural History*. Liverpool: Liverpool University Press, 2008.

McDonagh, Patrick and Tim Stainton. 'Editorial: Chasing Shadows: The Historical Construction of Developmental Disability'. *Journal on Developmental Disabilities* 8.2 (2001): ix–xvi.

McDonald, William. 'The Fool-Stick: Concerning Tristan's Club in the German Eilhart-Tradition'. *Euphorion* 82 (1988): 127–149.

McMahan, Jeff. *The Ethics of Killing: Problems at the Margins of Life*. New York: Oxford University Press, 2003.

Metzler, Irina. *Fools and Idiots? Intellectual Disability in the Middle Ages*. Manchester: Manchester University Press, 2016.

Michie, Allen. 'Gulliver the Houyahoo: Swift, Locke, and the Ethics of Excessive Individualism'. In *Humans and Other Animals in Eighteenth-Century British Culture: Representation, Hybridity, Ethics*, edited by Frank Palmeri, 67–81. Burlington VT: Ashgate: 2006.

Miles, M. 'Martin Luther and Childhood Disability', *Journal of Religion, Disability and Health* 5.4, 2001: 5–36.

Mitchell, David T. and Sharon L. Snyder. *Narrative Prosthesis. Disability and the Dependencies of Discourse*. Ann Arbor: University of Michigan Press, 2000.

Mitchell, David T. and Sharon L. Snyder. 'Introduction: Disability Studies and the Double Bind of Representation'. In *The Body and Physical Difference: Discourses of Disability*, edited by David T. Mitchell and Sharon L. Snyder, 1–31. Ann Arbor: University of Michigan Press, 1997.

Mojsisch, Burkhard. 'Grundlagen der Philosophie Alberts des Großen'. *Freiburger Zeitschrift für Philosophie und Theologie* 32 (1985): 27–44.

Mojsisch, Burkhard. 'Seele'. In *Lexikon des Mittelalters* 7 [1675–77]. Darmstadt: Brepols, 2000.

Mojsisch, Burkhard et al. 'Seele'. *Historisches Wörterbuch der Philosophie*, edited by Joachim Ritter et al., 13–22. Darmstadt: Schwabe Verlag, 1995.

Müller, Jan-Dirk. 'Die hovezuht und ihr Preis. Zum Problem höfischer Verhaltensregulierung in PS-Konrads "Halber Birne"'. In *Mediävistische Kulturwissenschaften*, edited by Jan-Dirk Müller, 205–227. Berlin: Schwabe Verlag, 2010.

Müller, Jan-Dirk. *Höfische Kompromisse. Acht Kapitel zur höfischen Epik*. Tübingen: Max Niemeyer, 2007.

Munsche, Heather and Harry A. Whittaker. 'Eighteenth-Century Classification of Mental Illness: Linnaeus, de Sauvages, Vogel, and Cullen'. *Cognitive and Behavioral Neurology* 25 (2012): 224–239.

Neugebauer, Richard. 'Treatment of the Mentally Ill in Medieval and Early Modern England: A Reappraisal'. *Journal of the History of the Behavioural Sciences* 14 (1978): 158–169.

Nokes, David. *Jonathan Swift, A Hypocrite Reversed: A Critical Biography*. London: Oxford University Press, 1985.

Noll, Steven. *Feeble-Minded in Our Midst: Institutions for the Mentally Retarded in the South, 1900–1940*. Chapel Hill: University of North Carolina Press, 1995.

Noll, Steven and James Trent, eds. *Mental Retardation in America: A Historical Reader*. New York: New York University Press, 2004.

Novak, Maximillian E. 'The Wild Man Comes to Tea'. In *The Wild Man Within: An Image in Western Thought from the Renaissance to Romanticism*. Edited by Edward Dudley and Maximillian Novak. Pittsburgh: University of Pittsburgh Press, 1972: 183–221.

O'Brien, Gerald. *Framing the Moron: The Social Construction of Feeble-Mindedness in the American Eugenic Era*. Manchester: Manchester University Press, 2013.

Oppenlander, Ella Anne. *Dickens' All the Year Round: Descriptive Index and Contributor List*. Troy, NY: Winston, 1984.

Perry, Lucy and Alexander Schwarz. 'Introduction'. *Behaving Like Fools: Voice, Gesture, and Laughter in Texts, Manuscripts, and Early Books*, edited by Lucy Perry and Alexander Schwarz, 1–13. Turnhout: Brepols, 2010.

Petryszak, Nicholas G. 'Tabula Rasa – Its Origins and Implications'. *Journal of the History of the Behavioral Sciences* 17 (1981): 15–27.

Porter, Roy. *The Greatest Benefit to Mankind: A Medical History of Humanity from Antiquity to the Present*. London: HarperCollins, 1997.

Porter, Roy. *Madmen: A Social History of Madhouses, Mad-Doctors and Lunatics.* Stroud: Tempus, 2006.

Pratt, Mary Louise. *Imperial Eyes: Travel Writing and Transculturation.* New York: Routledge, 1992.

Price, B. B. *Medieval Thought: An Introduction.* Oxford: Blackwell, 1992.

Rafalovich, Adam. 'The Conceptual History of Attention Deficit Hyperactivity Disorder: Idiocy, Imbecility, Encephalitis and the Child Deviant, 1877–1929'. *Deviant Behavior* 22 (2001): 93–115.

Rawson, Claude. *God, Gulliver, and Genocide: Barbarism and the European Imagination, 1492–1945.* Oxford: Oxford University Press, 2001.

Real, Hermann and Heinz J. Vienken. 'The Structure of *Gulliver's Travels*'. *Proceedings of the First Münster Symposium on Jonathan Swift*, edited by Hermann J. Real, 199–208. Munich: Wilhelm Fink, 1985.

Renaker, David. 'Swift's Laputians as a Caricature of the Cartesians'. *PMLA* 94 (1979): 936–944.

Roelcke, Volker. 'Biologizing Social Facts: An Early Twentieth-Century Debate on Kraepelin's Concepts of Culture, Neurasthenia, and Degeneration'. *Culture, Medicine and Psychiatry* 21 (1997): 383–403.

Rose, Nikolas. *Governing the Soul: The Shaping of the Private Self.* 2nd edn. London: Free Association Books, 1999.

Said, Edward. *Culture and Imperialism.* New York: Knopf, 1993.

Savarese, Ralph. *Reasonable People: A Memoir of Autism and Adoption.* New York: Other Press, 2007.

Scheerenberger, Richard. *A History of Mental Retardation.* Baltimore: P. H. Brookes, 1983.

Schnyer, André. '"Des Mönches Not" Mit Michel Foucault neu gelesen'. *Wirkendes Wort* 37 (1987): 269–284.

Schönberger, Rolf. 'Rationale Spontanität. Die Theorie des Willes bei Albertus Magnus'. In *Albertus Magnus. Zum Gedenken nach 800 Jahren: Neue Zugänge, Aspekte und Perspektiven*, edited by Walter Senner et al., 221–234. Berlin: Akademie Verlag, 2001.

Schulz, Armin. *Erzähltheorie in mediävistischer Perspektive*, edited by Manuel Braun, Alexandra Dunkel, and Jan-Dirk Müller. Berlin: De Gruyter, 2012.

Scull, Andrew. 'Contending Professions: Sciences of the Brain and Mind in the United States, 1850–2013'. *Science in Context* 28 (2015): 131–161.

Scull, Andrew. *The Most Solitary of Afflictions: Madness and Society in Britain 1700–1900.* New Haven: Yale University Press, 1993.

Scull, Andrew, Charlotte Mackenzie, and Nicholas Hervey. *Masters of Bedlam: The Transformation of the Mad-Doctoring Trade.* Princeton: Princeton University Press, 1996.

Sharp, Richard. 'Lynch, John (1697–1760)'. *Oxford Dictionary of National Biography.* Oxford: Oxford University Press, 2004.

Shorter, Edward. *A History of Psychiatry: From the Era of the Asylum to the Age of Prozac.* Chichester, NY: John Wiley, 1997.

Shorter, Edward. *What Psychiatry Left out of DSM–V: Historical Mental Disorders Today*. New York: Routledge, 2015.

Simpson, Murray K. 'Medicine vs. Psychology: The Emergence of a Professional Conflict in Development Disability'. *Journal on Developmental Disabilities/Le journal sur les handicaps du développement* 8 (2001): 45–59.

Simpson, Murray K. 'The Developmental Concept of Idiocy'. *Intellectual and Developmental Disabilities* 45 (2007): 23–32.

Simpson, Murray K. *Modernity and the Appearance of Idiocy: Intellectual Disability as a Regime of Truth*. Lampeter: Edwin Mellen, 2014.

Singer, Julie. '"*Une enroullure de sapience*": The Mechanics of Melancholy and Intellectual Disability.' Paper presented at Medieval Academy of America meeting, St. Louis University, St. Louis, Missouri, 22 March, 2012.

Singer, Peter. *Animal Liberation: A New Ethics for Our Treatment of Animals*. New York: Random House, 1975.

Smith, Roger. *Being Human: Historical Knowledge and the Creation of Human Nature*. Manchester: Manchester University Press, 2007.

Smith, Roger. *Between Mind and Nature: A History of Psychology*. London: Reaktion Books, 2013.

Smith, Roger. *Trial by Medicine: Insanity and Responsibility in Victorian Trials*. Edinburgh: Edinburgh University Press, 1981.

Spyra, Ulricke. *Das 'Buch der Natur' Konrads von Megenberg. Die illustrierten Handschriften und Inkunablen*. Köln: Böhlau Verlag, 2005.

Stainton, Tim. 'Reason's Other: The Emergence of the Disabled Subject in the Northern Renaissance'. *Disability and Society* 19.3 (2004): 225–244.

Stock, Brian. *The Implications of Literacy: Written Language and Models of Interpretation in the Eleventh and Twelfth Centuries*. Princeton: Princeton University Press, 1983.

Strässle, Thomas. *Vom Unverstand zum Verstand durchs Feuer. Studien zu Grimmelshausens 'Simplicissimus Teutsch'*. Bern: Peter Lang, 2001.

Summers, David. *The Judgment of Sense: Renaissance Naturalism and the Rise of Aesthetics*. Cambridge: Cambridge University Press, 1987.

Szasz, Thomas. *The Myth of Mental Illness: Foundations of a Theory of Personal Conduct*. New York: Hoeber-Harper, 1961.

Szasz, Thomas. *The Manufacture of Madness: A Comparative Study of the Inquisition and the Mental Health Movement*. New York: Harper Row, 1970.

Szasz, Thomas. 'Mental Illness as a Metaphor'. *Nature* 242 (1973): 305–307.

Szasz, Thomas. *Psychiatry: The Science of Lies*. Syracuse: Syracuse University Press. 2008.

Thompson, Carl. *Travel Writing*. London: Routledge, 2011.

Thomson, Mathew. *The Problem of Mental Deficiency: Eugenics, Democracy and Social Policy in Britain c. 1870–1959*. Oxford: Oxford University Press, 1998.

Thomson, Mathew. *Psychological Subjects: Identity, Culture, and Health in Twentieth-Century Britain*. Oxford: Oxford University Press, 2006.

Thorndike, Lynn. *A History of Magic and Experimental Science*. Vol. 3. New York: Columbia University Press, 1934.

Tobin, Rosemary Barton. 'The Cornifician Motif in John of Salisbury's *Metalogicon*'. *History of Education* 13.1 (1984): 1–6.

Todd, Dennis. *Imagining Monsters: Miscreations of the Self in Eighteenth-Century England*. Chicago: University of Chicago Press, 1995.

Trent, James. *Inventing the Feeble Mind: A History of Mental Retardation in the United States*. Berkeley: University of California Press, 1994.

Turner, Ralph V. *The English Judiciary in the Age of Glanvill and Bracton, c.1176–1239*. Cambridge: Cambridge University Press, 1985.

Turner, Trevor, Mark Salter, and Martin Deahl. 'Mental Health Reform Act'. *Psychiatric Bulletin* 23 (1999): 578–581.

Turner, Wendy J. *Care and Custody of the Mentally Ill, Incompetent, and Disabled in Medieval England*. Cursor Mundi, 16. Turnout: Brepols, 2013.

Turner, Wendy J. 'Silent Testimony: Emotional Displays and Lapses in Memory as Indicators of Mental Instability in Medieval English Investigations'. In *Madness in Medieval Law and Custom*, edited by Wendy J. Turner, 81–96. Leiden, Boston: Brill, 2010.

Turner, Wendy J. 'Town and Country: A Comparison of the Treatment of the Mentally Disabled in Late Medieval English Common Law and Chartered Boroughs'. In *Madness in Medieval Law and Custom*, edited by Wendy J. Turner, 17–38. Leiden, Boston: Brill, 2010.

Turner, Wendy J., ed. *Madness in Medieval Law and Custom*. Later Medieval Europe, 6. Leiden, Boston: Brill, 2010.

Turner, Wendy J. and Tory Vandeventer Pearman, eds. *The Treatment of Disabled Persons in Medieval Europe: Examining Disability in the Historical, Legal, Literary, Medical, and Religious Discourses of the Middle Ages*. Lewiston: Mellen, 2011.

Tuveson, Ernest. 'Gulliver's Travels'. In *Swift: A Collection of Critical Essays*, edited by Ernest Tuveson, 101–110. Englewood Cliffs NJ: Prentice-Hall, 1964.

van Deusen, Nancy. 'Cicero through Quintilian's Eyes in the Middle Ages'. In *Cicero Refused to Die: Ciceronian Influence Through the Centuries*, edited by Nancy van Deusen, 47–64. Leiden: Brill, 2013.

von Bernuth, Ruth. 'Aus den Wunderkammern in die Irrenanstalten – Natürliche Hofnarren in Mittelalter und früher Neuzeit'. In *Kulturwissenschaftliche Perspektive der Disability Studies*, edited by Anne Waldschmidt, 49–62. Kassel: Bifos, 2003.

von Bernuth, Ruth. 'From Marvels of Nature to Inmates of Asylums: Imaginations of Natural Folly'. *Disability Studies Quarterly* 26.2 (2006), no pagination. Accessed 1 August, 2014. www.dsq-sds.org.

Wailes, Stephen L. 'Konrad of Würzburg and Pseudo-Konrad: Varieties of Humour in the "Märe"'. *The Modern Language Review* 69.1 (1974): 98–114.

Waldschmidt, Anne. 'Paradoxien des Normalismus: Normalitätsvorstellungen im heilpädagogischen Diskurs.' In *Zeichen und Gesten. Heilpädagogik als Kulturthema*, edited by H. Greving, C. Murner, and P. Rödler, 98–112. Gießen: Psychosozial-Verlag, 2004.

Weddige, Hilkert. *Mittelhochdeutsch.* München: Beck, 2001.

Weiner, Deborah B. 'Foreword'. In Philipe Pinel, *Medico-Philosophical Treatise on Mental Alienation* [1800, 1809]. Translated by Gordon Hickish, David Henly, and Louis C. Charland. Chichester: Wiley-Blackwell, 2008.

Weisheipl, J. A. 'Classification of the Sciences in Medieval Thought'. *Medieval Studies* 27 (1965): 54–90.

Wendell, Susan. *The Rejected Body: Feminist Philosophical Reflections on Disability.* New York: Psychology Press, 1996.

Wertz, Spencer and Linda Spencer. 'Some Correlations Between Swift's *Gulliver's Travels* and Locke on Personal Identity'. *Journal of Thought* 10 (1975): 262–271.

Robert G. Weyant, 'Introduction'. In Etienne Bonnot de Condillac, *An Essay on the Origin of Human Knowledge: Being a Supplement to Mr. Locke's Essay on the Human Understanding.* Translated by Thomas Nugent, v–xvii. Gainsville: Scholars' Facsimiles and Reprints, 1971.

Williams, David. *Deformed Discourse: The Function of the Monster in Mediaeval Thought and Literature.* Montreal: McGill-Queen's University Press, 1996.

Worsley, Lucy. *Courtiers: The Secret History of the Georgian Court.* London: Faber, 2011.

Wright, David. *Mental Disability in Victorian England: The Earlswood Asylum, 1847–1901.* Oxford: Clarendon, 2001.

Wright, David. 'Mongols in Our Midst: John Langdon Down and Ethnic Classification of Idiocy, 1858–1924'. In *Mental Retardation in America: A Historical Reader,* edited by Steven Noll and James W. Trent, Jr, 92–119. New York: New York University Press, 2004.

Wright, David and Anne Digby, eds. *From Idiocy to Mental Deficiency: Historical Perspectives on People with Learning Disabilities.* London: Routledge, 1996.

Yolton, John W. 'Locke: Education for Virtue'. In *Philosophers on Education,* edited by Amelie Oksenberg Rorty, 173–189. London: Routledge, 1998.

Zall, Paul M., ed. *A Nest of Ninnies and Other English Jestbooks of the Seventeenth Century.* Lincoln: University of Nebraska Press, 1970.

Zirker, Herbert. 'Horse Sense and Sensibility: Some Issues Concerning Utopian Understanding in *Gulliver's Travels*'. *Swift Studies: The Annual of the Ehrenpreis Center* 12 (1997): 85–98.

Index

EU authorised representative for GPSR:
Easy Access System Europe, Mustamäe tee 50,
10621 Tallinn, Estonia
gpsr.requests@easproject.com

www.ingramcontent.com/pod-product-compliance
Lightning Source LLC
Chambersburg PA
CBHW051957270326
41929CB00015B/2683

9 781526 151643